Towards a Digital Ecology

Towards a Digital Ecology
NHS Digital Adoption through the COVID-19 Looking Glass

Victoria Betton

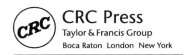

CRC Press
Taylor & Francis Group
Boca Raton London New York

CRC Press is an imprint of the
Taylor & Francis Group, an **informa** business
AN AUERBACH BOOK

First edition published 2022
by CRC Press
6000 Broken Sound Parkway NW, Suite 300, Boca Raton, FL 33487-2742

and by CRC Press
4 Park Square, Milton Park, Abingdon, Oxon, OX14 4RN

© 2022 Taylor & Francis Group, LLC

CRC Press is an imprint of Taylor & Francis Group, LLC

Reasonable efforts have been made to publish reliable data and information, but the author and publisher cannot assume responsibility for the validity of all materials or the consequences of their use. The authors and publishers have attempted to trace the copyright holders of all material reproduced in this publication and apologize to copyright holders if permission to publish in this form has not been obtained. If any copyright material has not been acknowledged please write and let us know so we may rectify in any future reprint.

Except as permitted under U.S. Copyright Law, no part of this book may be reprinted, reproduced, transmitted, or utilized in any form by any electronic, mechanical, or other means, now known or hereafter invented, including photocopying, microfilming, and recording, or in any information storage or retrieval system, without written permission from the publishers.

For permission to photocopy or use material electronically from this work, access www.copyright.com or contact the Copyright Clearance Center, Inc. (CCC), 222 Rosewood Drive, Danvers, MA 01923, 978-750-8400. For works that are not available on CCC please contact mpkbookspermissions@tandf.co.uk

Trademark notice: Product or corporate names may be trademarks or registered trademarks and are used only for identification and explanation without intent to infringe.

ISBN: 978-1-032-10866-7 (hbk)
ISBN: 978-1-032-10974-9 (pbk)
ISBN: 978-1-032-19879-8 (ebk)

DOI: 10.1201/9781032198798

Typeset in Garamond
by SPi Technologies India Pvt Ltd (Straive)

Contents

Preface ix
Author xiii

1   **Introduction** 1
      Where It All Started 3
      What Even Is Digital Health? 5
      A Perfect Storm 7
      Backdrop to Broken 7
      Necessity Is the Mother of Invention 8
      Relative Advantage 8
      When People Drive Digital 9
      Context Is King 10
      The Social Determinants of Digital 10
      The Jeopardy of Trust 11
      Bending the Curve on Digital Mental Health 11
      The Theatre of Tech – A Study in Solutionism 12
      We Get the Market We Deserve 12
      Momentum – Towards a Digital Ecology 13

2   **Backdrop to Broken** 15
      A Minor Inconvenience 18
      Ill-fated Plans 18
      Central Ambitions 20
      Changes You Can See from Outer Space 21
      A Competent Workforce 24
      X Is for Experience 27
      Diktat and Determination 29
      Between Rhetoric and Reality 31

3   **Necessity Is the Mother of Invention** 35
      An Outbreak of Pragmatism 37
          Logging on 39
          A Hospital in Your Home 42

v

vi ■ *Contents*

	The Clinical Entrepreneur	46
	Data Quality Rules Ok!	48
	Attending Anywhere	50
	Fighting Fires of the Future	54
4	**Relative Advantage**	**59**
	Relative Advantage	60
	NHS Care Is a Relational Business	64
	Saying Goodbye	65
	Looking Forward	68
5	**When People Drive Digital**	**73**
	When People Drive Digital	73
	Command and Control	78
	First Responders	81
	We Are Not Waiting	84
	A Software Ecology	86
6	**Context Is King**	**91**
	In Celebration of Mess	91
	Theorising Non-adoption	92
	Context Is King	94
	Thinking about Design	96
	What Happens in the Margins	101
	Culture Eats Digital for Breakfast	102
	Thinking Systems	105
	Nurturing a Habitat	109
	Put a Dictator in Charge	111
7	**The Social Determinants of Digital**	**113**
	The Wellness Myth	113
	Hello Inequality, Let Me Introduce You to COVID-19	115
	The Drum of Progress	117
	One Condition. Two Tales	118
	Pay-as-You-Go	119
	One Hundred Percent Digital	120
	The Law of Inverse Care	121
	Designing for Everyone	123
	Data Shadows	125
	Who Leads Digital Health Matters	128
	Just as Vital as a Food Parcel	130
	Beyond the Stats	133
8	**The Jeopardy of Trust**	**139**
	The Boundaries of Health Data	140

	The Data That Didn't Care	142
	A Cautionary Tale	143
	WannaCry	145
	Amazonian Challenges	147
	The Internet of Health	148
	One London	149
	The Controversies Continue	154
	A Social Contract	157
9	**Bending the Curve on Digital Mental Health**	**163**
	Introduction	163
	A Mental Health Pandemic	164
	A Salutary Lesson	165
	Cinderella Services	167
	The Fruit That Hangs the Lowest	168
	The Detractors	170
	A Faster Horse	170
	In Search of the Gold Standard	173
	A Digital Mental Health Pandemic	175
	Bending the Curve on Digital Mental Health	177
	To Save the NHS Click Here	178
	An Open Future	180
10	**The Theatre of Tech – A Study in Solutionism**	**185**
	There's an App for That	187
	Silicon Valley Style Hubris	189
	Do Something. Do Anything	190
	We Don't Have an App for That	191
	Checks and Balances	192
	In Love with Ada	193
	A Masterclass in Mismanagement	197
	The Beat of the Drum	199
	A Footnote	201
11	**We Get the Market We Deserve**	**205**
	How the Money Flows	205
	A Founder's Story – Fixing a Simple Problem	207
	The Scissors of Doom	209
	The Elusive Return on Investment	212
	Who Buys?	214
	But Does It Even Work?	215
	The Dark Art of Procurement	216
	Who Holds the Purse Strings?	220

viii ■ *Contents*

The Imperative Gap 220
A Static Market 221
An Open Future... 224
You Don't Win by Designing for Health Outcomes................ 225
What Business Models Actually Work?................................... 229
Lessons Learned 232

12 Momentum – towards a Digital Ecology 235
Towards the North Star 238
Entrepreneurs of the Future 240
The Characteristics of a Digital Ecology 242
Creating Curiosity... 243

Index.. 247

Preface

At first, it didn't seem like such a big deal. I had passively absorbed the coronavirus news from China, but only insofar as it formed part of my daily intake of Radio 4 news, as I got ready for work. Even when cases reached the UK, it still seemed quite remote with no particular personal salience. When my boyfriend and I went away for a seaside weekend mid-March break, we happily stood at the bar next to fellow customers and walked along the bay bustling with people taking in the chilly spring sun. Government ministers were still debating whether to permit large gatherings, and the official position determined that closing schools or sporting events could do more harm than good.[1]

As I started writing this book less than a month later, a BBC News alert popped up on my mobile telling me that the UK's daily death toll of 980 has surpassed that of Italy and Spain. The newsreader announces that gatherings of not more than two were banned. Shit got real. But just as it took a while for the penny to drop in our personal lives, so did the enormity of the implications for the digital health sector and the National Health Service take some time to sink in. As I began to write this preface, the pandemic was in full force and its implications beyond the immediate days and weeks, still very much unknown. As I concluded the final chapter, one long year later, the impact of the pandemic on technology adoption in England's NHS has been the subject of much debate, both within the sector and in any number of policy and research papers.

Having worked in and around the NHS for most of my working life, I am endlessly fascinated by its culture, organisation and idiosyncrasies. I have always been drawn to knotty problems, and it is probably for this reason I have found myself working in digital health. Digital in the NHS is still immature and emergent (we'll come back to that as a core theme in this book) but with the NHS engulfed by the biggest public health challenge of its 70 years, it appeared to come into its own. After personal protective equipment (PPE), a term most of us had never heard of before, digital appeared to be front and centre of rapidly shifting practices over the course of the first pandemic wave.

However, this is not a book about the pandemic. The starring role for this tale is our National Health Service, a flawed hero whose imperfections we the audience are endlessly frustrated by, but ultimately forgiving of. COVID-19 is the villain of the piece, wreaking a path of destruction which forces an inflection point whereby our hero has no option but to address their deficits and imperfections. This story may not give us the happy ending we desire, but it does conclude with a note of

ix

x ■ *Preface*

optimism for a digital ecology that supports England's healthcare system to thrive in the 21st century and beyond.

The villainous pandemic created a watershed moment for many profound reasons. It is fair to speculate that life will never be the same again. Many more people beyond those first 980 have lost their lives. All of us were affected to varying degrees by isolation, loss and grief. The fragility of the world and the interconnected nature of our health and happiness were more keenly felt than ever.

Whether it be administrative staff working from home to keep the engine room running, GPs doing routine patient appointments or clinicians undertaking remote multidisciplinary meetings, video communications became as critical to the daily business of healthcare as running water and heated radiators. Video consultation companies that had been selling to mostly disinterested customers suddenly got sales in the stratosphere. COVID-19 is the perfect lens through which to understand the factors which influence how digital technologies get adopted in our healthcare system.

In the leisure and retail sectors, there were winners and losers from the pandemic. Netflix was a winner, with a massive demand as people stayed at home and their viewing habits shifted. Face-to-face activities such as book groups[2] and even choir practice and yoga classes shifted to video streaming platforms such as Zoom who announced that it brought in more active users in January to March 2020 than it had in the whole of 2019.[3] Digital-first companies such as Uber pivoted their business model towards delivery services in response to massive decreases in demand for their taxi-hailing service, whilst Uber Eats saw an increase in use as more people ordered food delivery.[4] In the world of business, companies redrew their technology roadmaps, accelerating plans to digitise services.[5] Similar trends emerged in digital health, and I explore what this meant both during the pandemic and what it means for life beyond.

I have many people to thank who helped me in writing this book. Anne Cooper and Roz Davies are amazing colleagues and friends who reviewed chapters, gave advice and made introductions. Sheldon Steed helped me understand the sector through the eyes of a start-up and brought lots of critical challenges and cause for reflection. Janak Gunatilleke did some background research for me and sent useful articles as I wrote this book. I have various digital health WhatsApp groups to thank as I asked questions and got speedy responses from some of the brightest people in the digital health sector. In addition to being interviewed, Andy Kinnear made lots of introductions to people who had interesting things to say. Jim Richie obliged in a similar way, and Ayesha Rahim and Phillipa Winters both helped shape my thinking. David Hancock, Richard Graham and Aidan Peppin all kindly reviewed chapters for me. Last but not least, I want to thank Louise Sinclair for picking me up when I was down and supporting me in many ways beyond my writing endeavours.

Preface ■ **xi**

Finally, this book is for my three children, Molly, Ruby and Asa who are the people in the world I am most proud of and whom I love to the ends of the earth.

Twitter conversation:

Complete the sentence. <Nerd face>
The three most effective drivers of digital transformation in the NHS are...

@lennyNaar

1. Financial year end
2. Knee jerk requirements
3. Ministerial good ideas

@NHSNewey

1. Covid
2. Covid
3. Covid

@AyeshaRahimCCIO

A pandemic
Burning platforms
Centrally set targets
not what I want to say but these tend to be the things that get financed....

@SarahBoydNHS

People with ideas
Organisations that understand the opportunities
Reasonable timeframes to deliver and see benefits

@ChorltonJim

If I was a cynic I'd say

— money (cutting cost/making more/funding)
— ego (becoming recognised/centre of excellence)
— friends (good network)

But I'm not so

— existing infrastructure
— passion
— permissive culture/leadership

@MustBeMistry

xii ■ *Preface*

Notes

1 BBC News daily 13 March
2 https://www.theguardian.com/books/2020/mar/26/the-perfect-time-to-start-how-book-clubs-are-enduring-and-flourishing-during-covid-19
3 https://www.cnbc.com/2020/02/26/zoom-has-added-more-users-so-far-this-year-than-in-2019-bernstein.html
4 https://techcrunch.com/2020/04/20/uber-adds-retail-and-personal-package-delivery-services-as-covid-19-reshapes-its-business/
5 https://wp.technologyreview.com/wp-content/uploads/2020/08/Amid-the-pandemic-shifting-business-priorities_083120.pdf

Author

An author and public speaker, **Dr Victoria Betton** specialises in digital strategy, policy and transformation for social impact. She is a qualified social worker and coach with 20+ years of experience in local government, third sector, digital health startups and the NHS.

She has a consultancy practice and is cofounder of digital health startup, LOOP. She has previously founded mHabitat, a successful NHS hosted digital health consultancy and Co>Space North, tech for good collaboration space.

Chapter 1

Introduction

This book is about technology adoption in the NHS, told through the inflection point of a disaster. Disasters, which affect millions of people around the world every year, are events that threaten harm or death to a large group of people.[1] In 2020, we lived through a disaster of epic proportions, devastating humanity around the globe. It took a microscopic virus to wreak havoc on our healthcare system and force the adoption of technology in a way that had never been seen before. This book tells the story of digital technology uptake in the UK's National Health Service through the lens of that disaster.

It was back in January 2020 that the first two people tested positive for COVID-19 in the UK – holidaymakers from China who were staying in a York hotel. I have a slight recollection of hearing about it in the news. Then in February the first transmission of COVID-19 was confirmed in the UK. I was mildly interested and noted instructions about vigilant hand washing. It was only when the prime minister announced a lockdown on 23 March, telling us to stay at home in a televised address to the nation, that the gravity of the situation began to really sink in.

The COVID-19 pandemic was the most significant global health crisis to occur since the advent of digital technologies, ubiquitous data and widespread use of mobile technologies. This book documents the use of technology in the NHS through the lens of the first pandemic shock. Our most precious healthcare system, paid for by general taxation and free at the point of demand, was conceived and developed in a firmly analogue world. Born out of a post-Second World War settlement in 1948, the NHS predates the invention of the World Wide Web by some 40 years. This is not a book simply about technology, it is a study of the painful process of reengineering a mammoth and byzantine system that was built for a different era.

That diminutive virus created an inflection point for two decades worth of effort to digitise the NHS. What happens next has implications for all of us, whether we

DOI: 10.1201/9781032198798-1

2 ■ *Towards a Digital Ecology*

are citizens, patients, health practitioners, policymakers and governments. It has almost become banal to state that we are living through unprecedented times, but it is in the extremes that we might find a moment of lucidity, an ability to see more clearly what has come before and an opportunity to imagine how we might shape the future ahead of us. We have a moment, a choice, to repurpose an NHS fit for the digital age.

This book is about more than technology. The digital health sector is a microcosm of the wider healthcare system, through which grand themes of social inequality, public trust, private in tension with public interests, values and beliefs are played out. The sector is a clash of multiple discourses – the *civic* and doing good for society; the *market* and wealth creation; the *industrial* creating more efficient and effective systems; the *project* expressed as innovation and experimentation; lastly, the notion of *vitality* and leading a happier, healthy life.[2]

Each of these discourses exists in a state of flux and tension with the other. Oscillating between them, this book is offered as a critique of the role of digital technologies within healthcare. It is an examination of competing interests, approaches and ideologies. It is a story of system complexity told through analysis and personal stories. Whilst each chapter explores a primary theme, it will become apparent that each laps over the other like a gentle wave or criss-cross of threads on a loom.

Despite a strong policy push from successive governments to digitise the NHS, the results have been underwhelming. The current buzz phrase for the role of technology in dragging the NHS into the 21st Century is *digital transformation*. Tom Loosemore, who wrote the first Government Digital strategy in 2013, defines digital transformation as: "applying the culture, processes, operating models and technologies of the internet-era to respond to people's raised expectations."[3] Over the course of this book, I make the case that we need a paradigm shift in how we conceptualise efforts to adopt technology if we are to see a flourishing healthcare system, rather than an impoverished one in which we double down on digitising analogue practices or with technology bolted on the side.

This book explores exploitation of the affordances of digital technologies to metamorphose the NHS from paper, pen and fax machines into practices that work well, are data-driven and networked. Put simply, it's about doing things better, making life easier for clinicians and improving how people experience care and the impact of that care on their health and well-being. Sullied by its association with budget cuts and efficiencies, the phrase *digital transformation* has the feel of a wrecking ball about it. We should no longer hard-code what is already broken in our systems and processes. There is plenty to love and cherish in our healthcare system and some of that will be forever analogue. I believe we need to re-conceptualise a *digital ecology* in which technology is a nutrient to facilitate and sustain our healthcare system, helping it adapt to the ever-changing environment that surrounds it.

Whilst so many of us, smartphones in our hands, routinely check our bank balances, do our grocery shopping, watch movies and connect with our friends online, we may wonder why our primary method of communicating with the NHS is still through the telephone and letters. We may find it strange that our healthcare system does not appear to be making the changes that we have become used to in other parts of our lives. Silicon Valley loves to talk about how digital technologies are *disrupting* our lives, but the idea of moving fast and breaking things sits uneasily in a service whose motto is *first do no harm*. In a global assessment of those industries which have been most disrupted by technology, healthcare ranks fourth from the bottom.[4] We clearly have a long way to go in creating a successful *digital ecology* for our NHS.

This book is about the NHS. But it is important to acknowledge that our national health service in England is part of a wider interdependent ecosystem of social care. If we think the NHS struggled during the pandemic, then it had things relatively easy compared to services such as care homes, social services and other care services provided by local authorities. Already buckling under systemic underfunding over many years, social care comprises over 25,000 businesses, some of which receive public funding and some of which don't. The pandemic threw into sharp relief the fragile relationship between this sector and the Government.[5] But that is a story for someone else to tell. This book is unapologetically about the sector that I have worked in and around for most of my career.

I am curious about what this exceptional time can tell us about why digital technologies have been so hard to implement in healthcare in the past and what we can learn about their rapid adoption during the pandemic for the future. Through interviews, analysis and my own experience of working in the digital sector for just shy of a decade, I explore these issues to understand what has gone before and endeavour to offer some insights for what might come, as the pandemic subsides and we learn to live with whatever comes next.

Where It All Started

What was swiftly to become a global pandemic, first came to the attention of the World Health Organisation's (WHO) China office on 31 December 2019, where reports of a previously unknown virus came from Wuhan in Eastern China.[6] Global deaths have now risen exponentially and in the UK, they are way over the 100,000 mark according to the Johns Hopkins University COVID-19 dashboard.[7]

Symptoms of COVID-19 or its official classification "*severe acute respiratory syndrome-related coronavirus*"[8] are fever, dry cough and loss of smell or taste; they are mild for some but can lead to serious respiratory tract illnesses which are particularly dangerous in older people and those who have existing health conditions. When I first checked out the online NHS COVID-19 symptom checker, I was struck by how such apparently banal symptoms could have such devastating consequences for some. It was terrifying. I am used to keeping up to date with the twists and turns of global events but never had they felt so personally relevant to myself, my friends and my family.

4 ■ *Towards a Digital Ecology*

Like many, I experienced mild virus-like symptoms in mid-April that wiped me out for a week. Without public testing, I will never know whether I was affected by the virus. At the time it seemed like COVID-19 was the only illness in town and I rather hoped I was one of the 81% of people[9] who experience mild symptoms and maybe go on to develop some prized immunity. But so little was known about the virus at this point, it was impossible to tell.

In contrast, Maneesh started to feel unwell on 11 April and began to record his symptoms and experience of the illness on Twitter:

> So yesterday I woke up and noticed occasional shortness of breath and a dry cough. I wasn't coughing a lot, more like I would cough for a few seconds a once or twice an hour. I wasn't feeling 100%, sort of 90% of normal, as if one is under the weather but no fever.

He reported trying the online NHS symptom checker which came back negative and then he began to try other symptom checkers to see what they might tell him. To his consternation, Maneesh quickly noticed both the disparity of symptoms in different symptom checkers along with inconsistency in information about prevention, treatment and isolation on different official sites. He quickly began recording his experiences via his Twitter account. At that moment he became a citizen journalist, sharing his account on the timelines of his 14,000 followers.

What makes Maneesh different from many people sharing their COVID-19 experiences online is hinted at by his Twitter moniker #DigitalHealthFuturist. He is an early adopter of all types of health-related technology. Our paths had crossed most recently at a Royal Society of Medicine digital health event earlier in 2020, but I have known Maneesh since I started working in digital health. "William Gibson's famous quote The future is here, it just isn't evenly distributed" has never felt more apposite when I think of Maneesh; he's my go-to person when it comes to considering the future of digital. He's always the one already testing out the latest wearable or piece of software or virtual reality headset.

As I write this introductory chapter, Maneesh is on day 300 of COVID-19 and reports experiencing ongoing symptoms of fatigue. Whilst he avoided ICU and a ventilator, he has been severely ill and continues to be badly affected. In an exchange on the Twitter direct message he remains concerned about a possible relapse which he tells me is not uncommon at his stage of recovery. Maneesh is afflicted by what has become known as *long Covid*, where symptoms persist and can have debilitating effects over a long period of time.

Maneesh reported his experiences daily throughout the course of his illness, sharing his use of online symptom checkers and other technologies he used to self-monitor and track the progress of the disease. I would love to have interviewed Maneesh for this book, and he initially agreed to my request, but as I write this chapter he is still too ill to take part. He nevertheless agreed that I could share some of his story, gathered from his tweets and our occasional messages.

Introduction ■ 5

Throughout the course of this book, I elucidate many trips, falls, missteps and outright disasters in the journey of digital health. However, Maneesh's story sets the scene in a more optimistic light. In a series of tweets on 24 June, he begins:

> We hear stories about how the NHS is bad with digital technology, but here's a story of how the NHS can be quite remarkable, from a patient's perspective in terms of accessing data that previously would not be available directly to patients.

He goes on to describe how his GP had ordered blood tests to identify signs of muscle damage as a consequence of the virus, which had been done the same day in a hospital setting. Maneesh reports that he was told to wait a few days for the results and to schedule a call to review them. However: "I opened the NHS App on my phone this morning, and I was blown away to see that I could see some (but not all) of my blood test results in my medical record. I am so impressed!" and it turns out they were uploaded just four hours after the tests were taken.

Maneesh has a technology background and only more recently has focused on its application to healthcare. As for myself, I accidentally stumbled across digital technologies through my postgraduate study, in which I researched people blogging about mental health, back in 2012. My journey into digital health is very different from that of Maneesh. With an undergraduate degree in English Literature, I went on to do a Masters in Social Work; then followed several decades in the NHS in a variety of roles, but with improvement and innovation at the core I have always held a fascination with working out how we make things better within large institutions and been perversely enthralled by navigating the many and never-ending barriers and constraints that I address in this book.

What Even Is Digital Health?

I will pause at this point to explain what I mean when I use the somewhat slippery and ill-defined word *digital* in the context of healthcare.[10] It is a word that is enthusiastically bandied about but often ill-defined. It means different things to different people.

Let's start with the basics. Like most sectors, the NHS has a range of systems that help healthcare practitioners manage their work: clinical systems, such as patient administration systems (PAS) enable hospitals to manage things like scheduling and referrals; secondly, electronic patient records (EPR) are a digital version of our healthcare record, which are often provided by massive companies like Cerner and Epic, but sometimes developed in-house at a local level; then we have clinical decision support tools that help healthcare practitioners assess your condition, give a risk score, make a diagnosis or triage you to the right bit of a service. These are just a few examples; the list goes on.

6 ■ *Towards a Digital Ecology*

There are a massive 23,000 IT systems that connect to the NHS Spine, which supports the IT infrastructure for health and social care in England. Anecdotally it is not uncommon for NHS trusts to have well over 100 official clinical systems across one organisation. However, there are also many *shadow IT* systems which might be a spreadsheet or database, and there can be anything up to 800 of those in place at any time. Add into this any number of services secretly buying systems without informing IT departments and it is a big spaghetti mess. One chief information officer (CIO) described trying to manage and reduce shadow IT systems as like playing a game of whack-a-mole – one goes down and another pops up.

With this siloed and fragmented muddle of systems, we have data that is similarly dispersed and locked away into these many and varied platforms. Across those platforms, data is defined and captured in a multitude of different ways and formats. Patient records in these systems are a mire of structured and unstructured data comprising everything from demographics, diagnoses, tests, procedures, medical images and outcomes. We should remind ourselves that paper records, that is file upon file of handwritten notes and scribbles, are still the backbone of many hospital systems.

Then we have digital technologies that enable healthcare practitioners to interact with patients at a distance. These are sometimes referred to as *telemedicine* or *telehealth*. Common telehealth tools are online consultation systems that enable us to interact remotely by for example, doing an online assessment; video consultations systems enable us to have appointments away from the clinical setting; personal health records are platforms through which we can see our information online, book appointments and interact with healthcare practitioners; electronic prescribing enables healthcare practitioners and patients to manage and collect prescriptions.

Increasingly, there is a whole range of mobile applications which make it possible for citizens to do various health-related activities such as track, monitor, set goals, access information and resources. It is not uncommon for people to create peer support communities around particular health conditions on consumer platforms such as Facebook. The term digital therapeutics (DTx) applies to digital technologies which provide therapies to prevent, manage or treat a condition. Wearables and sensors around the home enable the collection of passive data that we can use to measure our heart rate, movements or other key factors. Some of these technologies are part of clinical care, but just as many are consumer products bought and downloaded from commercial companies.

Increasingly, emerging technologies such as artificial intelligence (AI), virtual and augmented reality and robotics are being applied to healthcare. AI refers to machines that can perform tasks generally thought to require intelligence. Most AI systems employ a technique known as machine learning, in which computers learn how to perform a specific task from examples, data and experience.[11] Amongst other things, AI can be deployed in decision support for assessing imaging (for example, x-rays) and predicting disease. The data that emerges from these technologies holds great promise in informing the planning of care at a population level, as well as enabling a shift in focus towards prevention and planning in addition to treatment and care. However, as we shall see, their application in healthcare is still early and the hype often overshadows the reality.

A Perfect Storm

Digital health is the perfect storm of small and nimble entrepreneurs and start-ups bumping up against established IT vendors and lumbering NHS providers; a collision of private interests in tension with public health priorities; and an immature sector that is only just beginning to find its feet. Throw in a global pandemic and suddenly business as usual is out of the door and possibilities emerge for doing things very differently, along with risks of reinforcing the worst that technologies can bring. This is the core of my inquiry throughout this book.

The Government has ambitious plans for the digital transformation of healthcare, and they exist within a wider societal context in which technology shapes our lives for better or for worse. The majority of us think that it has improved our lives but many of us also have doubts about whether it has been so good for society as a whole. Only half of us feel optimistic about how technology will affect us in the future and under a quarter of us believe that tech companies have our best interests at heart.[12] This is not a particularly compelling starting point for an effort that needs to galvanise the biggest employer in the country, with a workforce of around one and a half million people.[13]

Over the course of the first wave of the pandemic, I tracked changes that happened in the sphere of digital health, interviewing IT leaders (often called CIOs) GPs and other healthcare practitioners coping with the initial tsunami and then the aftershocks as the immediate crisis abated. I spoke with patients, volunteers, digital health companies, researchers and policymakers to elicit varied insights and opinions as the pandemic unfolded. I am grateful to the various WhatsApp groups where friends and colleagues shared insights and experiences and answered questions I posed as I sought to explore and understand what was happening in the sphere of digital health.

Backdrop to Broken

In the first part of the book, I take us back to basics and a world of clunky technology, paper records, siloed data with systems that refuse to interoperate. Despite a dollop of hyperbole and any number of national and local initiatives, the NHS has remained stubbornly resistant to the sorts of digital transformation experienced by other sectors.

The shadow of unsuccessful national IT programmes looms large in the collective memory of those who have worked in the field for some time. Initiated by the Labour government in 2002, the National Programme for IT was eventually dismantled ten years later by the Conservative and Liberal Democrat coalition after any number of delays, implementation issues and opposition by stakeholders.[14]

8 ■ *Towards a Digital Ecology*

The backdrop of shapeshifting government policy and a slow-motion merry-go-round of national control versus local determination have all played their part in frustrating efforts to modernise our beloved health system. Plans and policy documents come and go, along with celebrity doctors brought in by the secretary of state for the day to write their particular prescription of the day. Whilst the white noise of policy chatters in the background, intransigent challenges remain and people at a local level do their best despite the system rather than because of it.

Through interviews with NHS IT leaders and clinicians, I find out about the barriers that have hampered digital transformation and have led to high levels of frustration and scepticism about what might be achieved in the future. Digital promises to transform the experience of care for patients and improve staff morale by helping them become more effective and productive. However, it often seems like it is creating the reverse – an additional world of complexity and fragmentation. How do we avoid creating the legacy IT systems of the future? This book is an exploration of these challenges and the opportunities that sit alongside them.

Necessity Is the Mother of Invention

The use of digital technologies in the first wave of the pandemic crisis is just one lens through which personal and societal impacts were experienced and which I explore in the second half of the book. There was a sudden rash of technology improvisation – contact tracing applications for infected people, data analytics tools to detect potential outbreaks, web-based information and self-assessments, telehealth solutions for remote appointments. This was the largest health crisis since the advent of digital technologies and so their use to help curb and contain its effects was novel, without precedent and at times, contested.

Any number of reports purport mass adoption and profound digital transformation which they claim was accelerated through the pandemic. It is true that necessity forced the uptake of technologies that had been available for decades but which had been resisted by patients and clinicians alike. But the story is not quite as straightforward as it might seem.

In Chapter 3, I scratch beneath the rhetoric and through stories from health professionals on the frontline of NHS services, I seek to understand how those displacements and reworkings of clinical practice were achieved. I question whether the pandemic heralded a heyday for digital – a coming of age for technology in health. Or was it the case the pandemic simply prompted the NHS to spread some very basic but useful technologies that most of us take for granted in our everyday lives? The truth, as we shall find, is somewhere in between.

Relative Advantage

In the course of a year, the NHS delivers around 120 million hospital outpatient appointments in hospitals around England. These visits account for a whopping

85% of all non-emergency hospital-based activity. In March 2020, at the beginning of the pandemic, outpatient appointments delivered via phone call or video almost tripled from the number recorded the same time the previous year. Something had changed.

Whilst the hype of digital transformation favours an emphasis on AI and robotics, it is actually suppliers of the humble video consultation that had the most profound impact on the NHS in the first wave of the pandemic. With the fear of contagion keeping patients out of the consulting room, and clinical staff working from home wherever possible, audio and video communications came into their own.

In Chapter 4, I tell the story of this shift through first-hand experience from people who experienced it on the ground. I dig beneath the surface to really understand what this shift in practice meant to patients as well as clinicians. I draw on theories of diffusion of innovation to explain why this update managed to happen so quickly despite decades of non-adoption in healthcare services.

Through interviews with GPs, hospital consultants, junior doctors and a primary care receptionist, I find out the everyday realities, upsides and downsides of video consultations and consider what their role might be in a healthcare system with a thriving digital ecology.

When People Drive Digital

The NHS is a service for all of us, as patients and citizens, there for when we most need it. Many of us watched the US crime series Breaking Bad when it came out on Netflix. The story of a chemistry teacher who starts making and dealing in crystal meth to fund his stage three cancer treatment was spellbinding. But the idea that one has to turn to crime to pay for healthcare treatment is a curious anathema to those of us benefiting from a single-payer publicly funded system.

We may have open access to healthcare in the UK, but patients and citizens have not been routinely involved in digital transformation efforts which directly affect how we receive our care. Chapter 5 tells compelling stories of people who have innovated from their experience living with chronic conditions. They shine a light on frustration with the NHS's slow progress in digital uptake and show how some have decided not to wait but go off and solve those problems themselves.

Much of this book focuses on how the healthcare system, riddled from the top down and back up again with paternalism and inertia, is attempting to flip itself into the digital age that surrounds it. However, this chapter also explores the power of networks, of communities and of people who are not bound by the control and hierarchy of the system. It explores the constant flux between central diktat and local control and asks how we can best make change with people at the heart; how the healthcare system can both scaffold and enable this to happen.

10 ■ *Towards a Digital Ecology*

Context Is King

Culture and contextual factors are poorly understood by those entrepreneurs who harbour a sincere belief that their technology can save the NHS. Time and again I have seen digital health companies flounder when they come up against the hard reality that, without appreciating context, culture and complexity, their technology is doomed to the dustbin.

Just why has the NHS been so stubbornly intransigent when it comes to adopting digital technologies? In order to understand this most contemporary dilemma, we have to subsume ourselves in a jumble of complexity. To understand the non-adoption of technology is to steep ourselves in a very particular quagmire of culture, context and identity that any wide-eyed innovator should ignore at their peril.

In Chapter 6, I draw on compelling empirical evidence, my own experience born out of decades working in the NHS and stories from those trying to navigate complexity in their everyday working lives. Beguiled by technology, too often we treat digital transformation as a product to be implemented or a software license to be procured.

Human factors such as professional identity, team culture, organisational capacity to absorb innovation and the ability of people in leadership roles to persuade and cajole are woefully underestimated. I explore the emerging profession of user-centred design in the health service which brings a rigorous focus on seeking to understand the problems people are trying to solve and the goals they are trying to achieve. I consider whether a new cadre of professionals may hold at least part of the answer to transforming services so that we better meet people's needs.

The Social Determinants of Digital

If the pandemic showed us anything, it is that we depend on each other. Each of us was only as protected as the person who decided to wear a face mask at the supermarket or chose to self-isolate when they had a positive test. The Government persuaded, begged and cajoled us to follow the advice of public health officials and make personal sacrifices for the greater good. But COVID-19 made it impossible to escape from the harsh reality that inequality cuts deep into our society, and it was people from poorer backgrounds who paid the heaviest price.

In Chapter 7, I consider how digital poverty, literacy and inclusion are all factors that can no longer be downplayed by the NHS, as it endeavours to shift its many face-to-face interactions onto digital platforms. Through interviews with a digital inclusion worker, a policy expert, a clinician entrepreneur and a social change activist, I explore the dark world of data bias and why having a diverse team matters.

It is clear that digital exclusion is the symptom of deep inequality and lack of opportunity experienced by the very people the NHS most needs to reach out and support. A modern NHS must meet their needs first and foremost. We need to help

Introduction ■ 11

our septuagenarian NHS keep those core founding principles at its core – meeting the needs of everyone, free at the point of delivery, based on clinical need, not ability to pay. I explore how we can create a digitally inclusive ecology in healthcare.

The Jeopardy of Trust

Interoperability is the technical challenge of systems being able to seamlessly share data between them. But there is a human challenge too. That is the challenge of trust. It is not just the spectre of NPfIT that looms over efforts to digitise the NHS. There are a number of high-profile data debacles that cast a long shadow over endeavours to use data for what is known as *secondary purposes*, that is to improve care, for research, and to develop new products and services.

Health data is valuable. Despite the fragmentation of the NHS, our healthcare system remains the single largest integrated healthcare provider in the world, with primary care patient records covering the entire population from birth through to death.[15] Electronic patient record systems in hospitals are less well established, but nevertheless house around 23 million secondary episodic patient records. A 2019 report by global consultancy EY estimated that the 55 million GP records held by the NHS have an indicative market value of several billion pounds to a commercial organisation. The data stakes are high.

Digital innovation can't outpace trust. And the NHS can lay claim to the most valuable prize of being a highly trusted institution. But that trust has taken some data-shaped dents in recent times. With digital transformation comes a cascade of personal data about each of our lives and any aspect of our treatment and care. This data has to be safely managed, securely held and used with care and respect.

In Chapter 8, I explore just how the NHS can maintain its social contract with patients and the public in a digital age. I consider the increasing volumes of health data propagated from wearables and other consumer devices. I explore a novel approach to involving the public in making hard decisions about how healthcare data is used, not just for individual care, but to plan services and carry out medical research. I appraise some of the more promising approaches to data custodianship that might help rebuild public confidence so that we can reap the undoubted benefits of advancing our diagnosis, treatment and care at scale.

Bending the Curve on Digital Mental Health

In Chapter 9, I shine the spotlight on secondary care therapy services as a case study for technology adoption in the NHS. With comparatively mature digital flora and fauna, I wonder what it can tell us about the factors we need in place for digital to prosper. Struck by the pervasiveness of private companies in this arena, I am troubled about what this might mean for the future of the NHS. It is clear to me

12 ■ *Towards a Digital Ecology*

that there is an imperative for NHS services to adapt and evolve into this digital habitat if it is going to save itself; the question is how?

Like every other part of the NHS, secondary care therapy services were shaken by the pandemic, tripped into making rapid adjustments to how they were delivered out of necessity. Some of these changes may have eased the way for therapy services to embrace technology. If they can capitalise on the tactics they had to make and manoeuvre them into embedded practices, then maybe that could unlock their survival.

The Theatre of Tech – A Study in Solutionism

It would be remiss to write a book about the part digital technology played in the pandemic and omit to include the contact tracing app. It is easy to forget just how, in the very early days of the pandemic, governments all over the world pounced on the pleasing idea that a contact tracing app could be the answer to its tectonic viral spread.

Desperate to show that they were doing something, anything, the UK Government made a big deal about how a contact tracing app would save the day. Then it went quiet. Not a whisper. When the app did finally emerge from its secretive recesses and on to the app stores, its role in the pandemic had been diminished from headline act to supporting role. To be fair, this was the caste position it should have always held and so it is instructive to understand whose interests this misplaced role happened to serve.

In Chapter 10, I chart the sorry tale of the contact tracing app and consider its parallels with previous large-scale IT projects that have had similar fates. I mull over what we can learn from this particular tale about how to avoid the hubris and hyperbole that seems to be endemic with these sorts of grand initiatives.

We Get the Market We Deserve

Whilst ambitious programmes, massive structural change and political uncertainty are all part of the picture, there is another facet of digital transformation that is less well understood. In Chapter 11, I investigate the marketplace in digital health along with how money moves. How digital health products and services are bought and sold is confoundingly complicated when compared other gadgets, fixtures and consumables that our healthcare system buys.

The NHS is a big customer of everything from mattresses and hospital beds, through to kitchen equipment and MRI scanners. Digital health is the newborn baby of that marketplace, stretching out its arms to make sense of its surroundings. In contrast to established manufacturers selling tried and tested equipment to healthcare, digital health is characterised by small start-ups who often have untried and untested technologies.

In this chapter, I traverse a landscape that takes us on a journey from NHS budgets and procurement, along the muddy bog of evidence and regulation, and into the dense woods of investors and venture capital. I endeavour to detangle the many threads and lay them out so that we can begin to grope towards a means to create a flourishing marketplace.

Momentum – Towards a Digital Ecology

In the final chapter, I delineate the characteristics of an NHS fit for the 21st Century and beyond. Rather than attempt to narrowly define, I open up possibilities of what could be. I begin by setting out where we are heading in respect of the demographic contours of our country. I then ask powerful questions that people working in the sector might consider shaping whatever comes next. I don't purport to have the answers, but I believe we need to begin by making sure we are asking the right questions.

I develop the concept of a *digital ecology* and argue that we need to make a paradigm shift if we are to nurture an adaptive healthcare system fit for the digital age that nurtures equality and trust. It is possible to create a digital ecology in the NHS. It will not be linear. It will be complex. Our approach to a digital ecology should be to not only recognise and tolerate emergence but embrace it. A strategy is something that more often than not sits in a PDF within a forgotten folder on an un-navigable intranet.

An ecology takes a strategic approach to digital that blends the tactical and the visionary, the here-and-now with the possible. It works with assets and relies on relationships. It measures the right things. A digital ecology is a metaphor that embraces emergence and eschews the reductive nomenclature of Taylorism. It is carefully co-designed by using tools that facilitate cooperation and collaboration. It has agility and it is continuously learning.

I employ the metaphor of a digital ecology to provide a counterpoint. The way in which we currently conceptualise the labour of digital adoption is mired in normative and reductive technocratic language. Efficiency. Targets. Cuts. Effectiveness. You get what you put in. How we frame digital matters. The pandemic showed us, if we didn't know it already, that our fates are inextricably intertwined. A digital ecology assumes this to be fact and clasps it to its chest as an advantage rather than a handicap. A digital ecology is fair and it binds people together.

Notes

1 https://www.annualreviews.org/doi/full/10.1146/annurev-publhealth-032013-182435#_i1

14 ■ *Towards a Digital Ecology*

2 https://d1wqtxts1xzle7.cloudfront.net/58056169/When_digital_health_meets_digital_capitalism.pdf?1545655387=&response-content-disposition=inline%3B+filename%3D When_digital_health_meets_digital_capita.pdf&Expires=1612536727&Signature=Wv FwRLChzGYl90C4k9E4L6jCjAGiuINsie-zTdR-yO8MTosG3xPE61adn0xTwVLbx7j eJE-skzCLWT8qMdOp49E8b067lP2kRXGw8eKS3ECOo22oDQegqrlrH50HJ-doYTCRB4Q2w-1ouQLnoZypF3Vq82m3put1XeobOHEoLzBuHjRSNe4mz00i-grq27MJjhpo58hBoewZy9NUHXV10MYG1CtuNMbIEOzBaT7aUykSWiCB-3gqRq5VtsknLQKV6RVeaF9eCYZFyghWu-cMUl2uHuSqzIb9ejhF-P5hgKNk18RHr Ji3Yc8Mrth8tj25Z7rDB71SGBQXS57b07yataVg__&Key-Pair-Id= APKAJLOHF5GGSLRBV4ZA

3 https://nhsproviders.org/a-new-era-of-digital-leadership/what-is-digital

4 https://leadingedgeforum.com/media/1328/the_myths_and_realities_of_digital_disruption_-_an_executives_guide_executive_summary.pdf

5 https://www.cqc.org.uk/sites/default/files/20201016_stateofcare1920_fullreport.pdf

6 https://www.wired.co.uk/article/china-coronavirus

7 https://www.arcgis.com/apps/opsdashboard/index.html#/bda7594740fd 40299423467b48e9ecf6

8 https://www.nature.com/articles/s41564-020-0695-z

9 https://www.wired.co.uk/article/china-coronavirus

10 https://medium.com/@e17chrisfleming/an-introductory-guide-to-digital-healthcare-products-f467e3dc6b91

11 https://www.thersa.org/globalassets/pdfs/reports/rsa_artificial-intelligence---real-public-engagement.pdf

12 https://www.doteveryone.org.uk/wp-content/uploads/2020/05/PPT-2020_Soft-Copy.pdf

13 https://www.nuffieldtrust.org.uk/resource/the-nhs-workforce-in-numbers

14 https://www.cl.cam.ac.uk/~rja14/Papers/npfit-mpp-2014-case-history.pdf

15 https://assets.ey.com/content/dam/ey-sites/ey-com/en_gl/topics/life-sciences/life-sciences-pdfs/ey-value-of-health-care-data-v20-final.pdf

Chapter 2

Backdrop to Broken

> One of the greatest challenges in healthcare technology is that medicine is at once an enormous business and an exquisitely human endeavour; it requires the ruthless efficiency of the modern manufacturing plant and the gentle hand-holding of the parish priest; it is about science, but also about art; it is eminently quantifiable and yet stubbornly not.
>
> (Wachter, 2017, ps. 17)

Owing to the chaos of different systems, and the absence of any attempt to standardise ... co-operation between neighbouring authorities is difficult and expensive.[1]

Anyone familiar with the sluggish state of NHS digital transformation might read the above quote and guess it is from one of the barrage of reports tussling with how to accelerate technology adoption. However, they'd be wrong.

This is an extract from a report to the House of Commons by Liberal politician Sir Archibald Williamson, who was tasked with making recommendations for improving the supply of electricity all the way back in 1908.

Over a century ago, the electricity supply was a mess, with around 600 electricity power generators in the UK. In London alone, there were 70 suppliers of electricity with the same number of generating stations, 50 different types of systems, ten different frequencies and 25 different voltages. The report describes the system as chaotic, expensive and ineffective. Nothing connected to anything else. Even the erection of overhead wires could be vetoed by a local council.

Fast forward 100 years and another Parliamentary Committee was tasked with making recommendations for improving a different sector, similarly characterised by intricacy and complexity. The state of digital technology in the NHS bears all the hallmarks of the country's electricity supply a century before. In 2020, Labour MP

DOI: 10.1201/9781032198798-2

15

16 ■ *Towards a Digital Ecology*

Meg Hillier took on a similar task to Williamson, assessing the state of NHS digital transformation.[2] Her report begins with a sanguine analysis of the landscape we find ourselves in today:

> NHS's digital estate comprises an enormous number of out-of-date 'legacy' systems that cannot easily interact with each other and some trusts are using up to 400 different IT systems .... [there are] systemic issues within the NHS with broadband connectivity and outdated hardware, and a lack of funding and resources to train staff to use the technology available to them.

It seems that Williamson's electricity report is strangely prescient. In 2020, England was characterised by fragmented patient record systems, spread across thousands of local NHS organisations, with huge variation in the digital maturity of NHS organisations and their staff. Digital transformation is a mire of heterogeneity along with a tussle between local fiefdoms and central control.

This state of affairs has real-life consequences for patients and clinicians every single day in GP practices and hospitals around the country. A typical hospital worker has to log in to up to 15 different systems to treat just one patient, and it can take up to ten minutes to log in each time.[3] Just think of the frustration and time wasted in remembering all those passwords.[4] Lack of access to accurate information has material ramifications for patients too – less effective care, more tests and even medical errors.[5]

The issues raised in the Parliamentary Accounts Committee report took me back to an uncomfortable moment at the beginning of my career in digital health. I had invited myself to speak to a committee of psychiatrists about the use of digital technology in mental health. Having only just started out in the digital sector, I was chock-full of enthusiasm. I had prepared a PowerPoint presentation bursting with the promise of the latest technologies. I wanted to wow them into buying into my enthusiasm that it could improve their lives and those of their patients. I was gloriously oblivious to the fact that for many clinicians, their primary exposure to technology is through the electronic patient record. Far from being convenient, those record systems have a reputation for being labour intensive in data entry and not always intuitive or easy to use.[6]

Arriving early to the meeting, the chairperson invited me to listen in as they finished their previous agenda item, which happened to be about the state of their local electronic patient record. As I listened to them vent their frustration about how this basic piece of infrastructure technology was impeding their work, I suddenly realised the talk I had planned would at best seem irrelevant and at worst completely alienate them. I mentally overhauled my presentation as I sat and listened. If the everyday technology they used was not able to free them from their drudgery, they certainly would not be willing to listen to anything about the promise of my somewhat naive blue sky digital future.

My gut feeling back then is backed up by recent research from the British Medical Association (BMA). In a survey of their members, they found that deficiencies in basic technologies not only add to doctors' workload and stress, they result in 'disquiet at the increasing amount of attention being given to innovations such as AI (artificial intelligence), rather than to creating functioning, interoperable systems'.[7] Hype over reality has a habit of getting in the way of progress.

A survey of Royal College of Emergency Medicine members found that no electronic patient record system in the UK meets the internationally validated standard of acceptable usability for information technology.[8] In another survey of doctors, the BMA found that over a quarter report losing more than four hours a week because of inefficient hardware/systems. A few sums and this equates to approximately 4,870 full-time equivalent doctors working 37.5 hours a week over a calendar year. They conclude that the impact on other NHS staff may be similar. Not even the basics are yet properly in place for a digital technology-enabled healthcare system.

That meeting with a group of psychiatrists was pivotal for me. It alerted me to a dissonance between the promise and the reality of digital technology in the NHS. It drew me towards treating hype with suspicion and seeking to understand the lived reality of people working in the healthcare system. The path to digital adoption is not a smooth one, and the balance between local determination and central diktat is invariably problematic. This was never more so than for the NHS. Just as lack of standardisation hampered a national approach to electricity use across the country over 100 years ago, so lack of connectivity is impeding attempts for NHS organisations to work together across cities, towns and regions.[9]

Engaging in a never-ending dance of restructure and reorganisation, most recently the NHS is coming together in regions known as Integrated Care Systems (ICSs). The parliamentary report concludes that regional coordination of patient care requires data to move seamlessly between health and care organisations, and this simply can't be done with systems that don't speak to each other. The NHS requires a clear set of standards along with the right incentives for legacy IT systems to upgrade and improve. In May 2020, only three of the ten standards required for interoperability were ready. In evidence to the Parliamentary Committee, chief executive of NHSX, Matthew Gould conceded:

> We have an enormous legacy estate that is extremely complex and distributed. Even if we put in place standards, enforce those standards and ensure that all new bits of the estate are compliant, it will take years for that legacy estate to catch up with the standards. It would be replaced and sorted out bit by bit ... true interoperability across the system is a work of years.[10]

It is clear that the NHS has a long way to go. But what does that actually mean for you and me as patients and citizens? With 307 million GP appointments a year, the

18 ∎ *Towards a Digital Ecology*

NHS touches all of our lives to differing degrees and at different times.[11] The state of NHS digital adoption is materially relevant to all whether we work in the NHS, receive its services or contribute to its running as taxpayers. I wonder how this macro state of affairs affects the micro realities of our daily lives.

A Minor Inconvenience

Farhan hadn't ever consciously thought of it. He had always just assumed that his and his family's GP and hospital records could be seen by any health professional. It was only when he found himself in an accident and emergency department, whilst on holiday, that he realised this was not actually the case.

They were visiting family in Birmingham when his primary school-age daughter, Aaliya began struggling with her asthma. Farhan realised to his horror that they had run out of inhalers. Flustered and tired, they drove to the local hospital emergency department late that evening. It hadn't occurred to Farhan to bring his daughter's expired inhalers with him. In the past, the A&E doctor had no way of knowing which of the four variations of inhalers she uses; they would have had to rely on educated guesswork based on Farhan's recollection of the colour, size and shape of the inhaler. However, the good news is that the NHS Summary Care Record[12] means that the doctor did have access to the basic information she needed about Aaliya's condition and medication. Farhan's daughter got the treatment she needed, and the family was able to enjoy the rest of their family holiday.

The Summary Care Record is a game-changing development that supports continuity of care for patients. However, the lack of connectivity between clinical systems still has everyday consequences for patients and clinicians. The rich data which sets out the chronology of Aaliya's interactions with different services remain siloed in their separate systems, never to be connected. When combined together, they would begin to paint a rich picture of how Aaliya and her family manage her condition and help clinicians inform, advise and treat.

If that data is combined with data from other children such as Aaliya, it starts to tell a story about how we might better predict and treat asthma at a population level, spotting patterns in the data about factors such as where people live and the time of year when instances go up or down.

So why, when we can withdraw cash from an ATM in any part of the country, can we not access the totality of our healthcare information wherever we happen to be? It turns out we are still mired in the sorts of challenges the government of the time was tackling for electricity back in 1918.

Ill-fated Plans

It is not for want of trying. To understand why the NHS has remained so stubbornly resistant to digital adoption, we need to step back 20 years when the ill-fated

Backdrop to Broken ■ 19

National Programme for IT (NPfIT) was introduced in 2002. That same year saw the UK in the final throes of another devastating virus. Foot-and-Mouth disease cost the economy £8 billion, whilst decimating animal farming and related industries.[13]

The idea for NPfIT, a top-down and centralised approach to digital transformation in the NHS, had its genesis in a conversation between then Prime Minister, Tony Blair and Microsoft CEO, Bill Gates. So the story goes, a plan emerged for a formidable programme to create, amongst other things, an electronic patient record system across the whole of the NHS. This was Gates' solution to the issue of interoperability – create one big integrated system that every hospital would use and which would connect them to GP record systems across the country.

What seems like a sensible idea was eventually abandoned some nine years later after blowing its budget sky-high. It had failed to achieve its primary objective of creating a single electronic patient record. NPfIT turned out to be the most costly technology programme in the history of the NHS and the world's largest civil information technology endeavour.[14] It resulted in tectonic legal wranglings with some of the big companies who got involved, and it was ultimately unsuccessful.

NPfIT was blighted by a set of problems that will become familiar over the course of this book. We find them repeated over and again. Firstly, NHS chiefs completely underestimated the complexity of the endeavour. Secondly, there were many changes of leadership and too much haste to deliver at speed. Poor communication resulted in a lack of support from the very clinicians it was intended to benefit. Along with low buy-in, the changes required by clinicians to adopt a central system were woefully underestimated. Finally, there was the inevitable scope creep and costs began to escalate. As Joe McDonald, consultant psychiatrist and chief information officer recalls: "We signed contracts in blood with large IT suppliers without ever having consulted a clinician."

"We decided we would go big" explains Joe in a webinar on the topic "We didn't trial it anywhere, we would do the whole thing on a massive scale, unpiloted, untrialed, untested across the whole NHS."[15] Moving from one electronic patient record to another in just one hospital is a massive endeavour. Trying to do it for the whole country was just too much of a stretch. As well as casting a shadow over subsequent efforts to create a digital infrastructure for the NHS, it is a salutary case study for the current state of play in the pandemic-era of digital.[16] It turns out that previous mistakes are easily forgotten, and it is not uncommon to repeat errors of the past.

Having worked in the NHS for over 29 years in a variety of influential information technology and digital transformation roles, Andy Kinnear is well placed to comment on the £9.8 billion ambitious and ultimately doomed project to introduce a centralised integrated IT system for the NHS.[17] He reflects on the chequered history of digital transformation with an air of gloom: "When I look back at the last decade that we've gone through, I think we came into it under a real shadow off the back of the National Programme [for IT]."

"We had this major opportunity [with NPFit]" recalls Andy: "prime ministerial patronage, more money than we could ever possibly imagine, and ultimately we

20 ■ *Towards a Digital Ecology*

didn't succeed." There were some notable exceptions, including the creation of a national infrastructure (the Spine) to enable sharing electronic information between organisations, a single patient identifier (the NHS number) and electronic prescribing in primary care.[18] These have become important technology building blocks of our contemporary healthcare system. Even where there is an apparent failure, there is still learning to be had and each challenge builds part of the bridge towards a digital future.

When I speak to Andy, we are in the first lockdown and so our conversation takes place in our respective makeshift home offices via Google Meet. There is a certain joyful irony to the fact that Andy's Wi-Fi gives up at various points during our chat, competing as it is with other members of his household's streaming activities along with bad cable connectivity. Just like the National Programme, I think our call is ill-fated as the call drops out, but we manage to reconnect just long enough to finish our conversation. Andy is a key figure in NHS IT, having held a range of influential positions, including chair of the British Computer Society Health and Care Executive Committee. When he describes his experience of digital technology over the last 20 years as *largely frustrating*, I know he is not alone. The benefits and potential gains are immense, but the basics are still not evenly in place and the complexities daunting.

No one wants to be in charge of a digital transformation project that fails. With the backdrop of NPfIT, the perceived risk of failure bears heavily on NHS digital leaders. It might be better to stick with what you know than take the plunge to make the big changes we need to see. The time and headspace taken up with managing legacy systems make it hard to be strategic and furrow a new path.[19] We have a rocky climb ahead, but the destination is one in which our systems work better, clinician's lives are easier and patients get better care and treatment. It is worth the hike.

Central Ambitions

As NPfIT tripped and stumbled its way to an ignominious end, the Whole System Demonstrator was launched as a two-year research project which sought to provide definitive evidence that what is known as *assistive technologies* are cost-effective and improve quality of life for patients. Focusing on people with long-term conditions such as Type 2 diabetes, COPD and coronary heart disease, the demonstrator programme is another pothole in the bumpy ride of NHS digital transformation.

The Whole System Demonstrator hoped to prove that technology could "support people to live independently, take control and be responsible for their own health and care."[20] This was going to show once and for all that digital technologies were capable of transforming the NHS. The demonstrator was less about standardising systems and more about patients having technology in their hands to manage their own care. Advocates believed that technology-empowered patients would not only have a better quality of life, but it would say the NHS money too. However, the evidence turned out to be underwhelming.

Published in the British Medical Journal,[21] a randomised control trial with around 3000 participants compared the costs of assistive technologies with those of standard support and treatment alone. The term telehealth is a bit old-fashioned these days but refers to the remote exchange of data between a patient and health-care professional to assist in the diagnosis and management of a healthcare condition. This might mean a patient collecting and sharing vital signs (for example, blood pressure readings using a cuff) from their home, along with clinicians sending them online information, resources and being available on the telephone to give support when needed. This was in addition to their standard care and treatment. The intention was for people to manage their own conditions at home, reducing the need for clinic visits and hospital stays; clinician time would be freed up and they could focus their efforts on remote support via the phone, messaging and video.

The largest trial of its kind in England, the researchers concluded that adding telehealth to standard care actually *increased* costs by about 10% for only minimal gains in quality of life. They concluded that telehealth was not a cost-effective intervention for these patients, which means that the costs didn't weigh up with the benefits.

This was a massive body blow to those wanting to make the case for patient-facing digital transformation. The research cast doubt on the potential of technology to achieve its promise in the minds of clinicians and policymakers alike. It is another part of the complex tableau of digital health that forms the backdrop to the challenges we see today.

Changes You Can See from Outer Space

Attempts to transform the NHS through technology have taken place amongst real term cuts to public budgets and substantial structural change and reorganisation. A recent report from the NHS regulator, the Care Quality Commission, shows challenges in all parts of the NHS, including problems in accessing routine GP appointments and rising numbers of people waiting for treatment just before the pandemic struck.[22]

In particular, the controversial 2012 Health and Care Act, led by conservative Health Secretary Andrew Lansley, saw a major structural reorganisation of the NHS and an orientattion towards competition and privatisation.[23] At the time, the Health and Care Act was described by then NHS Chief Executive David Nicholson, as a reform programme so big that it could be seen from outer space.

In Andy's opinion, the fallout from this, along with other structural changes, has resulted in what he describes as the most broken version of the NHS that he's ever been part of. In a reflective mood, he bemoans how a backdrop of real term cuts and

22 ■ *Towards a Digital Ecology*

instability has made the job of digital transformation so much harder: "The projects we've been trying to deliver are at their heart collaborative," but the system has got in the way rather than helped:

> The NHS that we've been in post-Lansley has been a really challenging environment to be honest … I think it's rewarded a lot of the wrong behaviours in the system – organisation-centric thinking and this pseudo competitive environment doesn't lend itself to the kind of [collaborative] technology challenges we've been facing.

Constant reorganisation and restructuring have become a feature of our National Health Service. Every restructure swallows up people's capacity to do anything else other than manage each change imposed upon them. It is hard to get anything else done. A new Health and Social Act on the horizon will reverse the 30-year trend towards competition within healthcare and undo the fragmentation caused by the previous Lansley reforms.[24] However, some are concerned by its intention to strengthen ministerial control and therefore the likelihood it will become even more of the political football it has always been.

The last 30 years of constant structural tinkering has resulted in barely any benefit, whilst creating huge costs and distraction.[25] Anne Cooper, former Chief Nurse at NHS Digital, reflects on her 20-year career as a nurse in technology:

> I can't remember how many NHS reorganisations [organisational] I have gone through in my career … and change is disruptive, it distracts everybody … we experience a slowing down, having to work out the impact before picking up pace again, you get a lag and a slowing of everything, everyone is really distracted by whether they're going to be in work or not.

This backdrop of massive structural change, fragmentation and reduced finances has meant that attempts to make a gear-shift in technology adoption have faced an uphill struggle. The fact remains that only half of NHS trusts in England report that their staff can rely on digital records for information they need, when they need it.[26] What this means in practice is that healthcare practitioners develop workarounds to manage the everyday frustrations of bad IT. It is not unheard of to leave computers logged on in open work environments and to share patient information over personal email or WhatsApp to get a colleague's opinion. These small actions may solve the immediate problem, but they create all sorts of cyber security and information governance risks along the way.

Whatever political persuasion, ministers seek to make their mark, and I have worked in and around the NHS for long enough to observe for myself that ideas and initiatives come and go, get repeated and often don't quite deliver. Over the last ten years, digital health has been no exception to this rule. As the dust settled from NPfIT, a new Secretary of State for Health, Jeremy Hunt, went about reviving government ambitions for digital transformation. He confidently set an objective for the NHS to become paperless by 2018. That meant the paper records that we see piled in trolleys on hospital wards and stacked in hospital back offices would become a thing of the past.

However, such an apparently simple objective proved elusive, and the target was extended to 2020.[27] As a new decade approached, the target was downgraded to a diminished ambition for the NHS to be *largely digitised* by 2024.[28] This ambition receded even further when it was replaced by a commitment that in ten years the NHS will offer a *digital first option for most*.[29] Such shape-shifting policy illuminates the complexity of the challenge and how difficult digital transformation has been to achieve. One initiative gets replaced by another as it becomes apparent each is impossible to achieve within the often ambitious timescales set.

When American author and celebrity physician, Bob Wachter, was asked by Jeremy Hunt in 2015 to advise the government on NHS digital transformation, there was a frisson of optimism in the air. A regular on the conference circuit, I recall a keynote in which he recounted the story of a recruitment ad for a physician, in which one of the big selling points to work for this particular American hospital, was the *absence* of an electronic patient record. For Wachter, this was an indictment of the extent to which technology is experienced as clunky and distracting for medics wanting to get on with the job of treating patients. It was his call to action to improve this woeful state of affairs not only in his home country but in the UK also.

Author of *The Digital Doctor*, a bestselling book on the progress of technology in the US healthcare system, Wachter was asked by the government to lead a review and give recommendations for NHS digital transformation. In his 2016 report, he advocated for a measured approach in which digital transformation should be done *right* rather than in a *rush*. With a more measured assessment than a health minister trying to make their mark, he argued that the benefits could take ten years or more to be fully realised. We must be patient and do things right.

The start-up mantra of *move fast and break things*[30] was a founding principle of Facebook and may play well in Silicon Valley, but it doesn't translate so comfortably into the byzantine provinces of the NHS. Under the headline: "Can digital revolution save the NHS?" a Guardian newspaper article[31] at the time called out the "digital razzmatazz" in which too much is expected of digital, too quickly, with big promises made, quickly followed by a damp squib of delivery. This cycle of hype and disappointment only serves to knock the confidence of everyone involved and make each mountain seem that much steeper to climb.

The narrative of efficiencies and savings in Government plans to digitise the NHS is not necessarily compelling for clinicians who are ultimately responsible for enacting the desired change. Big promises and aspirations balanced on precarious foundations of retracting budgets is a familiar one. It is like trying to fix a battered old engine while it's still running with a mishmash of metric and imperial tools – the moving parts never quite fit together and the system fails to ever fire on all cylinders.

24 ■ *Towards a Digital Ecology*

A Competent Workforce

It was an operation that carried a 1–2% risk of death. But 69-year-old Stephen Pettitt tragically died during surgery for his heart condition.[32] So what went wrong? Back in 2015, it was the first time a new approach to surgery had been tried using a robot assistant. The inquest reported that the surgeon who performed the operation had received no training and there was an absence of local or national guidelines for him to follow in the use of robotics.[33] It was a death that need not have happened.

This cautionary tale illustrates a significant challenge; digital technologies will only realise their true value (and avoid harm) if they are properly used by healthcare professionals who have had the requisite training to do so. The BMA puts it starkly:

> getting new technology into the system is only the first step. Over-stretched GP practices or hospital departments will not benefit from being sent expensive new devices if staff do not have time to learn to use them. If they are to commit to change, it must be evident to users that there will be clear benefits within a reasonable period, timely upgrades and suitable training and integration, with time built into medical training and job plans. All of this must be part of any procurement and implementation plan.

Hot off the heels of the Wachter review, the Secretary of State for Health commissioned another American physician and academic, Eric Topol, to lead a review of the workforce implications of a digitally transformed NHS.[34] Given that one key factor in NPfIT's failure was the lack of engagement of clinical staff, it was encouraging to see a focus on the very people who will make the difference between transformation taking hold or dying in a ditch.

Topol's report paints a picture of an NHS workforce with variable digital skills and competence, right the way from the hospital porter to the board-level executive director. Used to dealing in hardware and infrastructure, the advent of digital technologies and data has proved a challenge to more traditional IT teams in the NHS. Topol looks forward 20 years to a digital future in which he argues the clinical workforce will need a whole new set of skills and competencies.

When I first started out in digital health, I could barely have a conversation with a clinician without them sharing their pet project for a new mobile app. Some of them would teach themselves to code; others would have a friend or family member who was a developer and off they would go. I observed a mounting graveyard of enthusiastically initiated but quietly abandoned projects; small amounts of money, goodwill and dedication never properly translated into digital products that would see the light of day.

At the other end of the spectrum, I recall running workshops for clinical teams where we would hand round an iPad with pre-loaded apps to reluctant staff who found it hard to see beyond the barriers of learning yet another new thing to add to their work and cognitive load. One occupational therapist was so nervous that she refused to hold the smart device, convinced she would break it (or maybe it would break her).

Anne knows better than most the challenges of convincing clinicians that it is in their interests to care about technology. She spent a significant chunk of her career working for NHS Digital, the national body charged with delivering large IT projects and custodian of patient data: "How many times have I gone out and spoken to nurses about using technology! Literally hundreds [of times] and it's only now that I'm starting to feel things are changing, and that's two decades." Anne recognises that change takes time: "This is a long game. It's not a short game" she reflects.

Anne believes nurses *must* engage with digital so they can mould technologies to their needs and working practices. This means being involved in the design and development of technology itself:

> Technologists would come in to talk to us to understand nurse's require-ments. They were lovely, there was no animosity, they wanted to help; but they needed answers and if we didn't answer them and help them to get it right for nursing, then they would have to do it anyway and we would get what we were given.

Now a non-executive director for an NHS trust, Anne sees some green shoots but she acknowledges that things are slow to move in this behemoth of a system:

> We are starting to see more board and executives talk about technology because they're starting to feel like it's part of the future ... but it's a bit like those nurses that I used to talk to, they haven't got the experience to vision what that might look like and they're cautious.

Having gleaned insights from an impressive array of experts, Topol made a series of recommendations for improving the digital competency of the workforce. He advocates that as well as senior roles responsible for advising boards on digital technologies, the NHS must develop a whole range of skills including an understanding of ethical considerations and critically appraise new technologies. Topol concludes that accounting for a five-to-seven-year time lag, there is an urgent need to upskill the workforce, which he believes will catalyse digital transformation: "There is no time to waste" he urges.

A 2020 inquiry into healthcare data by Imperial College London[35] concludes that the NHS simply does not have the knowledge or skills to deliver large complex IT programmes. Their assertion that lack of leadership in the NHS is a consequence of slow digital transformation over the last decade, rings true in my conversations with CIOs around the country. Some have either left or are thinking of leaving the NHS, frustrated by how little they are able to achieve, hampered by the fact their

26 ■ *Towards a Digital Ecology*

department is perceived as an overhead to be chipped away at, rather than a resource to be invested in. They do not have the resources to make the step-change we need.

It is also the case that the NHS struggles to compete with the private sector on salary and benefits when it comes to recruiting digital specialists.[36] One ex-senior IT leader, who now works in the commercial sector, explains to me why she eventually bailed on the NHS:

> I didn't feel like I could do a good job. I felt like I could do an average job ... you know there's not a lot to be proud of, because you're constantly patching stuff up; you're not the boy with the finger in the dyke, you've got your arm over here and your foot over there and you actually end up playing some game of Twister where you know you're holding back all of this stuff.

The increasing use of digital technologies in healthcare is creating the need for new types of specialist roles to work with the data we collect at a local and population level to create insight so we can improve what we do. In a paper entitled *Untapped Potential*, the Health Foundation makes the case that the NHS should do more to employ data analysts who can turn the data that patients generate and clinicians record into insight that can be used to improve services.

Those analysts need to be able to work with clinicians and improvement specialists to turn that insight into measurable change that improves treatment and care. The analysts who are employed in IT services in NHS trusts and Clinical Commissioning Groups across the country spend too much time doing low-value work, creating reports that aren't read and fail to make an impact on care. If the NHS does not invest in its own analytics and data science workforce, it will continue to be at the whim of private companies who do, and the knowledge and expertise will be lost as soon as they leave.

The good news is that there are efforts to stimulate and support the professionalism of people coming into IT roles. Health Education England has a heap of programmes to equip a digital-ready workforce.[37] Andy Kinnear has led the charge in professionalising the IT workforce as chair of the health and care section of the British Computer Society Health and Care and the force behind The Federation of Informatics Professionals (FEDIP) which has brought together five professional bodies representing people with informatics careers into a single entity to manage the professional standards and professional registration of all its members. Andy explains why this matters:

> The equation is pretty simple. The more professional people are, the better invested in educationally and the higher recognition they get, then the better able they are to do their job properly. As we improve the delivery of digital services then the trickle down to our clinical professionals and ultimately our patients grows and grows. It's that simple.[38]

There are similar steps to harness the digital and entrepreneurial skills of clinicians.

The Clinical Entrepreneurs programme endeavours to create a space for entrepreneurial clinicians to experiment with their ideas. The NHS Innovation Accelerator has fellowships for entrepreneurs to bring their innovations to the healthcare system. The NHS Digital Academy aims to equip the next generation of leaders for digital transformation, and an evaluation of the first two cohorts is encouraging. However, as a mentor on the Digital Academy programme, I am not surprised to see that participants have struggled to identify the direct impact their participation has had on their organisation. Unless the context in which they return to is a permissive one, it will only lead to leaders becoming frustrated and looking outside the NHS to develop their skills further.

Rachel Dunscombe is the rock star of CIOs. She is also the chief executive of the NHS Digital Academy. I first properly got to know her on a surreal day trip to Area 51 with a group of hapless digital health professionals, slightly lost in the Nevada desert. But that's another story. "They tried to kill me so I came back to sort them out," says Rachel as she explains how an accidental insulin overdose after a caesarean section was what drew her to the NHS. "I was absolutely confused as to how care was so disjointed," says Rachel as she tells me how she chose to leave the corporate life of yachts and Range Rovers for our public healthcare system. She found her initiation discombobulating: "Holy cow! We were so behind where I thought we would be."

Even though she has had her fair share of infrastructure challenges, Rachel believes that technology is not the biggest problem:

> Everything [else] is dwarfed by capacity, capability, humans and skills. Our biggest rate limiting factor will be people … getting people skilled up in designing the future properly, systemically, creating the solutions for the future, creating convergence and platforms people can build on, and working with our citizens to co-design and co-own.

For Rachel, this is about people and trust, at scale. This is a marathon, not a race.

X Is for Experience

In February 2019, the Government announced the creation of NHSX to drive digital transformation with what could be argued is a reverse ethos of NPfIT, orientated towards national standards but a local approach to implementation. A *unit* rather than an organisation, NHSX was tasked with strategic responsibility for setting the national direction on technology across the NHS.

This attempt to galvanise the system towards digital transformation was the brainchild of then Secretary of State for Health, Matt Hancock. The MP has a moniker of *Matt the App* on account of the *Matt Hancock MP* app he developed

28 ∎ *Towards a Digital Ecology*

to engage with his constituents when he was Culture Secretary. The app hit the headlines[39] when people noticed system alerts such as "Matt Hancock would like to access your photos" and "Matt Hancock would like to access your camera" which caused all manner of hilarity at his expense. Not the most auspicious start for a minister with his sights set on digital transformation as his legacy to the NHS.

It is widely thought that the creation of NHSX was Hancock's attempt to get a grip on the digital transformation of the NHS. However, some have argued that this latest kid on the block actually compounds the very problems it is meant to solve: "Forming just the latest part of the constantly shifting layers of complex and confusing national governance on digitisation, involving multiple often overlapping agencies, including but not limited to: NHS Digital, NHSE/I, Department of Health, the Care Quality Commission, Health Education England."[40] Without any statutory footing, this unit is another layer of confusion in what is already a crowded marketplace of arm's-length bodies.

Over the course of my conversations for this book, there has been a consistent sense of confusion about who is responsible for what. One senior clinician I interviewed summed up nicely:

> All these organisations, I still have no idea what they all do to be honest. They all have NHS and a letter at the end of them. It's all a bit of a mystery to me. We've worked our way through [NHS] E [NHS] I and now it's gone up to [NHS] X.

This opacity came into sharp relief during the pandemic. James Norman, a CTO for a global IT company and ex-NHS CIO is damning in his assessment:

> You can't rely on the centre ... it hasn't worked out how it works together ... it has become very confusing, a nightmare to know who is coordinating, who is going to make the decisions, who to believe, conflicts in messaging.

The National Audit Office is more measured, but similarly describes a "complex governance arrangement" that creates confusion for people within and external to the system who are trying to contribute to the underlying policy intent to digitise the NHS. Even senior people *within* the system admit to it being bewildering. In an interrogation by the Parliamentary Accounts Committee, then chief executive of NHS Digital, Sarah Wilkinson admitted: "... it is a work in progress. It is very complicated to insert a new organisation into a structure that is already very complicated ..."

In an attempt to get a grip on the complexity that he has contributed to, Matt Hancock controversially paid global consultancy McKinsey's nearly half a million pounds to carry out a seven-week review of NHS digital transformation in late summer 2020.[41] The deckchairs are shifting again, and NHSX is to be merged back into NHS England/Improvement and the Department of Health and Social Care. Whatever the corporate story that is told, each reorganisation, however small, carries a hidden cost of distraction and delay. The merry-go-round continues.

Diktat and Determination

"There has historically been this national versus local antagonism," explains Indi Singh as we chat to each other in the heat of the pandemic summer. Indi knows this better than most, having worked in a range of senior technology roles in NHS central bodies. "It's going to be hybrid, it has to be a hybrid between the two," he argues, a proponent of national bodies positioning themselves in a serving role whereby they do what's needed to help things work rather than acting as dictators to the localities.

Central NHS bodies have introduced a range of national programmes to accelerate digital transformation. The introduction of the LHCREs in 2018 resulted in many a bad dad-joke on the theme of tight gym wear. But beyond the wry smiles, the Local Health and Care Record Exemplar programme was a meaningful endeavour to get the many and disparate NHS IT systems to talk to each other across regions.[42] Badly burned by the NPfIT centralised model, this approach provided central funding to a number of local geographies to try different ways of connecting care records. The plan was to learn at a local level and then create blueprints that others could follow and national standards for everyone to abide by. The nomenclature has more recently moved to *shared care records*, and the newest acronym is ShCR with every region expected to have them in place by the end of 2021.[43]

Wachter recommended that more digitally advanced NHS trusts should receive central funding in order to demonstrate what could be achieved. The Global Digital Exemplar (GDE) programme saw 27 NHS trusts each receive a cash injection, with the expectation that they matched the funding from their own coffers.[44] Each GDE trust had a *fast follower* trust who would partner and learn from their experience. A Digital Aspirant programme was announced in early March 2020, with 23 NHS trusts who were digital laggards receiving £28 million between them to progress their digital ambitions.[45] In a second wave, seven trusts received up to £6 million over three years to progress their digital ambitions in 2021.[46]

One more sceptical lead within a GDE explained his concern about big chunks of one-off capital money landing in an NHS trust which has sparse revenue to keep things going once the cash has run out: "If the money lands in a puddle of red ink then how are ongoing budgetary impacts going to be managed?" He also confessed that in an NHS trust with a backlog of basic IT issues that needed sorting: "throwing money at unstructured innovation tends to go in the service of remedial action."

30 ■ *Towards a Digital Ecology*

The jury is out as to whether innovation trickles down and if blueprints and processes for sharing learning have an impact in practice. It could be argued that concentrating digital efforts in a small number of NHS trusts simply increases the digital divide between geographies.[47] National programmes give kudos to local initiatives that can get buy-in from clinicians but the burden of reporting acts as a negative counterbalance.[48] The reality is that cash strapped NHS trusts look to the centre for handouts as a means of progressing digital and it is an uphill struggle achieving much without it.

The array of initiatives on the part of the Government are in themselves confusing to many, not least those entrepreneurs and start-ups developing digital products for use in the health sector. A 2016 review of how technology can be better adapted in the NHS resulted in the Accelerated Access Collaborative with a top-down supply-driven push for a small number of well-evidenced technologies along with an Innovation and Technology Payment to pump-prime reimbursement. Along with the LCHREs and GDEs, there have been various grant funding initiatives such as Innovate UK's Digital Health Technology Catalyst Fund aimed at small companies developing health technologies.

Indi likens the constant churn of national initiatives to an archaeological dig whereby it is possible to discern strata upon strata of projects which layer on top of each other, each superseded by another before they are complete. A senior clinician, who shall remain nameless, once said to me: "The thing is, none of us ever believe these initiatives will actually get implemented anyway." It turns out we all conspire in this innovation performance, whilst secretly suspecting that change will probably not get followed through. Despite being well-intentioned, we know that it is only a matter of time before our heads are turned by another initiative. And ministers go on to their next government position and patients and the public see little tangible benefit.

Going back to the 2020 Parliamentary Accounts Committee, the most recent assessment of NHS digital transformation. Not mincing its words, the report states that despite being recognised as essential to managing patient care, there has been a lack of progress of interoperability as well as in developing and implementing consistent standards. The committee says it is "alarmed at how little progress has been made against current ambitions." Finally, it notes how the use of digital services has increased during the pandemic and how there is "substantial potential" for acceleration of digital technologies to do things better for patients, healthcare professionals and the NHS as a whole.

NHSX is to be incorporated into NHS England and Improvement, and it is not clear what footing a policy push for digital adoption with a new Secretary of State for health. There have been eight ministers for health and care since the advent of the National Programme for IT. They don't stay around that long. The new Health and Care Act is in the offing and the cycle of restructure and reorganisation will once again begin. Operating with the white noise of policy churn in their ears, clinicians, managers, chief information officers and chief clinical information officers will continue their endeavours to improve the system as they have always done.

Between Rhetoric and Reality

Farhan's daughter Aaliya, is just one of 5.4 million people in the UK with asthma. Whilst the Government and the NHS wrangle with the intransigent problem of digital transformation, she like many others are not able to benefit from the latest advances in technology. Farhan's daughter's condition is mild, but for Tamara Mills, a teenager from Newcastle, lack of data sharing was fatal. She died despite 47 separate visits to primary and secondary care over four years. The Coroner's report[49] concludes that each episode was treated in isolation and lack of interoperability between systems meant that the patterns were not able to be spotted. Data could have saved her life if it had been combined and analysed to create a rich picture of her deteriorating health over time.

A report by charity Asthma UK digital technology[50] describes how tragic deaths, such as Tamara's, could be prevented by connected clinical systems that enable good quality data to be shared. As it stands, the quality of data is often poor and we don't always even have standard ways of coding clinical terms, data is not routinely shared and we don't have the data scientists who can create algorithms for analysing data and spotting patterns that could predict an asthma attack.

Farhan is expected to take his daughter for an annual asthma review. Their GP practice is keen that they do it, not only because the evidence says it will help them manage her condition better, but because they are incentivised by a payment each time they undertake one.[51] The reality is that Farhan and Aaliya very rarely attend that review. They know that they should go. Farhan knows his GP practice needs them to go so that they get paid. He knows that the letter (yes letter!) he receives from the GP practice will have taken up the administrator's time and incurred the cost of paper, envelope and stamp.

But the reality is that there are too many minor barriers that make the effort of booking and attending the appointment greater than the benefit for what is essentially a mild condition that barely affects them day-to-day. Farhan has to find space in the working day to ring the doctor to make an appointment; it will invariably be engaged so this will take some time. He has to book time off work and take Aaliya out of school and drive her there and back. Once they are in the surgery they have no idea how long it will take, and sitting in a busy waiting room full of sick people is hardly their idea of fun. Basically, this analogue, siloed, paper-based system is completely out of step with Farhan's life and that of so many people like him.

There are all sorts of innovations popping up despite, rather than because of the system. We are increasingly seeing consultations such as asthma reviews being done remotely; smart inhalers connected to smartphone apps can send reminders and help people improve their inhaling technique; apps that provide self-management information and give weather and pollution data can help prevent attacks; predictive algorithms can help people identify patterns and take steps to avoid their conditions worsening. These are only a few examples and only for one condition. Just think of the possibilities!

32 ■ *Towards a Digital Ecology*

But there are too many barriers for these innovative start-ups, often led by patients or clinicians, who have identified a problem they are driven to solve. A clinical team implementing new digital technology will often create challenges downstream to the IT department. The CIO may well be supportive, but they will be worried about ongoing licensing costs from a non-existent budget, not to say the fact that the data will be siloed because the digital tool does not interoperate with the main electronic patient record. Digital becomes part of the problem – any number of separate systems that the clinician has to login to on top of the 15 systems they already use per patient. It is just not scalable without the basics in place.

Digitising the NHS requires these sorts of innovations to happen at scale in a consistent and sustainable manner, with standardisation at the core. This requires a combination of centrally driven measures like the ones we saw that changed the face of electricity back in 1918 and the ability for entrepreneurs to develop new technologies that can add value to both patients like Aaliya, as well as clinicians and the wider system.

The promise of digital is to transform the experience of care for patients and improve staff morale by helping them become even more effective and productive. However, at the moment it is creating the reverse – an additional world of complexity and fragmentation. How do we avoid creating the legacy IT systems of the future? This book is an exploration of these challenges and the opportunities of creating a digital ecology with the right conditions so that our National Health Service can thrive in the 21st Century and beyond.

Notes

1 https://archive.org/stream/reportofcomelec00grearich/reportofcomelec00grearich_djvu.txt
2 https://publications.parliament.uk/pa/cm5801/cmselect/cmpubacc/680/68004.htm
3 https://wpi-strategy.com/site/wp-content/uploads/2020/08/Caring-for-the-NHS-Workforce-Final.pdf
4 https://wpi-strategy.com/site/wp-content/uploads/2020/08/Caring-for-the-NHS-Workforce-Final.pdf
5 https://bmjopen.bmj.com/content/9/12/e031637
6 https://bmchealthservres.biomedcentral.com/articles/10.1186/s12913-019-4790-x
7 https://www.bma.org.uk/media/2080/bma-vision-for-nhs-it-report-april-2019.pdf
8 https://emj.bmj.com/content/early/2021/03/02/emermed-2020-210401
9 These are known as Sustainability and Transformation Partnerships or Integrated Care Systems.
10 Question 50 https://committees.parliament.uk/oralevidence/880/default/
11 https://digital.nhs.uk/data-and-information/publications/statistical/appointments-in-general-practice/oct-2018
12 https://digital.nhs.uk/services/summary-care-records-scr
13 https://en.wikipedia.org/wiki/Foot-and-mouth_disease
14 https://www.nuffieldtrust.org.uk/files/2019-05/digital-report-br1902-final.pdf

Backdrop to Broken ▪ **33**

15 https://www.youtube.com/watch?v=NEVhvP8E48c&feature=youtu.be
16 https://www.cl.cam.ac.uk/~rja14/Papers/npfit-mpp-2014-case-history.pdf
17 https://www.nao.org.uk/wp-content/uploads/2019/05/Digital-transformation-in-the-NHS.pdf p.13
18 https://www.nao.org.uk/wp-content/uploads/2019/05/Digital-transformation-in-the-NHS.pdf
19 https://wpi-strategy.com/site/wp-content/uploads/2020/08/Caring-for-the-NHS-Workforce-Final.pdf
20 https://www.gov.uk/government/news/whole-system-demonstrator-programme-headline-findings-december-2011
21 https://www.bmj.com/content/346/bmj.f1035
22 https://www.cqc.org.uk/sites/default/files/20201016_stateofcare1920_fullreport.pdf
23 https://kar.kent.ac.uk/71495/1/64VidCalovskiThesis.pdf
24 https://www.gov.uk/government/publications/working-together-to-improve-health-and-social-care-for-all
25 https://www.health.org.uk/news-and-comment/blogs/big-picture-a-closer-look-at-health-system-reform?utm_source=charityemail&utm_medium=email&utm_campaign=feb-2021&pubid=healthfoundation&description=feb-2021&dm_i=4Y2,79CMF,18YGUJ,TFH3K,1
26 https://www.nao.org.uk/wp-content/uploads/2019/05/Digital-transformation-in-the-NHS.pdf, p. 7
27 https://www.digitalhealth.net/2017/04/nhs-will-not-be-paperless-before-2027/
28 https://www.digitalhealth.net/2016/09/wachter-calls-for-extension-to-paperless-2020-target/
29 https://www.england.nhs.uk/long-term-plan/
30 Originally one of Facebook's company values
31 https://www.theguardian.com/healthcare-network/2016/oct/03/can-digital-revolution-save-nhs
32 https://www.judiciary.uk/wp-content/uploads/2019/05/Stephen-Pettitt-2019-0037_Redacted.pdf
33 https://www.bbc.co.uk/news/uk-england-tyne-46143940
34 https://topol.hee.nhs.uk/the-topol-review/
35 https://spiral.imperial.ac.uk/bitstream/10044/1/76409/6/Imperial%20-%20NHS%20Data%20-%20Maximising%20impact%20on%20health%20of%20UK%202020.pdf
36 https://www.nuffieldtrust.org.uk/files/2019-05/digital-report-br1902-final.pdf
37 https://www.hee.nhs.uk/our-work/future-digital-workforce
38 https://www.bcs.org/content-hub/three-years-of-change-and-more-to-come/
39 https://www.theguardian.com/technology/2018/feb/01/matt-hancock-mp-app-released
40 https://www.digitalhealth.net/2020/06/nhs-digital-transformation-remains-tough/
41 https://www.digitalhealth.net/2020/10/mckinsey-pockets-600k-for-seven-week-review-into-nhs-tech-leadership/
42 https://www.england.nhs.uk/wp-content/uploads/2018/05/local-health-and-care-record-exemplars-summary.pdf
43 https://www.computerweekly.com/news/252498076/NHS-will-get-shared-care-records-by-September-2021-says-Matt-Hancock
44 https://www.england.nhs.uk/digitaltechnology/connecteddigitalsystems/exemplars/
45 https://www.digitalhealth.net/2020/03/exclusive-first-wave-of-digital-aspirants-announced/

34 ■ *Towards a Digital Ecology*

46 https://www.digitalhealth.net/2021/03/exclusive-second-wave-of-digital-aspirants-announced-at-rewired/
47 https://bmchealthservres.biomedcentral.com/articles/10.1186/s12913-019-4790-x
48 https://www.nuffieldtrust.org.uk/files/2019-05/digital-report-br1902-final.pdf
49 https://www.judiciary.uk/publications/tamara-mills/
50 https://www.asthma.org.uk/f29019fc/globalassets/get-involved/external-affairs-campaigns/publications/connected-asthma/connected-asthma---aug-2016.pdf
51 https://www.nice.org.uk/standards-and-indicators/qofindicators/the-percentage-of-patients-with-asthma-on-the-register-who-have-had-an-asthma-review-in-the-preceding-12-months-that-includes-an-assessment-of-asthma-control-using-the-3-rcp-questions

Chapter 3

Necessity Is the Mother of Invention

> The coronavirus is coming to you.
> It's coming at an exponential speed: gradually, and then suddenly.
> It's a matter of days. Maybe a week or two.
> When it does, your healthcare system will be overwhelmed.
> Your fellow citizens will be treated in the hallways.
> Exhausted healthcare workers will break down. Some will die.
> They will have to decide which patient gets the oxygen and which one dies.[1]

All our lives changed in a heartbeat. In just the space of a week, our everyday realities became a distant fantasy from a faraway land. In those early days, the enormity of the pandemic was hard to wrap our heads around; no one was left untouched, although there is no doubt that the hardest hit were those whose lives were already the most precarious.

Required to isolate in our homes, our previous lives felt like a dream. The aftershocks continued to reverberate. Just as we emerged from the first crisis, we were catapulted into a second. As we sought to adjust our personal lives, the social, technological, economic, environmental, legal and political consequences began to unfold. The use of digital technologies in the first wave of the pandemic crisis is just one lens through which personal and societal impacts were experienced and which I explore in this chapter.

Necessity is the mother of invention as the proverb goes. When there are no other options available, we recourse to the unthinkable. And digital transformation has sat firmly in the *too hard* box for just shy of two decades. Any number of reports

DOI: 10.1201/9781032198798-3

36 ■ *Towards a Digital Ecology*

and editorials have enthused about the apparent mass adoption of technology and profound transformation over the first crest of the pandemic.[2] This narrative favours those whose role it is to promote innovation, and it suits a health minister who has bet on digital as his legacy. But to what extent is this tall talk borne out of reality? Stories from the ground illuminate a somewhat more nuanced story.

Like many others, my working life shifted from meetings, conferences and travel, to endless video conference calls from my makeshift sitting room office. By early afternoon my teenage children surfaced from the bleary consequences of late-night TikTok and movies. I would retreat to my bedroom with my laptop, whilst they took up residence in the sitting room, the television blaring in the background. With more time on our hands, our consumption of TV series and Netflix grew exponentially. Whilst others were losing their jobs or being furloughed, myself and my colleagues had never been busier.

The insidious spread of the virus was accompanied by a substantial drop in NHS referrals along with a sharp rise in people waiting for diagnostic tests. Planned surgery was cancelled as the NHS braced itself for an influx of COVID-19 patients. As staff succumbed to the illness or had to self-quarantine, pressure on the system rapidly simmered its way towards boiling point. With systemic underfunding and long-standing inequalities already in the mix, there was fear and trepidation in the nurses and doctors who recognised what was just over the horizon.

"The prevailing culture has been that if one person in a group of ten says no, then the no carries it, the risks of making change have always seemed to be higher than the risks of staying the same," explains Beverley Bryant, a chief information officer for a group of London NHS trusts "there's never been enough of a compelling reason to drive the change."

However, things did start to change. After an initial paralysis, COVID-19 started to speed everything up, corralled by a shared purpose to hold back the danger of an overwhelmed NHS. Red tape fell away and what had been suffocated by inertia, suddenly became possible with barely the blink of an eye. Connected together by a common objective born out of necessity and a shared purpose, health practitioners, NHS organisations and industry began to respond at pace.

There was a sudden rash of technology improvisation – contact tracing applications for infected people, data analytics tools to detect potential outbreaks, web-based information and self-assessments, telehealth solutions for remote appointments. This was the largest health crisis since the advent of digital technologies and so their use to help curb and contain its effects is of note.

Did this moment herald a heyday for digital – a coming of age for technology in health? In a techUK speech, Lord Bethnell, parliamentary undersecretary of state for innovation at the Department of Health and Social Care claimed that the pandemic *colossally* scaled the capability of the system in respect of data and digital.[3] But is it rather the case that the pandemic prompted the NHS to spread and adopt some very basic but useful technologies that most of us take for granted in our everyday lives?

The pandemic was certainly an accelerant for well-understood technologies and it forced many of us, whether we be patients, clinicians or administrators, to use them whether we liked it or not. But the most seismic shifts may have been in attitudes rather than in innovation or invention.

An Outbreak of Pragmatism

Thursday, 26 March 2020, was an unremarkable day, with cloudy early spring weather in my lockdown city of Leeds. That evening my daughter and I opened the French windows to the back garden as what seemed like a faint rustle grew louder and more persistent. As we peered out into the evening darkness, we realised that we were hearing clapping from windows and front doors up and down our street. In what was to become known as Clap for Carers, this clapping was the collective chorus of households showing their appreciation for NHS staff. In the unreality of that early phase of lockdown, this show of solidarity felt nothing less than quite extraordinary. My daughter and I were captivated.

The brainchild of Dutch Londoner Annemarie Plas, the weekly clap every Thursday at 8 pm became a way for people to show their appreciation for key workers over those early virus-infected months. Despite the enthusiasm from many, and its undoubted positive intent, I had a rising sense of unease about this mid-week ritual. All the talk of NHS heroes belied the fact that those staff (often underpaid and definitely overworked) didn't have much of a choice about going into work and managing the personal stress and risk of exposure. One newspaper opinion piece tagline put it well: "We're standing on our doorsteps and balconies to cheer a system that is broken, encouraging health workers to pay for it with their lives."[4]

Whilst NHS workers had justifiable reason to feel conflicted over the moniker of *hero*, the pandemic was a testament to resourcefulness and ingenuity as many sought to find solutions to unprecedented circumstances. It wasn't just key workers who did amazing things. Suddenly, the IT department went from being the team that everyone moaned about, to the team that everyone looked to for help and support. Rachel Dunscombe, ex-chief information officer and a big hitter in the digital health space, is full of admiration: "During covid our citizens have trusted us, and I have to say our professions have done an amazing job with what they've had." Almost all of the IT leaders I interviewed confessed to secretly enjoying this new-found popularity.

What did it feel like in those very early days when the virus had only really encroached on our lives through news reports from distant countries? As a chest physician, Dr Matthew Knight tells me he is particularly alert to any illness characterised by respiratory symptoms. I came across Matthew in one of the many NHS webinar YouTube recordings which aimed to share and spread novel working practices. I messaged Matthew via LinkedIn and he agreed to an interview from his temporary residence in Spain, where he was working remotely – an unexpected but

38 ■ *Towards a Digital Ecology*

welcome fringe benefit of the pandemic to those lucky enough not to be furloughed or out of work.

Recalling the very early days of the pandemic, Matthew recalls how he had been following the COVID-19 story since early in the new year of 2020. It became apparent to him, as the virus crept from China over to Europe, that the impact on his patients was going to be serious. And he was worried.

I was curious about what it felt like to be a clinician in those early days when the pandemic had hit our news feeds but not our lives:

> We were scared to be honest with you … I was scared for my family, scared for myself, scared for my patients, I knew a lot of my patients were likely to be extremely vulnerable to getting pretty sick and dying if they got [the virus].

Matthew describes a deep fear and a sense of concern about the enormity of the contagion that was hurtling towards us, barely checked and wildly infectious. "When you sit there and you're facing a humongous challenge you just think the worst, your job is to prepare for the absolute worst case scenario … so we were trying to predict the impact and the likely numbers were quite scary," he recalls. Despite a recent visit from the prime minister and the promise of a shiny new £400 million hospital, Matthew knew that his hospital premises were not up to the challenge. They had struggled to even cope with the previous winter pressures, never mind a pandemic ripping through the country like a wrecking tornado. "We knew our armoury was weak," he tells me.

It was this fear, combined with a sense of urgency and common purpose, that released an flood of entrepreneurialism that swept the NHS in a way I have never seen before. "One of the positive things about Covid," Matthew explains, "is there was this can-do attitude – can do, we must do, we have to, attitude." Highly tactical, it was a frame of mind born out of urgency and an absence of any other option. Doing nothing would have spelled disaster.

Beverley describes this stimulus as an "outbreak of pragmatism" that saw a blank cheque which drove a level of digital technology use that she is keen to capitalise on: "instead of the governance and the lack of money just being the blocker, suddenly all the paths have been opened." She is optimistic about the future: "people who would historically been scared about making decisions have suddenly stepped up and said 'yes just do it, do it.'"

Beverley found herself energised by this unexpected break from business as usual:

> A lot of people aren't used to making fast decisions, but there's a new sense of energy, people are literally energised and empowered to get on with stuff and have really risen to the challenge … the IT workforce

stepped into the opportunity rather than stepped back from it and it's been brilliant to watch.

There are so many stories to tell, from so many different parts of the NHS. I cannot hope to do them all justice. There are many that will be left to others to recount. There is the story of massively increased uptake of the NHS.UK website and NHS 111 online.[5] The story about when Guys and St Thomas NHS Foundation Trust created a round-the-clock 3D printing factory to produce face shields to be worn by hospital staff is compelling.[6] The tale of Kettering Hospital using Robotic Process Automation to automate COVID-19 reports that would otherwise have had to be crunched by the IT department is neat.[7] There are countless more.

This chapter shines a light on a small select few. I tell stories from key workers, entrepreneurs, IT Departments and people working in central NHS organisations that give a flavour of what became possible, whilst shining a spotlight on the gaps and deficiencies which came into sharp relief. Cumulatively, these stories start to paint a picture of the current state of affairs in technology use, and what a future NHS that makes good use of technology to do things better, might look like.

Logging on

In those very early days of the pandemic, anyone running a public or private organisation was first and foremost concerned with how to keep the show on the road. With office doors slammed decisively shut, doing the most straightforward tasks – logging into your computer – suddenly became fraught with challenges. The percentage of people working from home went from under 6% at the beginning of 2020, to just under 50% in April. A seismic shift.[8]

The NHS is a massive employer, with around 1.4 million staff.[9] As well as key workers, there are back-office staff within finance, human resource and facilities to name just a few. The NHS depends on all these staff, just as much as those delivering clinical care, to keep the wheels on the track of healthcare. And a big chunk of those people work from offices in ordinary times.

The immediate and most pressing need was for NHS staff to carry on their everyday work without the risk of infection. This meant that for staff who didn't have a clinical reason to see patients face-to-face, remote working became the new normal. The ability to work from home was a lifesaver for those staff who had to shield but who were still able to work, bolstering a workforce that had been quickly depleted through illness.

The extent to which this new normal represented a shift in expectations about what it means to be at work is profound. In my experience of working in corporate NHS services, it was frowned upon to not be sat at your desk, visible and available to your colleagues at all times. Working at home was the exception when there was an important report to write or a tight deadline to hit. The prevailing culture

40 ■ *Towards a Digital Ecology*

determined that you must be skiving if you weren't in the office. Despite pressure on the NHS estate and lots of talk of remote working, these ingrained habits and beliefs had created a deeply embedded torpidity. That changed in an instant. It had to.

NHS bosses made the decision to license and roll out[10] Microsoft Teams across the NHS, with the intention of making it easier for clinicians, supply chain specialists, IT technicians and senior management, to speak to each other quickly and securely. Teams provides secure instant messaging, direct audio and video calls and the ability to hold virtual meetings. In an impressive feat of mobilisation, Teams was rolled out to 1.3 million users over the course of four days in mid-March. Its uptake was exponential with an average of 132,000 users and just under half a million messages sent each day.[11]

Stephen, a healthcare executive at Microsoft, picks up the story, describing how Teams was made available free to the NHS for the first six months of the pandemic. An ex-chief information officer for a large London NHS trust, I turned to him to find out more. Stephen is keen for me to understand the context in order to better appreciate what happened during COVID-19. "When I came into the NHS I was presented with a burning platform," he tells me, "Our internal, on-premise email and everything else was on poor hardware, it was falling apart, it *did* fall apart pretty spectacularly just as I joined."

Stephen describes the situation he was faced with back in the early days of his new role.

> There was no vision, no real leadership, there was a bit of a blame culture, command and control, all the normal stuff … The hardware would go down and you would lose it, and you would have to restore stuff from backup, which meant you have to take everything offline, spend the next six hours restoring it, do it safely, then if something doesn't work you have to go back round the loop.

This was the grinding life of a chief information officer in an NHS trust: "It often took days at a time."

Stephen was faced with a choice. He could rebuild the in-house system, wait for a new national NHS mail system, or take destiny into his own hands and move over to Microsoft. "Not many people wanted to be the first," he explains: "but I had to make a decision, and I thought it can't be any worse than what we have now." As a result, he made a bold move, got rid of internal systems and servers, adopted Office 365 and moved to cloud hosting. The reason this is all relevant is that Stephen's choice set the context for the Trust's response to the pandemic.

By the time COVID-19 hit, there was already 95% adoption of Teams, and so the transition to remote working was far less painful than it might otherwise have been: "If Covid had happened maybe two years earlier, it may have been a different story. You may have seen some adoption, but you wouldn't have seen anywhere near the adoption [we got]." Stephen's story is apposite because it illustrates that

Necessity Is the Mother of Invention ■ 41

technology was able to be leveraged where there was already investment and embedded ways of working. This wasn't the case for everyone.

The experience of clinicians in those early days was mixed. Matthew describes how he set himself up in his study: "with a whole load of computer screens" that the IT department had set up for him "they had sort of gone under the stairs and found what they had, wires and adapters and so on. I had xrays on one screen and the hospital record on another." Dawn, a practice manager in a village GP surgery, resorted to Amazon to buy webcams so the doctors could carry out video consultations. There was a lot of scrabbling about for the necessary hardware to keep services moving. Even the basics just weren't in place for many.

Ibrahim is taking a pause in his medic training at a North Eastern hospital to undertake a PhD. As a 35 year old tech agnostic, he has a smartphone and Macbook "and that's probably as much digital as it goes," he tells me with a self-effacing smile. "I certainly see the value of digital," Ibrahim tells me, and he goes on to describe a referral app that is used on the renal ward he works on which has saved massive amounts of time by structuring and automating the referral rather than relying on phone calls and note taking. "But apart from that," says Ibrahim, "I just use my phone for general things, I wouldn't say I was tech savvy; I like the fact I can access social media and my emails quickly but that's about as much impact as it's had."

Previous to his role at his current trust, Ibrahim had always kept paper records at the hospitals he worked in:

> you spent all your time writing the notes, finding the notes, wasting time trying to decipher what people had written, wasting time trying to put your notes together in a meaningful way, wasting time having to go to the patient physically [on the ward] to access the notes.

Meetings with colleagues to discuss a patient would be undertaken face-to-face, and email, pager and calls via the hospital switchboard were the main channels of communication.

In those first weeks of the pandemic, Ibrahim recalls being overwhelmed with the number of patients he and his team were having to take care of. Having to put on PPE to treat each patient, remove it and then take notes was laborious and time-consuming. But in contrast, he found the shift to home working was in many ways lovely. Smiling, he tells me about his five-year-old daughter: "It gives me an opportunity to spend a bit more time with her … and still be able to be engaged and collaborate with my colleagues … I think that flexibility is very nice actually."

Whilst Ibrahim's experience has been largely positive, remote working has exposed yet another chasm of inequality. Professional and highly paid workers are almost twice as likely to be able to work from home as those who are least paid.[12] For people with less good broadband and comfortable home environments, at least the office creates a level playing field where you have equal access to amenities required to do your job.[13]

42 ■ Towards a Digital Ecology

Whilst I, like many others, moan about the tedium of homeworking, it is easy to forget that we are fortunate in having the choice to reduce our exposure to the virus.

For others, there is a trade-off between the relative safety of home working with the downsides of loneliness and social isolation.[14] Dawn, a receptionist and administrator at a GP practice, was clear from the outset that she wanted to work from the office: "I prefer working from the office, I enjoy my job and I enjoy the people and the contact, Being at home would drive me nuts. Too many distractions." Despite having a long-term condition in the shape of COPD, working from the office is important to her: "You learn something new every day, it helps keep your mind ticking over." Her bosses wanted her to work from home, but she tells me she refused.

That some companies, such as Microsoft, gave services away for free during the first six months of the pandemic is not without its critics. The pandemic presented an unusual opportunity for digital platforms to get unprecedented adoption that would not be possible in ordinary times. It isn't a big leap to conclude that the long-term business benefits will have outweighed six months of free usage. However, not all Microsoft products came off scot-free when it came to media attention during those early contagious times.

One of the more bizarre things to happen during the first pandemic wave shone a light on the consequences of substandard infrastructure. Public Health England (PHE), responsible for collating public and private lab results during the pandemic, had to rely on phone calls, pens, paper and a spreadsheet in the early days of the pandemic, to get the job done. Microsoft's spreadsheet, Excel, has a million-row limit which appears to have gone unnoticed as various CSV files were cut and pasted into the master copy. It was only sometime later that someone noticed that 16,000 results had fallen off the edge of the sheet never to be seen again. 16,000 test results failed to be recorded which meant that around 50,000 infectious people could have been missed by contract tracers who would otherwise have been told to self-isolate.[15] The fact that PHE had to rely on a spreadsheet at all is quite sobering.

A Hospital in Your Home

The notion of a virtual ward might conjure up Dr-Who-esque images of nurse holograms or maybe an immersive zombie apocalypse meets Victorian hospital video game with dismembered gown-clad patients and overturned bedpans. However, it turns out that the reality is somewhat more pedestrian and entirely less sci-fi than its name may suggest.

The concept of virtual wards has actually been around for a long time and even predates the advent of concerted efforts to digitally transform the NHS. Over a decade ago, a primary care team in Croydon won multiple accolades and national awards for their pioneering work to first introduce virtual wards in their local area.[16]

So what problem does a virtual ward solve and how does it work? It became apparent to the Croydon team that they had a cohort of patients who were being regularly admitted to hospital wards. These patients were typically in their 70s with

Necessity Is the Mother of Invention ■ 43

one or more long-term condition, such as arthritis or diabetes. These people felt vulnerable, and they found a hospital ward reassuring. They felt safe. But hospital care is intensive and costly. The team wondered if this group of people could be caught before they got too ill, cared for at home with the right support and *still* feel safe.

The team developed an algorithm to predict who was most likely to be at risk of hospital admission in the local area. Then, rather than wait for them to turn up at A&E, the team went out to those people and offered them hospital care in their homes as an alternative. It's as simple as that. And it worked.

Despite what one may imagine, a virtual ward isn't about you having your clinical team at your bedside. Instead, the virtual model mimics a ward environment in an individual's home but with the clinical team at a distance. With a daily ward round for each patient, the ward clerk coordinates a patient's care from the office, with the clinical work being led by a matron. Back in those early days, the lowly telephone and home visits were the main ways for the virtual team and the patient to keep in touch. It worked well, but before the pandemic had not been rolled out at scale.

Fast forward to 2020 and COVID-19 created the perfect conditions to reinvigorate the concept of virtual wards. With hospitals straining at the seams, and fear of contagion making them feel a less safe place than before, being cared for at home had all the hallmarks of the perfect plan. Even better, advances in technology since the inception of virtual wards have turbocharged what was possible in the Croydon precursor to the contemporary COVID-19 virtual ward.

This is how it works. Virtual pandemic wards enable patients to stay at home under supervision and for health professionals to spot early signs of deterioration which might require more intensive treatment. Sometimes the wards avoid the need for people to go into hospital and other times they enable early discharge from a hospital stay. As with many apparently digitally enabled innovations – pen, paper and telephone calls are often the default – but technology is starting to play more of a role.

One district general hospital based on the outer edges of London was in the technology dark ages before Covid, according to chest physician Dr Matthew Knight. Still running Windows XP, which is so outdated it hasn't received updates since 2014, this was not a tech-savvy hospital. According to Matthew, the hospital even retained an outpatient desktop computer limping along on Windows 95 – a cyber security nightmare waiting to happen that would give chills to any IT department.

In a YouTube webinar,[17] Matthew describes how COVID-19 propelled his team from the technology slow lane. With the occupancy of hospital wards going through the roof and a combination of scared patients and frightened staff, Matthew and his team decided to take action. One evening in early March, when it was still possible to meet in person, a colleague dropped by on the way home from work, and they stood around his dining table with coloured pens, paper and a pot of tea and designed a virtual covid ward. "It was as low tech as that," smiles Matthew. With

44 ■ *Towards a Digital Ecology*

the usual steady and slow pace of change replaced by pandemic-fuelled urgency, the team accepted their first referral just four days later, and the virtual covid ward was born.

Matthew brings to life the urgency of the crisis:

> We knew we couldn't admit everyone who might need a hospital bed. We knew we'd collapse almost within a week based on relatively modest predictions … the mortality and admissions statistics looked absolutely dreadful and if you assume fifteen percent of your population are going to need oxygen, then you quickly realise that you're about fourteen hospitals too few.

With very little known about the virus or how to treat it, this was a big leap of faith for the team to take.

Having run it past his *would it work for my mum* test, Matthew describes in the early days of the virtual ward, patients were given what he and his team called a *party bag* which included a pulse oximeter to measure their blood oxygen, a single-use thermometer, a mask and information about how to use each gadget. Doesn't sound like much of a party, but if avoiding sudden death is your idea of fun, then perhaps the name is more apposite than first appears to be the case.

Time to pause for a quick lesson in blood oxygen. COVID-19 is a respiratory disease, and many people who die have a sudden drop in their blood oxygen level a few days before their lungs fail. However, this drop in blood oxygen doesn't necessarily come with the breathlessness that people associate with the virus. As a result, people with *silent hypoxia* don't get the help they need, they either get to the hospital too late or die at home. The way around this is to take a measure of their blood oxygen that can give them an objective measure, rather than relying on noticing viral symptoms.[18]

A daily telephone call on the virtual ward meant that professionals could take blood oximeter readings along with self-reported symptoms. As people were often feeling pretty rubbish and worried about the virus, Matthew describes how that objective reading was an important factor in providing reassurance to people who felt bad but who weren't actually deteriorating. Conversely, people who felt ok but had low blood oximeter readings could have quick treatment before they got worse.

The virtual ward was working well and keeping people at home and out of the hospital. However, it was only displacing the pressure. One day, over the course of the Easter weekend, the stress began to bite as a team of three found themselves ploughing through 180 calls to patients in just one day. The team, who were averaging 12 to 14 hour working days, started to think about whether technology could help them manage the volume of work any better.

It's not what you know, it's who you know goes the maxim, and it turns out to be just as true for the NHS as anywhere else. After watching Matthew's YouTube webinar with NHSX, I approached him for an interview. During our conversation, he recounts how the chief executive of NHSX, Matthew Gould, had visited his hospital the previous summer. They had ended up in what he describes as a long geeky conversation about technology. "He gave me his card and said to keep in touch and I popped it with all the cards of important people who say these things but probably don't mean them," recalls Matthew.

He goes on to describe how he sat at his desk thinking that his team couldn't carry on working flat out. Matthew decided to reach out to Gould "I thought it was a futile thing to do … but at least I could say I had done all that was in my gift." A late-night email was reciprocated within the hour, and they scheduled to follow-up the next morning.

With help from Gould's team, Matthew and his colleagues reviewed a number of products and eventually settled upon a remote monitoring application with an app for patients to upload their vital signs and a platform for clinicians to review the results. Over the course of the next few weeks, they worked with the company to bespoke certain parts of the product and roll it out at what he describes as "phenomenal speed."

This new approach, where patients inputted readings and symptom data and the professionals reviewed a dashboard that showed which patients were deteriorating, started to save time, slash calls and cut their workload in half. It wasn't just the clinicians who were getting overwhelmed by calls, it turned out that it was sometimes intrusive for patients and many preferred this new form of remote contact. A tick on the app showed the patient when a clinician had checked their information, and this turned out to be important for them to feel reassured that they were in safe hands.

The app wasn't for everyone, and about half of the patients for whom it was offered, turned it down. The same went for video consultations. "Most patients didn't want to see me and they certainly didn't want me to see them in their bed," chuckles Matthew, recalling how the telephone still often trumps more sophisticated technologies. Matthew describes himself as: "no lovey-dovey hand-holding" clinician but tells me that even he recognised that for patients who were so anxious and isolated, a call from a practitioner was reassuring.

The virtual ward was and is a roaring success – over 2,000 patients have been through the system at the time of our conversation at the end of November. Matthew tells me he hasn't received a single complaint. And given that he receives 20 complaints a year about the car park, Matthew reckons this is a good result. His patients have told him that the virtual ward gave them the relief and reassurance of being able to chat to a senior medic. They tell him that this was critical to them getting through the illness. It may not be the story that makes the headlines, but according to Matthew, "reassuring a lot of people a little bit" was the main success of the virtual ward.

Virtual wards save lives. The mortality rate of patients cared for on virtual wards in England to date is just 2%.[19] However, their use during the pandemic highlights that we are still in the foothills of digital transformation – despite the hype of

46 ■ *Towards a Digital Ecology*

emerging technologies, it is clear that patients and staff are still relying on mostly basic technologies such as the telephone. They do the job, and they are ubiquitous.

Matthew bemoans the fact that whilst the remote monitoring app enables patients to send clinically useful information, it is limited by its inability to integrate with the main electronic patient record that they use day-to-day. This means the data remains siloed and clinicians have to log in and out of different systems. Interoperability is what he sees as the next stage of maturity of such products if they are to be really useful to clinicians coming out of the pandemic. A familiar refrain.

With this increase in virtual wards and home monitoring, apps which enable people to take vital signs, such as oxygen in the blood and blood pressure, are highly appealing. There are lots of companies developing digital products to fill the gap. However, the promise of these applications is not always borne out by reality when scrutinised by experts. Some apps claim they can measure oxygen in the blood using a smartphone's flashlight and camera. A cursory search on the iTunes app store reveals a number of oximeter apps with mostly terrible reviews: "doesn't work, waste of time," says one. A rapid evidence review of smartphone pulse oximeters by experts came up with a similar conclusion, determining that the evidence is too weak for their accuracy to be confirmed and they cannot be trusted.[20]

Virtual wards were nothing new. They have been around for a decade. But what the pandemic facilitated was a scaling up of this approach, taking it from the margins to the mainstream. As of January 2021, all regions received a letter from NHS England instructing them to set up COVID-19 virtual wards.[21] This is the real story of the digital pandemic – getting what we already know works out there for wider adoption.

The Clinical Entrepreneur

"No-one cares about the boring stuff," Dr Rizwan Malik says with a sigh: "but that's the stuff that has the most value … boring is stopping me doing repetitive tasks."

In his role as lead radiologist for an NHS trust, Rizwan is a self-certified geek and early adopter who is prepared to spend his evenings and weekends on the lookout for new technologies that can make life easier for his team and improve outcomes for his patients. Wanting to make life better for this radiology team and the patients they treat, his mantra is: "boring is good." With a 33% shortage of radiologists, his quest for technology to make life easier for clinicians and better for patients is not trivial.

"The basics don't sound sexy … and there is too much junk AI out there that wants to be seen as useful," he tells me. But with COVID-19 came an opportunity for Rizwan to ride on the wave of technology optimism and move forward projects that he had spent years of frustration trying to get off the ground.

"[COVID-19] is such a massive seismic change we need to capitalise on it," says Rizwan, keen to circumvent colleagues who he believes are keen to invent excuses to curb innovation. A deputy chief information officer in his NHS trust, Rizwan seized the opportunity to introduce two innovations he'd been trying to get started for the last seven years, but always hit the inevitable roadblocks of inertia and disinterest.

A bugbear of his was the fact that he and his colleagues could only do their work from the confines of the hospital. He had been trying for years to get the technology in place and the management support for radiologists to do their work assessing x-rays from home. What now, in a post-Covid world seems evidently sensible, Rizwan describes it as "maverick stuff" resisted by managers who sucked their teeth at the cost and wanted to know what they were going to get for free in return for licensing the requisite software.

There was a prevailing view that staff can't be trusted to be doing work if they are doing it from home. Rolling his eyes Rizwan explains "there's a lack of recognition that your time is valuable," and so his arguments for flexible home working fell on deaf ears.

When the pandemic hit, Rizwan seized the opportunity and dug out the business case gathering dust at the back of his office shelf. Before you couldn't get sign off for anything costing more than £5,000 but with COVID-19, where 30% or 40% of the workforce were either ill or shielding, it suddenly made sense. "In the first week, we had three of our twenty strong radiology team self-isolating and two with symptoms. Suddenly, the change I had been arguing for made sense to everyone else too."

With the inertia that typically characterises decision-making in the NHS supplanted by a sense of urgency, Rizwan describes how he got the £350,000 business case approved by his finance director in the space of an hour. It took a week of testing £10,000 worth of kit in his house to work through glitches and niggles and the home working system was good to go.

On the day of our interview, Rizwan is on call, which means he has to be available to review scans as required. He tells me he has made a decision to not go into the hospital to perform this role because he doesn't need to be there – his office extension number rings through to his mobile phone alongside messages from hospital systems: "basically there is no barrier to working as duty radiologist without me being there." Rizwan's persistence has meant that the show could be kept on the road despite the ravages of the pandemic.

As well as seizing the opportunity to get the basics of home working in place, Rizwan had his eye on some serious innovation in the often overhyped field of artificial intelligence. He had spent the last year trying to collaborate with a number of promising AI companies, but two of them left the UK over the course of their early conversations, finding that the amount of effort it was taking them to engage with the NHS wasn't worth their time and effort. Even the local body responsible for diffusing innovation was less than useless, says Rizwan: "I'm a little nobody from nowheresville." But once he had his chief executive hooked in, and they got involved, suddenly people wanted to listen.

Fortunately, one company was prepared to stay the distance and they decided to collaborate. "I was finding it nearly impossible to get things done from within the system, so I said, let's try and do it together." The irony is that the way I managed to

48 ■ *Towards a Digital Ecology*

get things done was to talk to the Department for International Trade and ask them if they could help a company outside the UK into the NHS. Even that was helpful and a few doors opened up, but it was still incredibly difficult. I was mindful that my hospital indulges me a little bit, there are so many opportunities but I have to focus in on one or two.

However, with COVID-19 everything once again accelerated and talk of a possible pilot shifted to deploying a live system. Within three weeks, he had a COVID-19 decision support tool installed, tested and live on his wards: "We'll be the first chest site in the country to do it," says a triumphant Rizwan: "Badabing badabong." The perceived barriers, the inertia, the bureaucracy all melted away, and Rizwan seized the opportunity to expedite things he had been dreaming of for years.

This is no small achievement, and Rizwan has seen his collaboration with AI company Quere.ai reported in the MIT Technology Review where he talks about the AI-based chest x-ray system which allows clinicians to triage people with more severe COVID-19 symptoms including lung abnormalities associated with viral pneumonia. With a significant reduction of staff in his hospital, this has become an important support tool for stretched clinicians, freeing up valuable time.

Despite the massive personal and societal costs of COVID-19, Rizwan believes the fact that it was more than a two-week flash in the plan crisis has been good for NHS digital transformation:

> had it been a few weeks, we would have had a great surge in interest and then it would have been all back to normal … because it's been such a seismic change … it's cut through the reasons people find for why they don't want to stuff, the perceived issues.

I reflect with Rizwan that his efforts have been pretty herculean, and he had to show grit and tenacity to achieve these changes. He agrees, reminding me that for the most part he has had to do this on top of his day job, with an inevitable toll on his family life: "being up until 1 in the morning trying to do this stuff and fit it around your weekends is very difficult and it takes a lot out of you."

Realising that this approach was unsustainable, he resorted to brinkmanship to persuade this hospital to give him a day a week to focus on digital innovation in his speciality of radiology, by threatening to stop the path he had started to take the organisation down. Even then, he tells me it is only agreed in three-month blocks, and Rizwan has to start making the case again. "It stops innovation and it stops people engaging," he tells me, "because everything is a battle."

Data Quality Rules Ok!

That early emergency response to COVID-19 brought gaps in data and the non-connectivity of digital platforms into sharp relief. It showed the best of what people can do when circumstances dictate. This is a story of heroic efforts by everyday people,

Necessity Is the Mother of Invention ■ 49

often hampered by inadequate infrastructure and the consequences of decades of snail-paced progress with technology adoption. The repercussions of bad quality data that is locked away in different siloed systems had material consequences for not only those people doing their best to respond to the pandemic but also for people's health, well-being and ultimately their lives.

Data quality counts. A humongous challenge facing the NHS as the pandemic began to sink its teeth into the nation was the ability to identify people who were clinically vulnerable so it could advise them to shield. The custodian of the country's data, NHS Digital, did not have this information readily to hand, and so it was forced to scrabble around and combine various datasets together. One source, hospital data, was seven weeks out of date and didn't capture sufficient detail about people's conditions. This not only led to 126,000 people being told to shield in error but also to 30,000 people who had died before 20 March being sent a letter advising them to shield. One can only imagine the distress this must have caused to families. Even the data that was available was riddled with gaps, including many NHS records which had missing or incorrect telephone numbers.

The ugly spectre of siloed platforms loomed heavy over frantic measures to reach the right people. This is one of the ripples caused by the legacy of the National Programme for IT that we explored in Chapter 2. A National Audit Office report on the Government's response to protecting vulnerable people concludes that the time taken to identify and communicate with the 1.3 million people they had managed to identify by 12 April "was largely down to the challenge of extracting usable data from different NHS and GP IT systems."[22]

Over subsequent weeks, it was down to local NHS trusts, GP practices and local authorities to review the data and draw on their local intelligence. The result of these colossal efforts was an additional 900,000 people added to the list who would otherwise have been left unsupported. There were material impacts for people who were left out in the original data trawl, insofar as they would not have been offered deliveries of food and medicine or been able to claim statutory sick pay if not able to work from home. There were also real and concrete impacts for healthcare and local authority workers at a local level who had to direct their efforts into painstaking data collection activities that would not have been necessary if the right systems with the right connectivity had been in place.

Dr Alec Price-Forbes is a consultant rheumatologist at a hospital in the heart of England. He was responsible for coordinating a number of hospital specialities that comprised patients who were immunosuppressed and should be shielding. He describes how it took seven weeks of manual effort using the humble spreadsheet to get the right data to help people most in need. "Things were fraught," he tells me, "because there is no infrastructure." Working with the local council it became apparent that there was substantial overlap between their spreadsheets and that of the hospital. "We merged NHS national datasets with what GPs have and what hospitals have and social care." Everyone was desperately gathering data in silos and then trying to merge it together. Alec describes it as "primitive population health

50 ■ *Towards a Digital Ecology*

management without the infrastructure and with spreadsheets." For Alec, this frantic situation illustrates the gaping gap in national connectivity and was a source of huge frustration, highlighting systemic challenges that he has been trying to address for many years: "I'm bored silly talking about [digital transformation] and not being able to deliver it," he tells me."

If we quantified the time, resource, personal effort and consternation in each locality and then multiplied it across the country, it would be unlikely to tell a positive story. Every region had to improvise and find a way to respond, making the most of its assets and doing its best to manage its deficits. The Norfolk and Waveney region reports how, after identifying 28,000 residents at risk of developing complications from the virus, they sent their own letters to each individual asking them to report their health and symptoms on a secure website that they created themselves to manage the response. In a newsletter, celebrating this great feat, they note that the letters they sent out to those vulnerable people "are in addition to the letters that patients may have already received from either local councils or the NHS." Presumably, some people might have received three separate letters, three separate stamps and three separate administrative efforts going on in the background.[23]

In the newsletter, Dr Anoop Dhesi, Chair of NHS Norfolk and Waveney Clinical Commissioning Group reports: "This initiative is unique to Norfolk and Waveney and uses technology designed by one of our local GP practices." Whilst the team at Norfolk were rightly proud of their efforts, we should not be proud of a system that is so flawed that it took herculean local efforts and the development of local systems to respond. One of the consequences that the system will have to accommodate beyond the pandemic is a whole ton of locally developed systems and data silos. More complexity and more flaws for the future.

Attending Anywhere

"Usually it's someone rushing around waving a stick, and that's the reputation we've got," smiles Jonny, reflecting on the reputation that NHSE/I (NHS England and Improvement) undoubtedly has got from the point of view of many of those NHS organisations working at a local level in towns and cities across the country.

It is all too easy to slam the centre, to blame central bodies when things go wrong. But I'd like to share a story that saw local, regional and national NHS organisations collaborating for the common good in the first weeks and months of the pandemic. This is the tale of the national roll-out of video consultation platform Attend Anywhere, to support hospital outpatient appointments switch to remote delivery wherever possible.

Jonny Brown leads a small team of three at NHS England, responsible for introducing the use of video consultations in secondary care. It was the summer of 2019 when thoughts of viruses and global pandemics were the last thing on Jonny's mind. Taking their lead from Scotland, his team had licensed Attend Anywhere and had been quietly working with various trusts who were interested in trying out the platform. Jonny describes it as "start small and find some interested trusts who might be up for giving it a go."

By December 2019, they had about 20 NHS trusts involved "The volumes were tiny, we're talking a few patients here, a few patients there," explains Jonny, "but there was lots of enthusiasm and lots of good feedback." Jonny and his team had set up a learning network and were busy running events to spread the word "trying to nurture the pilot along its way." As the Long Term Plan arrived that year, Jonny describes how his modest project got swept up in more ambitious plans for service transformation enabled by technology. He was not complaining. This new national priority meant that there was now money and momentum associated with his project.

When COVID-19 struck, his team was still in the formative stages of planning how to scale up their approach. Suddenly, Jonny found very senior people wanting to know how they could plug the pandemic free fall in outpatient appointments. "First of all they said can you do it in eight to twelve weeks," recalls Jonny, "then it was can you do it in four weeks." He describes what happens next as propelling the project nationwide on steroids. A superfast procurement using a government framework resulted in Attend Anywhere winning a 12-month contract. Jonny is at pains to emphasise how everything was done by the book, but with the usual sign-off processes speeded up and senior people making sure things were expedited quickly to move things forward.

Jonny's intention was to make it as easy as possible for local trusts who didn't already do video consultations to set them up and to remove as much pain as possible from them in doing so. NHSE/I bought a master license and then sub-licensed the platform to local organisations to make the process quick and simple. They found the funds, they did the procurement once so local organisations didn't have to and they licensed the platform that they believed would work. Once the platform was in place, Jonny's team set about doing as much as they could to reduce the workload on local organisations.

Firstly, they created a standard data protection impact assessment that could be adapted at a local level. Recognising that a limiting factor to taking up virtual consultations was not having the right kit in place, Jonny's team then managed to secure £20,000 per trust to buy laptops, webcams, microphones and speakers. Organisations did not have to license Attend Anywhere to use this money and indeed many of them ended up using the nationally licensed platform alongside other software they already had in place.

Not content to stop there, Jonny and his team did a deal with some of the mobile networks so that people using mobile data to access the platform would not be charged. "That was a big win," says Jonny, "and there's so much more we can do on the equality and digital inclusion agenda and trusts really appreciated it." This is where the centre really comes into its own, using its power and authority to negotiate good deals in a way that individual trusts or regions would find it much harder to do.

52 ■ *Towards a Digital Ecology*

As well as getting an agreement that trusts would receive funds to deliver consultations virtually in the same way as if they were face to face, the team also provided implementation support in partnership with regional systems and NHS Digital. With his tiny team of two staff, Jonny was able to make a massive difference through collaboration between the centre and local teams. He describes how they developed training materials, patient information leaflets, advice on devices, implementation plans and any other number of helpful tools. This was the centre at its best, providing an enabling role and taking the pain away from overstretched clinical services.

The team set up a help desk for questions and queries from clinicians and whilst they did try and set up one for patients too, Jonny says it proved too complicated amongst everything else they were trying to achieve. "Me and my team were literally answering help desk queries at the start because there wasn't anyone else to do it and we were getting maybe one hundred queries a day at one point," he recalls.

Beverley's trust was one of those which had been doing tiny pilots of the Attend Anywhere Platform. But with lockdown, everything changed. "On the back of having to cancel a load of outpatient appointments, the roll out went very fast," she recalls,

> so instead of us as a transformation and IT team pushing the outpatient teams to use it, they were pulling us, desperate to be able to run clinics. There's been a pull from the user base to the use of digital which has been refreshing.

However, it was not all plain sailing. "My mind's blocked it out," recalls Jonny smiling: "we had three incidents in the space of a week and two outages of around an hour and a half for the first one and two hours for the second one." He describes how this lapse in the availability of the platform led to criticism from trusts and quickly escalated to lots of senior people flapping around. "We never really thought beyond implementing," says Jonny, "we didn't have an appreciation that it could break and that we needed to be on top of these things and be in control of it."

After those early hiccups, the team managed to get on top of the operational side of things: "It made us realise that our response has to be sharp and it became clear that no one was ready for what we do if [the platform] goes off." It is now the case that trusts have contingency arrangements in place, they now know what to do if something goes wrong. Since those early days, the platform is more stable and how they manage things is much slicker: "all those things we never thought about in the early days but are important when you're running a patient service." The smooth-running operations they have today have come about through hard-earned and sometimes painful experience.

I ask Jonny what happens next. He has been keen to scope out how a continued national offer might work and what it would cost. However, it is clear that momentum is towards a devolved approach in which local regions do their

Necessity Is the Mother of Invention ■ **53**

own procurement. "I don't know where the rationale came from," he tells me and describes the decision to not continue with the model he developed as a body blow:

> I wanted to see, are there legs in keeping a national platform, replicating what Scotland have done? It was working, and people quite liked the fact that we took away all the pain of procurement ... and all the sort of stuff that goes along with when you have a relationship with a supplier.

Jonny's efforts have now shifted towards helping trusts' transition to locally procured solutions. This includes working out a standard set of requirements a trust would use to procure a video consultation platform. His team has reviewed the market to see what companies are out there and the procurement frameworks that can be used. A consultancy was brought in to interview clinicians, administrators and others to understand the characteristics of a good platform that met their needs. With an orientation towards making life as easy as possible for local organisations, his team has done all the work to make procurement as painless as possible.

Whilst he did not get his way on procurement, Jonny has successfully lobbied to keep dedicated funding for another year. He explains why this is important: "if we don't [give them funds] then trusts will use it as an excuse not to keep doing it. At the very least we should fund next year." For Jonny, the amount is a compromise but it is better than nothing. "If I'm still around next year then I'll go back to bat for more money for the year after," he laughs, "one year at a time."

I ask Jonny for his reflections after such a huge and unexpected undertaking that the pandemic rudely foisted upon him. "I'm really proud of what we've done," he tells me,

> I think we've made a difference ... I think video consultations would have happened anyway, but I think we've made it happen at a bigger scale and made it easier for people to do and I think we've shown them there's a way forward.

"The regions have played a huge part," says Jonny,

> they've held the [local] relationships, because it was too much for us, and regions have got scars like us. We worked all hours of all days for months, but they were doing the same. The reason why it worked, and I don't want to be too cliched about it, but it was because we were all working together – regions, trusts and national were pushing in the same direction ... it worked because we all had the same interests and goals.

I ask Jonny what comes next. He is worried that a sense of common purpose has been replaced by fragmentation of effort as regions take their own separate paths. He believes there still isn't sufficient headspace at a local level to maintain the

54 ■ *Towards a Digital Ecology*

momentum: "they're [too] busy trying to save patients from covid and a hundred and one other things, it's relatively far down the priority list, we've got to be honest."

"There will be a drop off … as we all go back to our old behaviours," says Jonny,

> this has been driven by doctors and hospitals telling patients 'you need to be seen and you need to be seen by video,' we need to flip it on its head and we need to convince a wider population of patients that you can still get great quality NHS care through these routes.

Jonny's personal ambition for the future has turned towards helping patients get the most from video consultations and he is keen to get a public help desk established that could then broaden its scope even further.

Jonny and I conclude our conversation musing about the rights and wrongs of centrally set targets. "Inevitably the national folk with turn to [targets]," Jonny says shaking his head. Sometimes referred to as *authoritarian drift*, what often starts as what appear to be good ideas on the face of it turn into the development of frameworks and guidelines, then become codified in targets and quickly become contractual requirements.[24] Jonny prefers to think of video consultations as just one of many tools that can be used to suit people's needs and preferences. He is interested in understanding the impact on carbon emissions and other wider factors stemming from remote consultations. Jonny's story is one of a tiny team making a big difference across the country as they cleared the path for local hospitals and community services to use video consultations. His tale is one whereby central bodies work to enable local services to deliver services and wrestle with the challenges of procurement and administration so that they don't have to. It is an example of how a digital ecology thrives best with a reciprocal interplay between the centre and the local, each doing what it does best.

Fighting Fires of the Future

"It was literally days," explains Nikki, a practice manager in a rural GP surgery, "we were being told one thing in the morning and by the afternoon we were having to do something different."

In the first shock, Nikki and her team turned to whatever they could put their hands on to keep the surgery going. Using the practice mobile phone, they used WhatsApp to keep in touch with patients and receive photos to diagnose a skin rash or guide treatment of a minor injury. She explains how they would send the photo from WhatsApp to the surgery email so it could be entered in the patient's health record. An impressive workaround. "It's something we'd never dream of in normal times," Nikki reflects. In those first few days, it was about keeping the service running while they set up clinical systems. She recounts how the Clinical Commissioning Group made funds available in an instant "it was just, get what you need and fill in a claim form and get it reimbursed."

Necessity Is the Mother of Invention ■ 55

As order reestablishes itself and we collectively adapt to the new emerging normal, this flurry of technology adoption has as yet unknown repercussions. For Nikki, the clinicians in her GP practice have got used to using Accurx, a communication platform made free by the venture-capital-backed company in the first wave. The Accurx revenue model is as yet unclear and with substantial adoption across the system, the company will need to start making money. Unfortunately for Nikki, the regional system has licensed another communication platform at a system level, so her clinicians will have to ditch the one they have got used to and start the learning process from scratch.

As a GP receptionist in a small village practice, Dawn has more immediate priorities than even video consultations,

> We don't have an answerphone. We are still in the dark ages. We have a new telephone system coming in January. We can't keep up, we only have two lines. So we're going to have a new system with twenty telephone lines.

While Nikki believes that remote consultations are here to stay, she is concerned about the impact on the doctors in her practice:

> From a clinician's sense of satisfaction with work, they need to have face-to-face as well, you need that balance. [I know] one clinician who is thinking about early retirement … they're actually very good with technology, it's just that they struggle with not having that face-to-face.

Nikki explains further, "they came into that profession to care, to see patients, and to see someone come in distressed and unwell and to see them leave with a resolution. That's why they came into the profession and it's what they thrive on." For clinicians less comfortable with remote care, their workplace has become more akin to a call centre, headset on and call after call after call.

For Nikki, diktats from the centre are as much of a hindrance as a help. "It's the red tape," she moans when I ask her to describe to me what the digital health landscape looks like from her position in a local village practice. "It's the hoops that you have to go through and the chopping and changing," Nikki warms to her subject: "The problem is that the people who make the decisions have not got a primary care background. They've no idea what it's like to be on the ground." Nikki and her GP practice team want to be able to make pragmatic decisions that make sense to them in their local context.

Beverley has been similarly frustrated by burdensome administration: "We have managed pre-Covid to turn professional meeting attendance into a career and it's got out of hand, suddenly through Covid we've managed to decimate all the meeting schedules, cancel cancel cancel." For Beverley, this creates an opportunity for the future,

56 ■ *Towards a Digital Ecology*

[we can] have meetings that half the length they used to be, still have a consensus with people involved, through MS Teams, agile fast decision making and all written down for the record and so one of the big things coming out of this is can we please have a really sharp eye, real discerning eye on what do we really need from a governance perspective for decision making perspective, what do we really need.

I ask Matthew for his views of the future digital adoption post-pandemic as we round up our early morning Zoom interview so we can start our respective working days. He pauses for a moment: "The NHS is inherently allergic to change," he laments, "imagine that you're a regional director and you've got twenty or forty hospitals all with bright ideas about how to do things; but your main job is to deliver today's targets today." Matthew becomes somewhat maudlin as he reflects on his conviction that the NHS can do *so* many things better than it does: "but there are always fires to fight and resources are always focused on fighting those fires, and if I was in one of those senior roles then my attention would be on fighting those fires as well."

"We have to make the last year count for something." These are the words uttered by a CIO at a digital health conference taking place exactly a year to the day from when we first went into lockdown. I wonder if COVID-19 really does create a once in a lifetime opportunity to rapidly accelerate the adoption of digital in the NHS. A veteran of NHS IT, Andy Kinnear has a cautious assessment of the future:

My slight fear is that what might happen, is the dial might slide quite a long way back once a level of normality returns and people are back in their buildings … once you [clinician] are up and running outpatients again, you'll be sending letters out like you always did, for appointment times that nobody chose, like you always have done … facing cancellations and DNAs [did not attends] at the same level you always have … and you'll still be expecting patients to come to the hospital and see a doctor face-to-face. I'm very sceptical that the change that they describe will actually truly embed itself.

As the danger of the pandemic subsides, a new danger of drifting back to the norm becomes ever more present.

I have captured and shared just a few stories from the many more that could have been told. I wonder what themes we can draw from them that give us an insight into the state of digital technology in the NHS along with the conditions we need for a *digital ecology* to flourish and grow. It is clear that investment in both people and infrastructure reaps benefits when the chips are down. We should not take lightly the importance of well-established relationships and trust when it comes to getting things done. The sense of common purpose around a crisis was a powerful, galvanising force that cut through self-limiting rivalries between national bodies and those

Necessity Is the Mother of Invention ■ **57**

working at a regional and local level. However, how to sustain and cultivate them remains a challenge as the panic subsides.

People working in the NHS surprised themselves at what they are capable of and perhaps the most profound change to come from the pandemic is that we have a new story to tell ourselves about digital adoption that might even release us from the gloomy sentence of NPfIT. If we can galvanise a new-found confidence, perhaps we can ride a wave of optimism that attracts talent and brightens the digital ecology. However, sustained intense pressure over months is also taking its toll and it seems unlikely that the NHS will create proper space to nurture its own recovery.

Beverley is nervous about the future:

> We need proper budgets for tech in trusts, what this [the pandemic] has enabled is free kit and some licenses, it hasn't given us proper budgets for a proper professional IT team to actually run and manage and be based in each department and that's what we really need.

According to the think tank Institute for Public Policy Research, our health and care service needs a boost of 12 billion pounds a year over the next five years if it is to bounce back from COVID-19. The think tank's figures include upgrading digital infrastructure across the NHS and care in order to improve productivity, care quality and drive further integration.[25] We can't expect a digital ecology to mature if we don't have the resources to tend and nourish it.

Finally, it is clear that there is no room for hype in a digital ecology that regulates itself through trust. Whilst it may be more novel technologies that got the limelight, there is no doubt that the telephone proved itself as the most useful and ubiquitous technology around. And finally, we should take time to applaud and appreciate the impressive efforts that the protagonists of the stories in this chapter made to help the NHS stay on its feet during unprecedented times. But a mature ecology should have the right conditions to weather a storm. We urgently need to nourish the ecology and build its reserves for whatever future challenges that it will inevitably have to encounter.

Notes

1 https://www.google.com/url?q=https://medium.com/@tomaspueyo/coronavirus-act-today-or-people-will-die-f4d3d9cd99ca&sa=D&ust=1587749222251000&usg=AFQjCNGzLYeEyv-DSoYxrTH9xmnk2OgVyQ

2 https://www.nhsconfed.org/-/media/Confederation/Files/Publications/Documents/NHS-Reset_Best-practice-and_innovation_FNL.pdf

3 https://www.healthcareitnews.com/news/emea/uk-health-minister-tech-has-made-huge-impact-our-battle-against-disease

4 https://www.independent.co.uk/voices/coronavirus-clap-carers-ppe-shortage-boris-johnson-nhs-a9525596.html

58 ■ *Towards a Digital Ecology*

5 https://www.hsj.co.uk/technology-and-innovation/demand-for-nhs-tech-services-rockets-amid-covid-19-crisis/7027275.article
6 https://www.thehtn.co.uk/2020/04/22/guys-and-st-thomas-launch-3d-printing-farm/
7 https://www.digitalhealth.net/2021/01/kettering-hospital-builds-mary-bot-to-automate-covid-reporting/
8 https://wiserd.ac.uk/sites/default/files/documents/Homeworking%20in%20the%20UK_Report_Final_3.pdf
9 https://wpi-strategy.com/site/wp-content/uploads/2020/08/Caring-for-the-NHS-Workforce-Final.pdf
10 https://www.nhsx.nhs.uk/blogs/tech-frontline-how-nhsx-partners-are-delivering-pace/
11 https://digital.nhs.uk/news-and-events/news/almost-half-a-million-ms-teams-messages-a-day-sent-in-the-nhs-during-lockdown?utm_source=Healthcare+Roundup&utm_campaign=63f68dd5a3-EMAIL_CAMPAIGN_2020_05_21_12_57&utm_medium=email&utm_term=0_78e7587464-63f68dd5a3-121741153
12 https://www.resolutionfoundation.org/publications/the-effects-of-the-coronavirus-crisis-on-workers/
13 https://news.gwsolutions.com/2020/11/25/inadequate-home-internet-speeds-during-lockdown/
14 https://www.totaljobs.com/advice/lockdown-loneliness-the-collapse-of-social-life-at-work
15 https://amp-theguardian-com.cdn.ampproject.org/c/s/amp.theguardian.com/politics/2020/oct/05/how-excel-may-have-caused-loss-of-16000-covid-tests-in-england
16 https://www.theguardian.com/society/2007/oct/02/publicservicesawards
17 https://www.youtube.com/watch?v=gcPg5TEwTSY&feature=youtu.be
18 https://www.ucl.ac.uk/news/2020/nov/analysis-how-virtual-wards-care-covid-19-patients-home
19 https://www.ucl.ac.uk/news/2020/nov/analysis-how-virtual-wards-care-covid-19-patients-home
20 https://www.cebm.net/covid-19/question-should-smartphone-apps-be-used-as-oximeters-answer-no/
21 https://www.england.nhs.uk/coronavirus/wp-content/uploads/sites/52/2021/01/C1041-letter-supporting-hospital-discharge-covid-virtual-wards-13-jan-21.pdf
22 https://www.nao.org.uk/wp-content/uploads/2021/02/Protecting-and-supporting-the-clinically-extremely-vulnerable-during-lockdown.pdf
23 https://www.norfolkandwaveneyccg.nhs.uk/publications/documents/93-covid-protect-briefing-updated-26-may-2020/file
24 https://www.jscimedcentral.com/CommunityMedicine/communitymedicine-6-1047.pdf
25 https://www.ippr.org/news-and-media/press-releases/12-billion-booster-shot-needed-to-make-nhs-and-social-care-fit-for-future-after-pandemic-landmark-report

Chapter 4

Relative Advantage

In the course of a year, the NHS delivers around 120 million hospital outpatient appointments in hospitals around England.[1] These visits account for a whopping 85% of all non-emergency hospital-based activity.[2]

In March 2020, at the beginning of the pandemic, outpatient appointments delivered via phone call or video almost tripled from the number recorded the same time the previous year.[3] Something had changed.

In April, Elaine was one of the people making up those numbers which, incidentally, are provided by hospitals to NHS Digital and reported in their monthly Hospital Episode Statistics (HES) publications. One of the many datasets collected across England and put into publicly available reports.

In preparation for her appointment with the breast cancer family history clinic, Elaine had already booked half a day of work. She knew she would need that time to drive to the hospital, making sure she got there early so she could give herself enough time to find a car parking space. She had resigned herself to the fact that it wouldn't be possible to predict how long she would be there, remembering that the waiting room, with its water cooler and frayed magazines, is always packed with people in a similar plight to her own.

All that changed with COVID-19. Elaine received a call from an administrator asking her if she was happy to do the consultation via the phone, and they booked it in the diary. On the day itself, she received the call at the exact time specified. She paused and sat in the back garden, soaking up spring rays as she answered a series of questions and discussed treatment options. The appointment was done and dusted in the space of half an hour. No car journey. No parking charge. No waiting. No half a day off work. Elaine's phone appointment even made a modest contribution to reducing greenhouse gases, with such travel journeys typically accounting for 5% of all traffic in England.[4]

DOI: 10.1201/9781032198798-4

60 ■ *Towards a Digital Ecology*

That simple phone call transformed Elaine's experience of outpatient care. Without the requirement for a physical examination, it turned out there was no need for her to visit the hospital at all. Her experience is not universal, but it is common enough to warrant a complete rethink of the traditional model of face-to-face outpatient consultations.

It is not just hospital appointments that have been catapulted into a massive channel shift. In May, during the early summer heat of the pandemic, half of GP appointments were carried out remotely. NHSX reported that, by 1 June, 87% of general practices were live with technology to enable online consultations and that more than two-thirds of practices had appointments booked online.[5] Whilst video consultations got the spotlight, it was actually text message and telephone that proved by far the most popular, perhaps because of their ubiquity and familiarity.[6]

Whatever the medium, there was a huge increase from pre-pandemic February, where the overwhelming majority of appointments had taken place in the doctor's clinic amidst the familiar lopsided posters peeling away from brittle Blu Tack on magnolia walls.[7] The NHS' Long-Term Plan's commitment that by 2023/24 all patients will have the option for a remote GP consultation was delivered rather unexpectedly ahead of schedule, a surprise policy gift from the coronavirus.

With almost all GPs across the country now offering remote consultations, I was curious about whether they are here to stay. I found at least part of the answer in a survey of GPs undertaken by the British Medical Association (BMA) in June. As we were emerging from the worst excesses of the first wave of the pandemic, a staggering 88% reported that they would like to see remote consultations remain.[8] It is hard to underestimate this sea change in an opinion given the glacially slow adoption of remote consultations over the last decade. So what on earth changed?

Relative Advantage

To shed light on the rapid uptake of remote consultations in primary care, we can do worse than travel back to pre-war America. Born on his family farm in Iowa, the young Everett Rogers observed with curiosity, his father's reluctance to take up a novel innovation that led to a stronger, more resilient corn. It was only during the devastating drought of 1936 in which thousands of Americans died that Rogers' father was persuaded to adopt this innovation into his farming practice, after observing the superior crop of his neighbour's farm.

Forever influenced by his experiences on the family farm during that heatwave, Rogers committed his academic career, as a rural sociologist, to studying what prevents uptake of innovation. Having coined the now familiar term "early adopter," his research has been highly influential in the field of technology adoption. It turns out, his thinking has also influenced the work of another renowned academic, Trish Greenhalgh, professor of primary healthcare sciences at the University of Oxford.

I first came across Trish when I stumbled across a paper entitled: *Beyond Adoption: A New Framework for Theorizing and Evaluating Nonadoption, Abandonment, and Challenges to the Scale-Up, Spread, and Sustainability of Health and Care Technologies*. NASSS[9] is an empirical framework for understanding the barriers to uptake of new health technologies. Since then we have collaborated on translating NASSS into a tool to assess complexity in health and care technology projects. In a Zoom conversation she recorded as a teaching tool for her students, I asked Trish to account for the stratospheric COVID-19 related adoption of remote consultations, she drew on another of Roger's key concepts, that of "relative advantage." She believes this concept is central to explaining such a rapid uptake of remote consultations.

Let me explain. We experience relative advantage when the benefit of a new innovation clearly outstrips the benefits of staying with the current way of working. This is exactly what Roger's father experienced back on that farm, and it is what we are experiencing now in both primary and secondary care. "It's not that easy to try software," explains Trish: "You have to buy it, you have to get it downloaded, you have to get permission, you have to learn it; so unless that software has a real advantage, you're not going to use it."

Trish's observation is born out in a separate conversation I have with Ibrahim, a junior doctor in a nephrology outpatient clinic. He reflects on the fact that pre-pandemic, remote consultations had never been taken up with enthusiasm in his clinic. I ask him why. "That is a very important question," he ponders, "It's probably a combination of things. It takes ages to get anything changed in my experience. When someone has had a good idea, or there has been an important recommendation [from a professional body] I've seen it takes time for practice to change. I don't know why. Maybe it's a point of being comfortable in what you're doing and carrying on with it; maybe it requires leadership to drive a lot of this stuff; I think [with the outpatient clinic] people just accepted it and got on with it … you just accept doing what you're doing," he says with a shrug of his shoulders.

However, COVID-19 created a relative advantage over face-to-face consultations simply because of the highly contagious nature of the disease. "Do you know what? I don't want to die examining a patient. And as a patient I don't want to catch an infection from my GP." Over half of hospital doctors[10] and GPs[11] reported not feeling fully protected at work during the pandemic, with personal protective equipment in short supply. "The thing that has changed more than anything," Trish tells me, "is that the relative advantage for both the patient and doctor has gone off the scale."

Trish is not exaggerating – of the 1.1 million primary care consultations that take place every day, telephone and video consultations used to account for 3%. During the first wave of COVID-19 they accounted for 95%.[12] She argues COVID-19 has created what she calls a triple novelty: it is a new disease that we know comparatively little about, its infectious nature has necessitated different ways of interacting with patients and services have had to organise themselves in a completely different way

62 ◾ *Towards a Digital Ecology*

to manage the risk of infection. It may be AI and blockchain that get the headlines, but some of the more basic technologies, telephone and video communications, have come into their own.

Whilst relative advantage may have persuaded primary care practitioners to adopt remote consultations, it has been down to the wider system to remove the barriers and create the infrastructure for its use to explode. This is because it still remains the case that many mundane things get in the way: internet speed, variable hardware and software, telecommunications infrastructure and a simple absence of training and support have all had an impact on many GPs, hampering adoption and creating everyday barriers.[13] A member survey by the Royal College of Physicians in May showed just over half did not have access to a webcam to carry out video consultations, even if they had wanted to.[14]

The rapid uptake of virtual consultation software has been enabled by a whirlwind of activity from central NHS bodies: two new purchasing frameworks cut down the procurement red tape, laptops were rolled out to staff and funding was made available for NHS organisations to purchase necessary hardware. Furthermore, resources[15] were made available for staff to help them optimise the use of video conferencing in practice. In their guidance, even The British Medical Association[16] softened their position on consumer products such as Skype, WhatsApp or Facetime which they concede: "can be considered where you urgently need to have a video consultation with a patient and if alternative channels are not available."

Whilst the relative advantage and a permissive infrastructure have been critical enabling factors, the quality of technology has also significantly improved. Back in 2009 when Trish was first researching video consultations, she recalls how bad the technology was. It wasn't just the camera and the audio quality, it was also that products like Adobe Connect and consumer Skype weren't fit for purpose: "It didn't look or feel like a clinical consultation." However, bespoke software has now come on the market that has been designed for medical consultations. With a virtual waiting room and a simple means of connection, the technology has become easier to use and more acceptable to clinicians and patients alike. This groundwork along with mature video consultation products has paved the way for the relatively painless uptake we have seen. This is a familiar thread. The technology explosion legend that is beginning to creep into the narrative of post-Covid NHS reports appears to be confined to technologies that were already in use but just hadn't had the firepower for wide adoption.

The final piece of the jigsaw puzzle is a more nuanced shift in how clinicians have adapted their practice to fit the technology. This is where human creativity and ingenuity come into play. Not only has the technology adapted to the requirements of the medical context, doctors and nurses are adapting their practice to optimise the technology. Trish describes how one doctor found a novel means of assessing breathlessness without the usual physical examination. The patient is asked to pace up and down the living room until they get out of breath and then instructed to put their hand on their chest whilst they breathe in and out in front of the camera. The rise and fall of the hand over the chest gives a clearer indication of breathlessness that could otherwise be objectively measured. Whilst this may appear fairly trivial, the adaptive nature of both technology and human practice is a facet of promising technology adoption.

It is still in the early days of lockdown when Sanjeev describes the new normal has taken some adjustment at his Birmingham-based GP practice. He chats to me via Google Hangout from his kitchen table. Over his shoulder, I notice the fridge door covered in children's paintings and I can discern the ambient sound of play in the background. "I haven't been in to my practice for three weeks," Sanjeev tells me. "It's good in a lot of ways. I've realised how much you can handle remotely. We can do 90% at home." However, even as a self-proclaimed early adopter of technology, Sanjeev has found some challenges in adapting to this new way of working: "Week one and my son, who is 2, rang into the room and shouted 'daddy I have a willy!' whilst I was on the phone to a patient," he says with a shrug of his shoulders and a wry smile: "working from home is like this."

Patients' experience of video consultations has varied widely during the pandemic, as illuminated by one story reported by the patient organisation, National Voices:

> As I was told by the receptionist that the doctor will call me sometime today. Not knowing when that 'sometime' will be. I was constantly looking at my phone, making sure I will not miss the doctor's call. However, after one hour of waiting, I stopped paying so much attention to my phone as I had to do something else. Unfortunately, I missed the call from the doctor and had to wait another hour to be called back.

In their qualitative study undertaken during the pandemic, National Voices found that people mostly had bad experiences when they were left uncertain or unclear about what would happen and how.[17]

In the midst of the pandemic, remote communications are meeting an immediate and urgent need. But what about the post-Covid future when they are no longer a necessity? "So many clinicians have had many consultations that have gone really well. They've ironed out the glitches that always happen when you're adopting a new technology, and they are confident and are able to deliver a professional service through video," says Trish. Sanjeev echoes this sentiment: "One of the partners in my old practice hates technology, it's another password to learn. He used to type a letter with one finger on the keyboard at a time. But even he has embraced it." The professional shame that comes with conscious incompetence was replaced by a new normal as the pandemic took its course.

64 ■ *Towards a Digital Ecology*

NHS Care Is a Relational Business

Any number of guides and how-to toolkits aimed at helping clinicians use video consultations tend to focus on the transactional aspects of care. However, there is less focus on helping them focus on the relational that is the bond of trust and mutual regard between clinician and patient. Research shows that a strong relationship between a doctor and patient contributes to improved health outcomes, particularly for people with chronic conditions.[18]

In a blog post[19] in which he reflects on his own shift from face to face to virtual, Hackney-based GP Jonathon Tomlinson reflects on the more subtle aspects of relating to a patient through a computer screen:

> If I look at her then I am gazing off to the left, if I look at the camera then it looks as if I am looking at her, but I'm not. If I look at myself (I can't help it) then I'm looking somewhere else. The concentration required is unnatural and exhausting.

Tomlinson is not alone in experiencing what has become known as "zoom fatigue." An article in National Geographic[20] resonates with my personal experience of countless virtual meetings throughout the working day, followed by the same with friends and family in the evenings. If I finish the day exhausted from this novel type of concentration, what must this be like for clinicians who are focused on the more important task of accurately diagnosing and treating a patient? I am curious about what it means for clinicians, often interacting with people at their most vulnerable and frightened, grappling with issues of fear and mortality, to have those conversations infiltrate their home environment. They can no longer leave trauma and distress at the office. The office is their home, and their days are no longer punctuated with the restorative variety of the bustle and conversation in a place of work.

Social interactions are made up of both verbal and non-verbal communications, barely registered by the conscious mind, but which form the foundations of how we relate to one another. In the urgency of the pandemic crisis, these factors seemed less relevant, but we may come to reflect more in the aftermath about how we maintain a healthy balance between the physical and the virtual.

It is not clear what the absence of physical proximity and the reduction in the senses to just sight and sound will mean for clinicians and patients alike. For some, convenience will be the most salient factor, and consultation from home will obviate the need to take time off work or make an extra trip. For some patients, remote consultation will reduce anxiety, but for others, it will do the opposite. Some healthcare professionals will miss vital information on a call while others will find that seeing a person in their home environment provides richness to the interaction. The downsides are real. Around a quarter of trips to the GP are for what are called *undifferentiated symptoms* whereby a discussion of wider social circumstances becomes important. It is unclear how easily this can be done when not in person.

An unanticipated finding during a physical examination sometimes catches something that saves a life.[21] There is some evidence that remote consultations can lead to increased prescribing or referrals to specialist services as GPs err on the side of caution.[22]

For some, those who struggle to communicate or women who are in an abusive relationship, the clinic may be a place of refuge. Sanjeev echoes these concerns:

> The danger is we are catering to a tech savvy group and we can't keep on ignoring inequalities and there are the people who are going to suffer. It's a double edged sword. I am concerned about overloading people with digital. We need to keep it simple and straightforward.

He is nevertheless sanguine: "but it's one of these things, we learn as we go along." All of these nuances and interrelated factors need to be carefully understood post-pandemic if we are to leverage a better NHS rather than an impoverished version.

Trish believes the effects will be long-lasting, and professional reservations about virtual clinical care will disappear over the course of the pandemic and beyond. She also concludes this will be the case for many patients. Not everyone will feel comfortable being examined remotely in front of a video camera, but Trish predicts that a new normal will see around 20% of consultations continue via video. A blend of in-person and virtual will be most effective when it is suited not only to the individual and preferences but also to the nature of the condition and the particular circumstances at that time. These decisions will be nuanced and contingent and must meet the needs of people requiring care and treatment.

Remote consultations will work for some and not for others. It will work in some circumstances and not in others. It is important that the Government's push towards a *digital first* NHS does not disadvantage the very people who depend the most upon its services.

Saying Goodbye

On 5 November 1887, an editorial in *The Lancet* proposed that the telephone could be used effectively as a companion for an individual afflicted by an infectious disease and their friends:

> All of us must have felt the heartaching anxiety of longing to hear the voice of a dear friend when either ourselves lying on, or the friend being confined to, a bed of sickness. The comfort of hearing the voice, with all its intonations, in such a case, does not need to be described in words.[23]

This bygone excerpt from one of England's most prestigious medical journals proves all too prescient for this contemporary pandemic. It is not just the doctor's clinic

66 ■ *Towards a Digital Ecology*

and outpatient appointment where remote communications have had a transformative impact. Video communications have played an important role on COVID-19 wards where patients, separated from family and friends, would not otherwise have been able to say their last goodbyes.

The risk of infection means that COVID-19 inpatients cannot have visitors or any contact with the outside world. A particularly distressing story that was splashed across newspapers on 31 March was of a 13-year-old boy who died in King's College Hospital of the virus all alone, without his parents by his side. It was a heart-rending example of the horror this virus wreaks on those affected most badly by it.

Alert to the plight of patients and their families, ward staff have found creative ways to connect patients and families together; and whilst commercial platforms such as Facetime might be suitable for some, one NHS London chief information officer (CIO) was unhappy with workarounds. Having recently declared a critical emergency due to lack of beds, London North West University NHS trust was struggling. Luke, chief technology officer for software company Made Tech, picks up the story.

"It was 10pm on a Tuesday night and I got a DM a text and an email all at once [from a colleague] saying: 'are you interested in the thing Sonia's talking about?'" With a smile, Luke recounts how it all started. Sonia Patel, the NHS trust CIO, put out a call for help on Twitter on the evening of 14 April for help to develop an application which would connect patients with loved ones via video call: "The challenge to SMEs we need an alpha version in the next 24–48 hours – time is precious" and then a follow-up tweet: "DM [direct message] me."

"At 5.30am the next day my phone starts going buzz buzz buzz and it woke me up and I looked at my phone and it was Sonia saying are you available for a call? I'm not a morning person," he smiles,

> and by 8am I was on a phone call to Sonia and I say: 'Yeah I'll get a team together in an hour's time' [laughs] and so I put a message out at half 8 saying: 'can I have a team by 9am?' And I got a message back saying: 'Luke I think you need to rephrase your wording a bit, it seems a bit like you're commanding something' And I was like: 'Well I sort of am, this is a 48 hour turnaround.'

On a mission to prove open-source technology and rapid development as a credible way of developing software for the NHS, it is evident that Luke is enjoying this most unusual endeavour. When I spoke to him over video call early one evening in April, his team were still actively in product development:

> So yeah that morning we did a mini discovery ... and by the afternoon we had – it was very basic, it was, just put a phone number in, sends a text and puts them [patient and loved one] together in a call. But the next day we built scheduling in and off the back of that we're into a second week of building that feature out.

Relative Advantage ■ **67**

Interviewed by *Wired* magazine, Sonia Patel reflects on why she had put this call out for help on her Twitter feed:

> We had some distraught nurses at one point, there were some patients at the end of life and they couldn't connect with their loved ones in the early days … For them to be gifted with that technology actually made a real difference.[24]

I was curious about the motivations of Luke and his team. They had created a technology with an open-source licence (meaning anyone can take the source code) and no interest in creating a revenue stream, Made Tech developed this product rapidly and entirely at their own expense. Luke explains:

> A success story would be handing this over to NHS Digital or NHSX or someone to look after it for the long term, and I think it's just a case study for open source, for rapid development, for taking a solution hypothesis and doing something.

Luke is also driven by a desire for the NHS to have good quality, purpose-built technologies. He expresses frustration at the plethora of what he sees as mediocre commercial products that the NHS either settles or tries to repurpose:

> From a data collection point of view [our product] is only storing data for as long as it needs; it's NHS branded; it does the scheduling for you rather than staff on the ward having to sort with paper or workarounds; it's a scalable process built into a product that's fit for purpose and you're not repurposing some other system; and your data's not going to places outside the NHS.

He, along with other advocates of open technology, believes this is the best route for digital in the NHS.

Now called *NHS Book*, the application has more features and has been picked up and used by other NHS trusts.[25] It is an example of how simple technology can facilitate humanity in exceptional circumstances. I have drawn on the academic work of Professor Trish Greenhalgh in researching this chapter and interviewed her to bring her work to life, but it is Trish's tweet on 10 December 2020 that brings home the personal cost of the pandemic, along with the essential role that technology is playing for so many of us in saying our last goodbyes:

> Goodbye Mum.
> You died of COVID-19, days before you were due to be vaccinated.
> You told them to give the ventilator to someone else.
> I said a FaceTime farewell from a hospital car park.

68 ■ *Towards a Digital Ecology*

You will have a Zoom funeral.
You are 2020.
Thanks to the devoted, exhausted #NHS staff.

Looking Forward

It was in 1879, some three years after the invention of the telephone, that the notion that it could be a useful tool for doctors was first made in *The Lancet* medical journal. An anonymous writer recounted an event in the US whereby a mother concerned that her baby might have the croup placed a midnight call to the family doctor. According to the story:

> Perhaps because of the lateness of the hour, the doctor "asked to be put in telephonic communication with the anxious mamma. 'Lift the child to the telephone,' he commanded, 'and let me hear it cough.' Both mother and child complied. 'That's not the croup,' the doctor declared, and declines to leave his house on such small matters.[26]

In this story, that telephone call got a doctor out of the inconvenience of an unnecessary home visit. However, this new talking instrument was not without its detractors. In 1892, concerns were raised about all manner of potential telephone-related maladies including cephalgia, vertigo, hyperaesthesia, insomnia and even "physical disturbances of a character which might become chronic." New technologies tend to be treated with suspicion, their negative impacts anticipated, their potential uses resisted. Our fears about the telephone may be consigned to history, but concerns about digital communication technologies prevail.

It is strange. In the dim distant past of the world before COVID-19, we worried that such technologies might lessen the humanity of our interactions. Now we rely on them to do the opposite. During the pandemic, technologies became a lifeline to our humanity, transcending spatial boundaries and facilitating the most profound connection in our most vulnerable moments. They have given cause for us all to rethink their role in healthcare.

We are left with an important puzzle to be solved about how the NHS takes the best of remote care during the pandemic and builds it into whatever normal we have ahead of us. Technology facilitated care will need to both anticipate and bear the brunt of choppy pandemic seas that we no doubt have ahead of us. Technology will need to make our lives easier, whilst deepening human connection, if it is to realise that elusive relative advantage.

It may have taken a pandemic to deliver remote appointments at scale, but it was only accelerating what many had been arguing for a long time. The Royal College of Physicians has been vocal in making the case for transformation of outpatients and a shift to remote contact where possible.[27] Back in 2018, a pandemic was

Relative Advantage ■ **69**

not uppermost in their minds, but they did make the case that technology would increase resilience in the face of weather-related travel disruption. Replace the word *travel* with *virus* and it becomes more than relevant today.

In the target fetishised, performance-driven, command and control culture of the NHS, it will be all too tempting for those at the centre to compel us to embed this change through a bludgeon of measures and metrics. This fear is felt deeply by Alec, a consultant rheumatologist and chief clinical information officer (CCIO) in the Midlands. An advocate of patient-centred care, he has a strongly held belief that we should use remote consultations "for the right reasons" and not simply because "some executives are saying face to face appointments should be the exception." "That's rubbish," he tells me, "it should be based on needs, where you will add value."

Alec gives me an insight into the depth of his relationships with patients, sometimes over the course of their lives: "I have relationships built up over many years with my patients, some have thanked me for saving their lives, I have diagnosed some with cancer, I have built up a relationship with them and their families." He describes to me how some tell him they like his smile and others that they enjoy the smell of his aftershave. It is a reminder that we are sensory beings, drawing on smell and touch as well as sight and sound. The relationship between patient and clinician, particularly built around a chronic condition over many years, can be a profound and meaningful one. It can mean the difference between a longer or shorter life.

Having introduced video consultations in his clinic back in 2017, Alec is an advocate for digital technology. But he is worried about what a target-driven future might bring: "There is too much transactional focus on bums on seats … but if you are getting the outcome for the person, *how* you do it doesn't matter." Alec wants to see a focus on people's experience of care and their health outcomes. In this new normal, he believes remote consultations should be deployed if they make the most sense for that person and aren't if they don't. Simple.

In an interview with the Health Foundation, GP and health policy expert Becks Fisher reflects on the impact of COVID-19 on GP practices:

> I think we'll look back on March 2020 and the start of the pandemic as a watershed moment in general practice. Some of the ways we're working now are positive, but some won't be – and there may be some consequences that we won't know about for some time.

She argues that the NHS must take stock and evaluate the impact of these changes to learn what we should keep and what we should discard.[28]

The COVID-19 crisis has created a demand for remote consultations out of necessity. But beyond its immediate utility, they may have been transformative in showing clinicians how they can successfully use technologies in practice. Clinicians have overcome the professional shame that many dreaded. It may be the case that this is the most salient impact of the pandemic on digital transformation in the

70 ◼ *Towards a Digital Ecology*

NHS. Remote consultations may be the NHS version of the gateway drug that leads clinicians towards a wider world of digital transformation. Many have become hooked and they want more.

Beyond the immediate emergency, there is an opportunity to galvanise ourselves to think imaginatively about the possibilities remote consultation technologies afford. We should pay attention to the transactional nature of how we embed them in the everyday practicalities of clinical care; we should work out how we deploy them to enhance and augment care and treatment for each individual patient and their family; we should think creatively about how we may make a step change that takes us beyond merely digitising an analogue process. We are only limited by our imagination.

Forward-looking clinicians are already working some of this out. For example, one US clinic is delivering group interventions online, blending peer education and support between patients with similar conditions with clinical expertise. Early learning from the Cleveland Clinic indicates that this shared care approach enables patients to spend more time with their clinician whilst also interacting with one another, both of which can be calming in the context of social isolation.[29]

Video consultations also have utility for the daily work of a hospital; the Massachusetts General in Boston has ditched the traditional medical round which usually requires clinicians to be huddled together around a computer screen looking at radiology reports or discussing test results. The authors anticipate that creating virtual teams may enable staff to experience:

> less psychological trauma caused by physical distancing and wearing personal protective equipment (PPE), and enable otherwise non-essential personnel and student trainees (who have been frequently removed from hospital settings during the pandemic) to rejoin the workforce, thereby creating a scalable platform for knowledge sharing and collaborative teams between facilities to help with load balancing as needed across health systems.

If clinicians and administrators are given good IT infrastructure, a permissive environment in which to experiment, along with the space and resources to do so, then we can build on the shift in business as usual that we saw during the first wave of the pandemic. It is in these shifts, born out of necessity, that the seeds of better ways of doing things could be realised. But we have to do so with people in our vision and targets out of sight.

Notes

1 https://files.digital.nhs.uk/5D/8AAEB1/HESF%20Monthly%20Report%20NHSdigital.pdf
2 https://www.rcplondon.ac.uk/projects/outputs/outpatients-future-adding-value-through-sustainability

Relative Advantage ▪ 71

3 https://digital.nhs.uk/data-and-information/publications/statistical/hospital-episode-statistics-for-admitted-patient-care-outpatient-and-accident-and-emergency-data

4 https://www.rcplondon.ac.uk/projects/outputs/outpatients-future-adding-value-through-sustainability

5 https://www.cqc.org.uk/sites/default/files/20201016_stateofcare1920_fullreport.pdf

6 https://www.digitalhealth.net/2020/06/text-and-telephone-consultations-trump-video-during-covid-19/

7 https://digital.nhs.uk/data-and-information/publications/statistical/appointments-in-general-practice/may-2020

8 https://www.bma.org.uk/media/2557/bma-covid-19-survey-results-for-gps-4-june-2020.pdf

9 https://asset.jmir.pub/assets/534442d84fd4d5f0a2b559a4594e0300.pdf

10 https://www.bma.org.uk/media/2555/bma-covid-19-survey-results-for-hospital-doctors-4-june-2020.pdf

11 https://www.bma.org.uk/media/2557/bma-covid-19-survey-results-for-gps-4-june-2020.pdf

12 https://www.bma.org.uk/media/2557/bma-covid-19-survey-results-for-gps-4-june-2020.pdf

13 https://www.bma.org.uk/media/2557/bma-covid-19-survey-results-for-gps-4-june-2020.pdf

14 https://www.rcplondon.ac.uk/news/giant-leaps-digital-progress-have-we-missed-small-steps-along-way

15 https://www.england.nhs.uk/coronavirus/publication/video-consultations-for-secondary-care/

16 https://www.bma.org.uk/advice-and-support/covid-19/practical-guidance/covid-19-video-consultations-and-homeworking

17 https://www.nationalvoices.org.uk/sites/default/files/public/publications/the_dr_will_zoom_you_now_-_insights_report.pdf

18 Find reference

19 https://abetternhs.net/2020/04/24/consulting-during-covid/

20 https://www.nationalgeographic.com/science/2020/04/coronavirus-zoom-fatigue-is-taxing-the-brain-here-is-why-that-happens/

21 https://jamanetwork.com/journals/jamainternalmedicine/fullarticle/2769550

22 https://www.nuffieldtrust.org.uk/news-item/a-digital-general-practice-what-have-we-found-out-so-far

23 https://pdfs.semanticscholar.org/ea46/5b2cecc1535ca330d8e6b6ae32ce4eb45354.pdf

24 https://www.wired.co.uk/article/nhs-coronavirus-technology

25 https://www.madetech.com/blog/evolving-the-nhs-book-a-virtual-visit-service-with-kettering-general-hospital

26 https://pdfs.semanticscholar.org/ea46/5b2cecc1535ca330d8e6b6ae32ce4eb45354.pdf

27 https://www.rcplondon.ac.uk/projects/outputs/outpatients-future-adding-value-through-sustainability

28 https://www.health.org.uk/news-and-comment/newsletter-features/a-gp-perspective-on-covid-19?utm_source=charityemail&utm_medium=email&utm_campaign=aug-2020&pubid=healthfoundation&description=aug-2020&dm_i=4Y2,70H7Z,18YGUJ,S9POH,1

29 https://www.thelancet.com/journals/landig/article/PIIS2589-7500(20)30101-1/fulltext

Chapter 5

When People Drive Digital

The way in which collectivity creates resilience is particularly clear in crises. It is when people think of themselves as 'we' rather than 'I' that they are most likely to accept measures that optimise the overall fight against coronavirus even if they personally are disadvantaged. And it is as a 'we' that people are coming together in innumerable mutual aid groups at street, town and national levels to give a level of support that the state could never provide. As so often in disasters, the real 'first responders' are the people themselves, way before any emergency services can arrive on the scene and the role of the state must be to scaffold, not substitute for that self-help.[1]

In the UK, all innovation is clinician driven, professionally driven; the role of the patient is not seen as useful. We are not valued in that way. The penny dropped only recently … The system only trusts health professionals.

Michael Seres[2]

When People Drive Digital

This chapter starts with a story, a very personal story. I know the story very well because I've heard it countless times, retold from many different keynote conference podiums over the years. It is a powerful story because it comes from the heart and the soul. It is the story of innovation that is wrenched from the gut of personal lived

DOI: 10.1201/9781032198798-5

74 ■ Towards a Digital Ecology

experience. I will do my best to recount this story, but it won't be quite the same as if it was told by the person for whom that experience is the closest. And I can't ask him to tell you for himself, even though I know without a doubt he would have loved to share it with you. I can't ask him, because he is no longer with us.

I first came across Michael Seres in 2014 when I was making my first hesitant steps into the digital health sector. I have to confess I can't recall quite how our introduction came about, but I do remember that I was organising a conference track at a Health 2.0 event and he was recommended to me as a good speaker. It turns out that that was an underestimation. Michael was an amazing speaker, and he had a powerful personal story to tell. But before I share that story, I want to explain why on earth I was running a conference track on a topic I had barely started getting to grips with myself.

Having already been to several digital health conferences, I was perplexed that the conference stage was invariably crowded by clinicians and industry speakers but rarely inhabited by the very people who were supposed to be reaping the benefits of technology innovation. We are all patients at some times in our lives, we also are citizens with rights and responsibilities, and of course, we are all people. But the voice, experience and insight of people as patients is routinely sidelined in favour of people as clinicians, researchers or engineers. The token patient is often an after-thought; window dressing to drive home a message or appeal to the heartstrings for just a moment so that the audience can be reminded why we are all here in the first place. To be honest, not that much has changed over the years.

This was the first event I had run and devised with my new friend Mark, a mental health activist I had met whilst undertaking postdoctoral research. We called the track *Citizen-Led Digital Health and Wellbeing* and the session description went: *in this track session you will hear examples of how citizens have made use of digital tools and developed mobile apps to solve problems that they were experiencing in managing their health and well-being*. I am proud, looking back, at the approach we were in our own small way trying to promote, against the grain of most corporate events. The programme information concludes: *The session will focus on principles of co-production and co-design with the guiding principle that better solutions are found when citizens are at the heart of mHealth innovation*. This was, and remains, my belief and a guiding principle in my work today.

Michael, with diminutive stature and a big open smile, arrived just before the conference track began, with a big woolly hat covering his head. He explained that he was mid-chemo, and he had taken a break to come and do the speaking slot and would be heading straight back to finish it off afterwards. The woolly hat was to cover his hair loss. This was typical of Michael. He was sweet and generous and kind, whilst being one of the most tenacious and bloody-minded people I have ever met. Alongside Michael, speakers included Sheldon who had devised Mumoactive, a mobile app to manage his children's diabetes, and Kat who brought her lived experience to mental health start-up BuddyApp. We were attempting to be disrupters in our own small way, advocating for a novel approach in which people as patients are at the centre of digital innovation.

When People Drive Digital ■ **75**

It was that small conference track with an audience of around 30 that set the path for *People Drive Digital*, a series of events that I went on to run with my friends Anne and Roz. It seems fitting to recount Michael's personal journey from a YouTube video of the 15minute talk he gave at one of those events back in the summer of 2015. Surrounded by a group of 100 or so delegates, Michael did what he managed to do every time he spoke, captivating the audience with his intrepid tale.

From the age of 12, Michael had lived with Crohn's disease, an incurable bowel condition which meant that his colon (part of the bowel) had been operated on to divert it through an opening of the tummy. Through this opening or stoma, his body waste (or crap as Michael liked to call it) was collected in a pouch which is often called a stoma bag. Regular hospital stays were an inevitable part of Michael's life, and it was during one of those stays that Michael had an idea. In his talk, he explains: "the doctors said to me, you need to measure your crap, we need to know when that output is, we need to know when it happens, because by knowing that we can tell whether your gut is functioning properly."

But this wasn't as straightforward as it might seem:

> So you're sitting in hospital … and you're trying to empty your crap into a bowl, write down that measurement, put it on a chart, give it to a nurse who can put it on a fluid balance chart. And it's not great.

Frustrated with this routine and embarrassed by the many times when the pouch would overflow, Michael did what he explains many patients do and turned to social media "for me, one of the greatest underutilised resources in healthcare is without a doubt peer to peer interaction and that ability to talk to another patient."

"So I went on to social media," he continues, "and I spoke to around thirty thousand patients around the world through various groups." Michael asked a series of questions that only people living with the same condition could answer. He wanted to know whether other people were experiencing the same problem as him and if so, what they were doing about it. He felt sure there must be some technology out there that could help. Michael was particularly eager to find a better way to measure the output from his bowel and avoid those humiliating overflows. But all he heard back was the same thing "we just guess, we just send it back to the nurse and we hope that they will deal with it."

Through his conversations with peers, Michael realised that this was a common problem that no one seemed to have solved. He tried to find out if there was something out there, but he found nothing. So Michael decided to invent it himself:

> Sitting in hospital I had an awful lot of time, so I'm staring at the bag attached to my body and going, so okay every time it fills it changes shape, so if I could get stuff to alert me when that bag starts to change shape I could stop it spilling.

76 ■ *Towards a Digital Ecology*

This was the beginning of his journey into digital health.

Michael describes how we started searching online and bought various bits of kit on eBay, including a Blackberry battery, an assortment of wires and a Nintendo Wii glove: "I found online this sensor strip from a Nintendo Wii glove and the principle of this strip was, when you put your hand in the glove and you bend the glove, it sends a signal somewhere." He got the various parts delivered to his ward and started prototyping from his hospital bed.

Without an electronics background, Michael commandeered the help of YouTube videos to create a prototype sensor, which he sellotaped onto the outside of his stoma pouch. Now his doctors became interested, and they asked if there was a way the sensor could automatically measure the volume. He realised he was on to something:

> So I went out to patients [on social media] and asked them, if you had a sensor would you use it? Would you pay for it? How much would you pay for it? What do you want it to do?

Once he had gathered feedback from people in similar circumstances to himself, he decided his idea was worth pursuing. This was a decision that was to shape the rest of his life and set him on his digital health start-up journey.

"So I pitched it to this guy who gave me some cash to make it into a proper device," explains Michael, describing how over the following year he developed his prototype into a working product. "Off I went to America to a big patient conference and said 'so here it is, what do you think?'" With positive feedback ringing in his ears, he trekked back to the UK to start wading through all the regulatory requirements that would make his innovation a fully approved medical device that could be recommended by a clinician and safely used by a patient both in the UK and the US.

Five years on from Michael's talk, with *People Drive Digital* as part of our shared history, we bumped into each other at a digital health conference in Helsinki. This time Michael was the keynote speaker to over 4,000 delegates. This was to be the last time we met. I recall our conversation in the hotel bar where Michael's urgency to create impact, knowing that time was limited, was almost visceral. Frustrated by the inertia in his country of birth, he had gone to live in California where he found he could develop a thriving business. With his product in major hospitals around America, he was finally realising his dream. But his heart was in the UK, where his experiences had been largely of frustration and disappointment. Why was this the case?

To answer this question, I will take us back to Michael's *People Drive Digital* talk. Michael was direct in expressing his frustration with digital health in the UK:

> The first thing you do is turn to the digital health team at NHS England and go 'help! How can I do this?' because there's no pathway to adopt patient-led innovation; there's no streamlined process that says follow A

to Z and you come out the other end and you either get it right or you get in wrong.

Michael did what was asked of him by the system. He made the health economic case. He proved his product improved people's quality of life. He participated in digital health accelerators. He ticked the boxes. But the NHS wasn't ready or able or willing to adopt his innovation.

As Michael finished that talk, he gave an anecdote that has always stuck in my mind. He recounts a story from a conversation with a physician when presenting at Stanford Center for Digital Health. "As a hospital we get thirty new innovations coming to us a month," explained one of the team,

> twenty nine of them are from companies who have developed tech and then come to us and say 'find us the health environment to put this tech on to'. And [for every thirty] one of them comes to us from a patient with lived experience who knows the problem and then builds tech around it ... and those are the ones we adopt, and those are the ones that get scale and traction.

Michael was a passionate advocate for the role of patients being involved in and even leading innovation. They can identify and even solve problems that, although they may be invisible to a clinician, will have the biggest daily impact on living with a chronic health condition. "When you think about adoption," says Michael as he finishes his talk, "the ones that succeed, are the ones where patients either develop them in partnership, or if the tech companies have brought in the users right at the very beginning."

"I was very lucky, I built a product to meet my needs, and it was very niche, and there was a market for it," concludes Michael,

> If I'm honest with you, sitting on a transplant ward watching a bag fill up and leak with crap all over me, I would have paid anything to have solved that problem ... but it would never have happened without social media, without other patients and without the ability to go out to real world users and ask them 'do you experience the same problems that I do?' and that for me is the power of patient-driven innovation.

Michael eventually succumbed to the condition that had been part of his life since the age of 12. Michael had survived three separate bouts of cancer, two transplants and had over 25 surgical interventions. It was finally a bout of sepsis that proved too much for his body to take.[3]

Universally well-liked, all of us who knew him and collaborated with him miss him terribly. His legacy is not just his thriving company, which he named 11 Health in honour of the fact he was the 11th patient in the UK to receive a bowel transplant;

78 ■ *Towards a Digital Ecology*

Michael's legacy is also the embodiment of the power of patients as partners and as innovators in the digital health sector. Michael was the first e-patient-in-residence at Stanford's medical-tech conference, Medicine X where he promoted the role that patients can and should be able to play, not only in digital innovation but also in their own care.

Michael leveraged the power of his peers and his phenomenal social networks to solve problems that would improve the everyday lives of people with Crohn's disease. Because of his warmth and his undoubted magnetism, Michael became the poster boy for people driven digital health. Even though he is gone, his philosophy continues in the work of many patient-led innovators and communities who, tired of waiting for the healthcare system to solve problems for them, have taken matters into their own hands. From the do it yourself *We are not Waiting* patient diabetes movement, to *Patients Like Me* which connects patients to each other, this is people exercising personal and collective power, deciding they are no longer content to wait for the system to transform itself.

Much of this book focuses on how the healthcare system, riddled from the top down and back up again with paternalism and inertia, is attempting to flip itself into the digital age that surrounds it. However, this chapter explores the power of networks, of communities and of people who are not bound by the control and hierarchy of the system. It explores the constant flux between central diktat and local control and asks how we can best make change with people at the heart; how the healthcare system can both scaffold and enable this to happen.

Command and Control

Michael took an entrepreneurial path and created a solution to his problem with which he went on to create a business. But what about those people working within the system who want to create change from the inside. Their path is a different one to Michael's, but in many ways, it is equally frustrating.

The NHS is riddled with not just bureaucracy but with hierarchy too. The particular idiosyncrasies of those pecking orders take various forms, from the managerial chain of command to the respective status and influence between different professional groups. A peculiarity of NHS vernacular is that people are routinely talked about in respect of their pay grade. People will make references to a band 6 nurse or an 8a practice lead without giving pause for thought. I used to do it too when I worked in the NHS. It seems to me that this somewhat dehumanising practice is about knowing your place. It is heavy with undertones of stick with your pay grade and defer to your seniors.

But the rigidity of hierarchy doesn't end there. Command and control culture permeates from the outside in. NHS trusts are held to account by NHS England and other national bodies, providing performance and reporting data to commissioners, regulators and inspectors. There is a constant tension between central control and local determination which operates in a state of constant flux. Hierarchy is expressed in clinical care too with a culture of paternalism that, whilst not universal, has been a feature of healthcare forever and a day. It is this culture of *doctor knows best* that Michael felt so dissatisfied with. As someone living with a lifelong condition, he fervently believed that he was an expert in his own care. He wanted to be round-the-table working collaboratively with his medical team as partners and enablers.

Anyone who has worked in the NHS will be familiar with the organisational chart. A series of boxes containing job titles (and sometimes Agenda for Change bandings) with arrows that connect job roles in respect of what roles then report to, and so on. In the many NHS job descriptions I have written over the years, I have been required to add one of these charts that illustrate the hierarchy in which a particular position is placed.

In a workshop on system leadership, Myron Rogers argues that these charts not only show how organisations attempt to organise themselves, but they represent a philosophy about how to best organise human endeavour. These charts embody an assumption that work is directed from the top downwards. According to Rogers, "if you reduce every activity to its smallest possible part, and have that part done superbly, and then connect it all together in a linear process, then you will get something out the other end." He argues that this orientation "works exceptionally well for machines, but not so well for people." [4]

Sam Shah understands these tensions better than most. A clinician and public health specialist, Sam has worked at NHS England and NHSX as well as within technology companies and delivering clinical services. Sam is concerned about central command and control where he sees an absence of empathy and orientation towards local communities. "The national decision maker thinks one size fits all, top down targets or top down decision making, well intended, assuming the data they have [applies] everywhere, but forgetting that locally those things will vary." Sam advocates for decision-making devolved to local communities, where he argues that the assumed efficiency of a single approach is traded for better population outcomes.

The big question is, does this dominant centralised, command and control orientation enable and facilitate the NHS to respond to the complex social, technological, environmental and political challenges it is facing? The answer is a loud and resounding *no*. In fact, it creates a rather bizarre paradox. The paternalistic and managerial preference for order, structure and bureaucracy gives the illusion of control but in fact, delivers the reality of waste. Lots of meetings take place and reports are produced, but very little is achieved.

We urgently need to find new and different ways to respond to the complexity of our contemporary reality that releases rather than constrains the Michaels of the world. We need to forget pay grades and seek out the person, wherever they may sit in an organisation, who spans boundaries, connects people together and catalyses innovation. We then need to release them from the shackles of bureaucracy and set them free to make a difference. I am not arguing to slash and burn governance and

80 ■ *Towards a Digital Ecology*

cut out the committee. They have an important and necessary role. But I am arguing for that which is proportionate along with a tolerance for emergence as much as for order.

Myron Kellner-Rogers has a long-distinguished history of working with organisations to help them manage change in complex systems. Seeking inspiration from life and nature rather than engineering and machines, *Myron's Maxims©* are a guiding set of principles for enabling change in a complex world: [i] people own what they help to create, [ii] real change happens in the real world, [iii] the people who do the work, do the change, [iv] we should connect the system to more of itself and [v] should start anywhere and follow everywhere.[5] These maxims are rooted in the concept of living and learning systems rather than notions of expert knowledge and positional power.

It is these principles that have been adopted by digital health consultancy, mHabitat in their model for *Inclusive Digital Transformation* which they are taking out to regions across the country. Their mission is to help the NHS and their social care and third sector partners, create a (digitally-enabled) comprehensive service, available to all. In a blog post, managing director Roz Davies sets out the challenge:

> So what we have is a 'wicked system problem'. This means it is complex and messy, there are interconnected factors and it is difficult to solve. There is no silver bullet or one route to solving the issue. This doesn't mean we can't and shouldn't act to improve the situation.[6]

Heavily influenced by Sheila McKechnie Foundation's social change project, mHabitat conceptualises digital transformation as social change rather than simply a series of technology projects. Roz and her team have a simple but elegant proposition. Local areas should begin by understanding their assets (which will be unique to each locality) and using them as their starting point, nourishing what is already starting to bloom. The team advocates that localities should then start with what matters to the people in a local area, where the energy is and grow from there. Regions should seek out good practice and insights from elsewhere to save time, resource and effort but that they should hold in mind Myron's Maxim *we own what we create*, the process of development is often as important as the end game. "Once you understand the need and priorities," Roz argues, "find out who are the touchpoints - who has the relationships of trust with the communities you want to engage and work with."

This notion of finding and building on assets is rooted in the idea that complex adaptive change is emergent and iterative. It is willing to adapt as it morphs to local contexts and conditions. It is a blend of planning with purpose and small acts of collaboration which may be distributed across a system.[7] mHabitat's approach couldn't be more different to the mega-programmes which aim to take a solution, cookie-cut and scale it.

Roz believes their approach, grounded in the emergence and an appreciation of complexity, "really lends itself to the nature of integrated care systems because it requires a partnership approach." They recognise that "No one partner, organisation or sector has all the answers or resources to tackle this issue. For example local governments understand the wider determinants, the voluntary sector is often rooted in specific communities, the NHS has resources and clinical expertise."

Within the world of chief information officers and IT departments, there is a growing appreciation of the social nature of digital transformation. Even what appear to be the most straightforward activities, such as implementing technical standards in a consistent manner, turn out to be largely about adaptive change. A research report by the Nuffield Trust on digital transformation, which interviewed many chief information officers, found that messages and direction from central bodies often conflict and create confusion at a local level, "[I]f you took all the advice and guidance in terms of the percentage of money that should be spent on different attributes of the service, unfortunately it comes to more than 100%. So the centre … in itself isn't joined up," exclaimed one exasperated digital specialist.[8]

How can the NHS shift from central diktat to a position where it can support, enable and scaffold? Sometimes it is an emergency, an unforeseen state of affairs, that fractures business as usual and creates a situation that one organisation, on its own, cannot contend with. Does the shock of the early days of the pandemic hold some clues as to how we may organise ourselves differently to respond to complex situations?

First Responders

A first responder is a trained specialist who is the first called to an emergency. They may be a paramedic or a firefighter. In the case of COVID-19, it was more often than not the neighbour or the local support group that came to the rescue.

It was the week after lockdown. A homemade flyer had been posted through my letterbox. A grainy photo of a man in his mid-30s smiling at the camera with his arm in a bear hug around who I guess is his nan. The flyer contains details of a Facebook group and his mobile number. Posted through all the doors on my street, the flyer implores me to get in touch if I need assistance during the pandemic.

I was not alone in receiving the flyer; there are now over 3,000 WhatsApp and Facebook groups binding local communities together for mutual support, from picking up prescriptions through to grocery shopping.[9] Whilst such community-led initiatives have captured the public imagination, eager for good news stories at a time of crisis, there are many other groups in existence beneath the radar. One such group has the moniker: CV 19 Suppliers Help.

82 ■ *Towards a Digital Ecology*

Over the last few years, I have moved away from public platforms like Twitter to semi-private WhatsApp groups. Whereas once Twitter felt like a place to converse, share and learn, it has become increasingly polluted with disagreements and polarised positions. I still use the platform to get news and information but limit my posts to sharing work-related information and news items. In contrast, I have found semi-private WhatsApp groups have become a safer space to connect and chat.

One such WhatsApp group has a membership of 30+ individuals all working in different parts of the NHS, small digital health companies and big tech firms. James, a CTO at a global tech company, was the instigator of this group, which has become a living and breathing microcosm of the digital health sector.

Sitting in his home office, speaking over a Google Hangout, James chats to me whilst managing the usual distractions of a dog whining to be let out into the garden and messages pinging from multiple platforms: "It was the easiest way of communicating … putting everyone in touch with each other," he explains. Over several years, the group has grown and morphed, becoming a space that is part information sharing, part memes, part personal updates and part collaboration.

As the pandemic began to gain momentum, the WhatsApp group turned to the discussion of COVID-19. James decided to take the members of this group and create a newly expanded group called *CV 19 Suppliers Help* and open it up to all his contacts. He explains the impetus behind his decision:

> There just seemed to be so many different conversations going on about technological solutions that were being bought or talked about by the centre, but no one really disseminating information out to the NHS.

In the absence of direction from central bodies: "Local NHS organisations were also posting on groups to me about how could we [tech companies] help them?"

James invited all his contacts from up and down the country to the WhatsApp group and gave it the following description:

> Group set up to capture and disseminate offers of support and help to NHS and healthcare organisations tackling the CV19 pandemic, from the private sector. Please invite people who would benefit or can add to the solutions list.

After a positive response: "All my NHS colleagues jumped on saying this is fantastic" it quickly became apparent that the single conversation thread afforded by WhatsApp was not sufficient to keep track of the requests and offers of help: "Within a day I couldn't cope with the traffic," says James. With a membership of 200, the group became impossible to manage and it was clear something else was needed.

One member of the group created a boards.net account for people to post offers and requests for help and another set up a Slack channel, a messaging platform that allows sub-channels for different topics. Each sub-channel was then linked to

When People Drive Digital ■ 83

a Google Sheet in which people could input their requests and their offers of help. As the first wave of the pandemic peaked, the Slack group had around 900 members posting requests for and offers of help, updates and the latest news. I observed people helping each other out with everything from supplies of laptops through to boxes of PPE. It was pretty astounding.

This group, and no doubt others like it, was filling the conspicuous absence of central direction from national NHS bodies. Perhaps those bodies were not sufficiently fleet of foot to respond promptly to the crisis. Some speculate that the layers of decision-making and lack of clarity about respective roles and responsibilities between NHS bodies slowed things down. Either way, it became apparent that distributed informal networks based on existing relationships between industry and local NHS organisations were valuable. The ability for people to connect via multiple fora helped people get the help they needed when they weren't able to find it through the usual channels.

With 800 or so people posting daily, James and a few others created a small group to put some checks and balances in place and to connect this informal network to central NHS bodies in partnership with industry representative organisation, techUK. This is just one naturally emerging group that sprung up out of established trusted relationships, galvanised by people who wanted to find a way to assist in the drama of a pandemic that had curtailed all our lives. However, in reality, the NHS didn't have an easy way to receive those offers and most of them were never taken up or realised. Anecdotally, I have spoken to a number of people who, try as they might, couldn't even get free offers of help accepted or translated into practice.

The pandemic saw a proliferation of community-led efforts to curate information and resources in order to help people use technology to respond to COVID-19 from citizens and civil society. For example, the Coronavirus Tech Handbook[10] is a wiki that curates technologies that can help with different aspects of the pandemic, from remote working through to tools for epidemiologists. With an impressive advisory board, including representatives from Wikipedia, Public Health England and the Open Data Institute, the site had 98,000 page views over the previous month when I visited it on 17 May 2020.

CovidX is an initiative by private consultancy Luminary which: "seeks to identify opportunities for government and the private sector to accelerate meaningful innovation that addresses this and future pandemics" and includes an index of resources. There are also semi-private communities like the Slack group called Open Tech Response where the open-source community have sought to collaborate and share learning. It is not easy to assess the extent to which these groups will have made a positive impact on our ability to cope with and respond to the pandemic, but there is no doubt that, at every level, people felt a need to contribute in some way.

Cross-industry collaboration was another feature of the compulsion of many to find a way to contribute to the national effort. Even the Mercedes Formula 1 team got in on the act, working round the clock with collaborators at University College London and University College Hospital to create Continuous Positive

84 ■ *Towards a Digital Ecology*

Airway Pressure (CPAP) devices to help coronavirus patients with lung infections to breathe more easily. In the North of England, a Sheffield Makers against COVID-19 Slack community sprung into life with 60 or so volunteers making hand sanitisers and protective equipment for health and care practitioners.

Investing in partnerships in the good times makes a difference when we hit the hard times. A review by the Care Quality Commission found that local areas with less established partnership working found the impact of the pandemic the most overwhelming:

> We found that the success of collaboration among providers to keep people safe was varied, often affected by the maturity of pre-existing relationships within the system. Understanding the needs of the local population, including cultural differences, was especially important. At times the pace of change felt overwhelming for health and social care providers.[11]

It is clear that investment in partnerships and relationships across sectors and with communities is not frivolous. It is in fact time well spent. The resilience that comes from trust built over time comes into its own when the chips are down.

The NHS needs to think of itself less as a castle and moat and more of a busy marketplace. But for patients whose lives depend on innovation, not everyone is prepared to wait.

We Are Not Waiting

This chapter began with Michael's story, which had a passion for patient-centred innovation at its heart. The heat of the pandemic created an urgency that meant patients and the public were bypassed in decisions that out of necessity were made on the fly.[12] As we see in Chapter 7, there is a big risk that technology can exacerbate as much as dissolve inequalities and so Michael's mission must be maintained. If we take our foot off the participation pedal, then it will far too readily slip backwards.

But some patients are no longer willing to wait. Dana Lewis was dragged kicking and screaming into what she calls *self-quantification* when she got a diagnosis of Type 1 diabetes at the age of 14. "It's really hard to empathise with until you've gone through your own health experience, but a data point to a person with diabetes can be the difference between life and death," explains Dana as she shows her continuous glucose monitor, which gives her an alert when her sugars cross a certain threshold so she can take action to bring them back in range.

"Who likes to sleep?," asks Dana to the packed auditorium where she is sharing her story.[13] It turns out most of us do. Dana explains that the problem she had with her glucose monitor was that those warning bleeps that occurred when she was asleep didn't wake her up. She recounts how she spent her teenage years knowing that sleeping through a bleep could be deadly. When she left her family after college

When People Drive Digital ■ 85

and moved into her own place "my biggest fear was that I would not wake up in the morning ... and I used to think I ought to text my mum and tell her I love her, just in case I don't wake up."

Dana had raised her concerns with the device manufacturer, but they had not shown any interest in the issue. As she wondered about how she might find a way to get the data off the device, she came across someone on Twitter who had found a way to do just that on his son's monitor. That person shared the software code with Dana and she fixed the problem, connecting the data to her phone so she could create a louder alarm.

Now she had liberated the data from that device, she became curious about what else she could do. She had an idea to alert her family if her sugars were below a certain threshold and she had not responded. She then started to create predictive alerts and named her innovation a *DIY Pancreas System*. Ever restless to improve life and those of others living with diabetes, Dana found someone else who had built another component that enabled her to push commands to her pump "I now have a raspberry pi that I bought on Amazon ... and it talks to my insulin pump ... and so this is a closed loop artificial pancreas."

Dana and her open-source community have created a movement called OpenAPS[14] which has the mission of getting the technology they have created out to as many people as possible in as safe a way as possible. Using open-source software and documentation that anyone can use, should they be confident enough to do so. It won't be for everyone but offers the possibility for people to free themselves from the constraints of what manufacturers have deemed appropriate for them. Not all patients are prepared to wait.

"Don't look at me as a patient and think, [this is] not a company, we have nothing to learn," Dana concludes,

> [this] *we are not waiting* movement ... all started because I didn't want to wait three more years for an artificial pancreas that might maybe come to market ... I don't want to die between now and then. I don't want my friends, my loved ones, the people in my community who I've come to know and love, to have that same fear of going to sleep at night.

Dana and her community are challenging the medical and manufacturing establishment, taking things into their own hands, because their lives and their futures depend on it.

Digital transformation is a contact sport. The field is muddy and full of potholes. The game is messy, and the winning team needs a blend of attack and defence and everything in between. The squad needs to be a diverse one if it is going to see the field for what it really is. Patients need to be at the centre. Some of them won't wait as we have seen already.

Not only do we need technology experts but we need people who embody mastery in organisational development and social change. We need philosophers and

86 ■ *Towards a Digital Ecology*

ethicists as much as we need legal experts and people with regulatory authority. Just like the *we are not waiting* movement, we should leverage online networks and communities as much as those who are geographically close. The boundaries of the NHS need to be amorphous and open to others, not least patients and citizens, with their particular brand of lived knowledge and expertise.

If we are to get this right, we need to foster a spirit of inquiry and a sense of agency and urgency that is not obliterated by hierarchy. We should nurture people to understand adaptive change and give them the headspace and protected time to work it all out. This is a luxury not often afforded in the NHS. We need to spend time creating a shared purpose that galvanises all the moving parts of a system towards a common goal. Someone once said to me that trying to innovate in the NHS is like a mechanic trying to fix an engine while it is still running. This is truer than you might imagine.

You may remember a definition of digital transformation that I introduced at the beginning of this book, which is "applying the culture, processes, operating models and technologies of the internet-era to respond to people's raised expectations."[15] This is not simply a linear process of deploying technologies into systems. In fact, if we take this approach, they will invariably fail. Central NHS bodies must see themselves as the enablers, putting the scaffolding in place and unblocking the pipes to allow innovation to germinate. This includes creating a small number of things at the centre which it doesn't make sense for local organisations to develop themselves. The future is modular and distributed but with common standards at the core. The centre should be facilitative rather than overbearing.

With this mindset, the illusion of predictability and control is capsized and assumptions that change happens at the level of policy, structure and procedure are exploded. In fact, according to Rogers, change actually happens at the level of meaning, action and trust which are produced from identity, information and relationships. If you impose change on people then they will filter it and remake it as their own, based on their identity and the meanings that emerge from that identity. Change has to be co-produced.

When we posit (as is often the case) that clinical staff are *resistant* to technology, this is a failure to appreciate the meaning of technology to their belief system and their identity. When we assert that we want to empower patients to take responsibility and they don't do what we expect, we should seek to understand rather than blame. We should resist the urge to push away what we don't expect but seek to understand and connect.

A Software Ecology

In the era of personalised medicine and wearable surveillance, our health is in danger of being reduced to an individual responsibility. As a responsible citizen, I must do my part in drinking less and exercising more to save the NHS and other public services from having to meet my needs when I get sick. But we know that social factors are by far the biggest influence on our health. Michael and Dana's stories are not just about individual agency but also about collectivity, situated peer knowledge and connection.

The same principles apply to how we develop software. Rather than centrally led mega projects such as NPfIT, we have to work at a local level with the assets that we already have and build out from there. This is a collective endeavour and a social process, co-created from the ground up. The basic infrastructure requires shared clinical nomenclature (terminology) and shared standards so that systems that run across organisational boundaries can connect together and data can flow. These can be described as common enabling and more generic components. Built on top and around them are more specific capabilities that may enable a patient to book an appointment or see their test results and so on. Just as we have networks of people that need to come together to facilitate change, we have networks of technology components that need to connect together rather than be locked in silos.

Margunn Aanestad, a professor at the University of Oslo, has been studying information technology in healthcare for many decades. Bringing a socio-technical lens, she is interested in complexities caused by the fact that digital technologies are not single, stand-alone entities but connected into vast webs of interconnected systems. She believes that these webs can create unintended consequences. With a similar conceptual approach to mHabitat, she argues that technology projects should seek to *cultivate* rather than *construct* that is, they should iterate in an incremental way, rather than start with big plans and tight management control. Even technology resists the grip of command and control.

Aanestad advocates that technology projects should start small and grow and should be led by people on the ground who have to work with the systems. In the way that mHabitat advocates identifying *assets*, she talks about working with the *installed base*, which is not only about starting from your existing IT infrastructure, but at a conceptual level is

> a sense-making tool to examine and reflect on the challenges faced in the development of infrastructures. It implies a process-oriented understanding where it becomes crucial to trace and analyse the historical sequence of events and decisions that shape the forming of infrastructures.[16]

The core message that Aanestad brings, from her many decades of research on digital technologies in healthcare, is that successful digital projects need more than a clear goal, technological capabilities and the right people. They require a deep understanding of context and a conscious approach for working with the foundations within any given context.[17] This is a conceptual shift from the linear towards the ecological.

None of what I am describing is easy. There is no clearly trodden path. But the good news is that there are some core principles that can provide the map for any

88 ■ *Towards a Digital Ecology*

journey we care to take. And this is not the map of NPfIT or grand project management schemes and plans. This is the map that requires us to lean in to what we already have, start where the energy is and find the people who have the qualities to make the change happen. Remember that those people may not sit at the top of the organisational chart, it is their orientation, credibility and networks we are interested in. Lean into the tide and surf the wave, building your confidence as you learn the particularities of your local context.

So much has changed since those early days when I was collaborating with friends and colleagues at a tangent to corporate and central command. We ran open space events where participants determined the topics to be discussed, we created *People Drive Digital* where the only voices on the stage were those of people as patients who were innovating from their lived experience. In our own tiny way, we were trying to create communities where people who cared about similar things could come together, share ideas and feel connected.

As well as any number of patient-led communities tucked away in Facebook groups, there is the Shuri Network that promotes black and minority ethnic women in digital health; then there are more formal programmes such as the Digital Academy that creates a space for people working in digital technology to learn and develop and the Clinical Entrepreneur Programme which harnesses the passions and interests of healthcare practitioners. These are just a few.

As my conversation with Sam draws to a close, he gives me his prescription for how the centre could best scaffold rather than control digital transformation: "Let local teams identify their problems, let local teams collaborate with each other to work out what solutions might work, take similar communities in different parts of the country to collaborate … share approaches, share suppliers." This locally determined picture requires central bodies to create a safe and permissive context: "Allow the national [bodies] to create a framework to operate in but don't set hard targets. Give the trust and the empowerment to local teams," says Sam: "allow that flexibility, so there's some governance about how the money is spent, but localisation over who and what they are going to spend it on to achieve the outcome."

An *ecological* orientation is explicit about the tension between the centre and the local. It recognises that people who have lived experience as patients with chronic conditions know things that are invisible to the clinicians who treat them. It understands that change is a messy, unpredictable social process that emerges through relationships. Creating and nurturing this ecology is not a one-off activity. Like a garden, it needs to be nurtured. With a gardener's trowel and fork, we tend to the soil of change. A thriving NHS is cultivated through relationships not only within its borders but in the habitat that surrounds it. A *digital ecology* is the path and the lawn of underpinning infrastructure as well as the shrubs and flowers of tools that enhance everyday practice and nurture patient experience and outcomes.

Notes

1 https://thepsychologist.bps.org.uk/two-psychologies-and-coronavirus
2 https://www.inhealthassociates.co.uk/uncategorized/you-have-to-be-three-times-as-good-michael-seres/
3 https://pifonline.org.uk/news/michael-seres-tribute/
4 https://www.youtube.com/watch?v=uKsTMNDjAVI
5 https://www.heartoftheart.org/?p=1196
6 https://wearemhabitat.com/blog/discovering-inclusive-digital-transformation
7 https://static1.squarespace.com/static/55c3fe0fe4b065156c5dba36/t/5cb0dc35e79c705cd0ddfe6b/1555094669728/organization-development-review-spring-2019.pdf#page=63 p.25
8 https://www.nuffieldtrust.org.uk/files/2019-05/digital-report-br1902-final.pdf p.30.
9 https://www.wired.co.uk/article/coronavirus-mutual-aid-groups
10 https://coronavirustechhandbook.com/
11 https://www.cqc.org.uk/sites/default/files/20201016_stateofcare1920_fullreport.pdf p.10
12 https://www.nuffieldtrust.org.uk/files/2020-08/the-impact-of-covid-19-on-the-use-of-digital-technology-in-the-nhs-web-2.pdf
13 https://www.bing.com/videos/search?q=Dana+lewis+video&docid=608044984634900643&mid=4BADD4EE1EA435B27BA74BADD4EE1EA435B27BA7&view=detail&FORM=VIRE
14 https://openaps.org/what-is-openaps/
15 https://nhsproviders.org/a-new-era-of-digital-leadership/what-is-digital
16 https://library.oapen.org/bitstream/handle/20.500.12657/27913/1002086.pdf?sequence=1
17 https://library.oapen.org/bitstream/handle/20.500.12657/27913/1002086.pdf?sequence=1

Chapter 6

Context Is King

The world we had been taught to see was alien to our humanness. We were taught to see the world as a great machine. But then we could find nothing human in it. Our thinking grew even stranger – we turned this world-image back on ourselves and believed that we too were machines.

Wheatley & Kellner-Rogers (1996, p. 6)

The experience of industry after industry has demonstrated that just installing computers without altering the work and workforce does not allow the system and its people to reach this potential; in fact, technology can sometimes get in the way. Getting it right requires a new approach, one that may appear paradoxical yet is ultimately obvious: digitising effectively is not simply about the technology, it is mostly about the people.

Wachter review, 2016

In Celebration of Mess

Birth is an excruciatingly painful and messy process; I can personally attest to this fact, having subjected it to myself more than once in my life. This was no different for the National Health Service, as it was propelled into being on 5 July 1948 by the Labour government of the day. The NHS gasped its first breath and cleared its lungs against a backdrop of challenge and discord. In an unruly attempt to prevent its genesis, the NHS was voted against 21 times by the opposition and with vigorous dissent from the British Medical Association, both of whom bitterly resisted its parturition.

Our National Health Service was born in and from an analogue era, with foundations of bricks and mortar. Its complex systems have been serviced by paper and pen which record, store and move information around a byzantine system. The

DOI: 10.1201/9781032198798-6

92 ■ *Towards a Digital Ecology*

internet era, which has engulfed almost every aspect of our lives, has yet to gain real purchase in the NHS. Even the foundations have yet to be entirely laid, and good ideas can all too readily fall between the cracks of its uneven terrain.

Just over 70 years from its creation, the NHS is finally succumbing to a rebirth of a digital nature. There are as many dissenters as there are proponents. Unlike companies born of the internet era, healthcare services have to take a different path, an adaptive one whereby they mould their analogue systems and processes to a web-based future. This is not as easy as it may seem.

Complexity and system inertia are only part of the story of digital health. Culture and contextual factors are poorly understood by those entrepreneurs who harbour a sincere belief that their technology can save the NHS. Time and again I have seen digital health companies flounder when they come up against the hard reality that, without appreciating context, culture and complexity, their technology is doomed to the dustbin. Tech solutionism is a road to irrelevance. Context is everything. Complexity is everywhere. Culture eats digital for breakfast. A digital ecology needs to be nurtured.

Theorising Non-adoption

I learnt about the critical nature of context the hard way. Having set up a digital health project back in 2014 and fortunate to have a budget to investigate the use of technology across the NHS in my then home city of Leeds, I set about finding clinical services that were willing to collaborate.

Confident in my own naivety, I started bringing software developers together with clinical services to work on what we named *projects* but in reality were more like experiments. I had a vague idea that if we developed compelling products that worked, then we could perhaps generate income by making them available to other parts of the NHS. The reality turned out to be completely different.

Over the course of that first year, we created five web-based applications. One was a smartphone app for an eating disorder platform; another was a mental health peer support platform; a text messaging service for an assertive outreach team; finally, a self-management platform for a chronic fatigue service. None of them ever saw the light of day. Not one of them was ever properly used in practice. They certainly never made it past the small team that had willed them into being. So what went wrong?

You might think this apparent failure was due to incompetence. But that's not quite the case. There were many reasons these experiments failed, but there is a common theme – we didn't appreciate or understand the contextual factors that would make the difference between success or failure. All our efforts went into developing the product, and we forgot to pay attention to what would come after. I recall a similar experience with the birth of my first child. During those nine months, everything was focused on the birth. The fact I would have a child to look after was somehow

Context Is King ■ 93

eclipsed in the drama of scans, tests and birthing plans. I have a sharp memory of a sinking realisation, at home with my baby for the first time, that this was just the beginning, not the conclusion. The journey was only just starting and I felt frighteningly ill-prepared.

I look back and wince at my ignorance. I thought a digital project ended at the point we handed over the technology. So why was no one using it? I quickly learnt what researchers in the field already knew – that contextual factors are everything, attempts at innovation often fail, NHS systems and processes are a mire of complexity. This is the point at which I want to bring in the mighty force that is Professor Trish Greenhalgh.

A few facts about Trish – she was a GP back in the day and is now a professor of primary health sciences at the University of Oxford; she wrote a bestseller book *How to Read a Paper* which is now in its sixth edition and retails at £24.01 on Amazon; she co-wrote a complete guide to breast cancer based on her own her experience; she has a marine biologist son and a predilection for free swimming.

You may wonder how I know all of this. With over 100,000 followers on Twitter, Trish is a master of blending professional content with the odd smattering of personal facts and insight. In some ways, Trish's Twitter persona exemplifies the core theme of this chapter – you get further by appreciating the human alongside the technocratic – you build trust, credibility and if you're Trish, quite a fan base too.

I was (and still am) one of her Twitter entourage as I scrolled through my timeline in 2017, I came across a link to a new paper she had produced: *Beyond Adoption: A New Framework for Theorizing and Evaluating Nonadoption, Abandonment, and Challenges to the Scale-Up, Spread, and Sustainability of Health and Care Technologies.* Despite the long-winded title, Trish and her team had created a brilliant empirically based schema for technology (non)adoption, synthesising a range of theoretical approaches into something pragmatic that can be applied in practice.

It is not an underestimation to say that her research has been a revelation to me. Trish's years of investigation into why technology doesn't get adopted in the NHS made sense of what I found out through my clumsy fledgling attempts to support digital projects within the NHS. Her work gave me an explanation, a language and even answers to how they might be approached differently, to get better results.

Employing a social sciences lens, Trish and her team combined secondary research with six technology implementations which they studied over three years across more than 20 organisations. The NASSS framework and the growing body of work that she has developed around it tell an almost identical story to that which I experienced in my first few years in digital health.

I contacted Trish at the height of the first pandemic wave for an interview for this book. At the time she was bouncing from TV station to radio, to a webinar, to Twitter to promote the wearing of pandemic masks. As a busy woman, she turned down the interview and suggested instead that we record a video conversation that she could use for one of her teaching classes. We recorded it in May when the pandemic was still in the early days of its pestilent hike across the globe.

94 ■ *Towards a Digital Ecology*

Trish explained to me how she came about developing NASSS,

> We developed the NASSS framework initially, I have to say it, to explain
> failed projects, or not necessarily failed projects, but technology projects
> which started off with a lot of enthusiasm and gradually over six, twelve,
> eighteen months or even longer, didn't get adopted in the way people
> anticipated.

Trish's paper was intended to try and explain what was going wrong: "we were trying to explain all the different interacting factors that explained effectually non adoption, abandonment and then lack of scale up, lack of spread, lack of sustainability." Trish's framework carves up this complexity into seven domains – the condition, technology, adopters (patient, carer and professional), value proposition, the organisation, wider system, embedding and adapting over time. She argues that any digital project in health or care needs to pay attention to all of these systemic factors if it is to succeed.

It is not always obvious what is going to scupper your project. It could be an enthusiastic clinician moving on to a new job, or it could be just as easily a team with too many other competing priorities. It may be that organisational imperatives change or it could be that the patients whose needs you had hoped to meet have goals you failed to anticipate. Complexity is the spear that most often tears into the heart of a digital health project, rendering it limp and lifeless, destroying the dreams of its creators.

Context Is King

Digital health frequently attracts entrepreneurs with a passion born out of personal experience. Often it is a clinician who is frustrated with a problem and wants to fix it. Sometimes it is a patient with a health condition who has seen a way to solve a problem and decides to do something about it. Occasionally, it is a company with a technology product that sees an opportunity to apply their product in healthcare. Wherever they come from, they all tend to make a common mistake, and that is that they design for the model patient (or clinician) behaving in the model way in model circumstances. They underestimate the complexity of people's lives and they are ignorant of the contextual factors of a fragmented and overstretched health system.

I recall many an uncomfortable moment in any number of committee meetings when our Trust chief financial officer would assert his favourite phrase: "cash is king!" to a group of eye-rolling clinicians. Needless to say, his motto didn't go down too well with professionals, whose primary motivation is to deliver clinical care. If he had instead asserted "context is king!" he might have not won any more friends, but at least he would have been correct. The message of this chapter is, ignore context at your peril.

Context Is King ■ 95

How much of the benefits realised from the introduction of new technology can be attributed to the technology itself? This is the question I asked seasoned digital health entrepreneur Sandeep when interviewing him for a series of masterclasses I ran for recipients of Innovate UK's Digital Health Technology Catalyst fund. "Fifteen percent," he said without hesitation. His answer has continued to reverberate in my mind because he was so precise and definitive in his response. The force of nature behind Medic Bleep, an alternative to the hospital pager, Sandeep is one of the small number of innovators who has a business that is successfully scaling in the NHS. So when he tells me that the contextual factors outweigh the technology itself, well, I believe what he says.

Innovate UK commissioned these masterclasses because they kept bumping up against the problem that providing grant funding for entrepreneurs was solving only part of the problem. The money got them so far, but contextual factors in the NHS had a tendency to kibosh their likelihood of success time and again. The fact that their new technology is only one factor in an improvement to a clinical service, is a salutary lesson for any wide-eyed innovator who believes they have the answer to the NHS's problems with their new product or service.

Sandeep's assertion is backed up by a report from the Association of British Healthcare Industries, a membership organisation for digital and MedTech companies. They commissioned research to explain why innovation adoption is so painfully slow in the NHS. With the sophic title, *Falling Short* the study concludes that innovation is overly supply-driven with an unhelpful emphasis on the product rather than more helpfully starting from the problem to be solved.[1] It's like trying to plug the screams of a newborn baby with a pacifier when what they actually need is their nappy changed. Maybe we are doing everything the wrong way round.

A recent report by independent think tank, The Nuffield Institute, criticises the Accelerated Access Collaborative (AAC) for also falling into this trap.[2] Established with the purpose of streamlining the adoption of new innovations in healthcare, the AAC incentives adoption of proven innovations using a payments system. However, these sorts of incentives are symptomatic of the supply-side, top-down approach that perversely have a tendency to impede the adoption of innovation.

Offering an NHS trust a free technology with proven benefits seems like a no-brainer. A cash-strapped NHS trust will grab the opportunity for a freebie without stopping to consider the opportunity costs associated with deploying them. What starts out as a good idea quickly fades into insignificance once clinical teams realise the effort involved in incorporating the product into their everyday workflow. I once worked with a team in exactly this position. Only around 30 of the 2000 free licenses they had been gifted got used. It quickly became apparent that onboarding a patient added 30 minutes to each consultation. Without the support or the headspace to spend time working out how to make the changes, they would need for the mobile app to give rather than take time, they abandoned it. This is not an unfamiliar story.

96 ■ *Towards a Digital Ecology*

That primary care community team's experience is reflected in yet another recent report[3] (there is no shortage of reports) analysing innovation in the NHS. The research finds that the effort that goes into stimulating entrepreneurial activities (for example, through investment and accelerators) is out of kilter with the incentives to promote the uptake of the innovation in the context it is intended for. This misalignment means that even the most promising technologies are anaesthetised if the support is not there to implement. To create that alignment means understanding who your stakeholders are, involving them from the outset right through to implementation and the embedding process over time. This is not an insignificant task.

Innovative companies in the private sector typically spend twice or three times as much on diffusing an innovation than developing it. But the NHS appears to do the reverse. We spend over £1.2 billion on research and development, of which only a tiny fraction is spent on dedicated spread activity. The traditional belief that once an innovation has been successfully piloted, it can be easily taken up by others, doesn't stand up to scrutiny. A technology may need to be refined, revised and reinvented in each context in which it is applied.[4] This takes time, resource and commitment on the part of the implementing organisation. For a start-up with an innovative product or service, the time and money required may mean that they can't stay the distance.

We are not dealing with simple projects. Trish asserts that *technology projects* are only suitable for assembly lines that are relatively predictable and repeatable. There is very little in the NHS that is either of those things. I learnt this to my cost. Beguiled by the promise of a mobile app for an eating disorders service in my local NHS trust, my first foray into digital was helping the enthusiastic service develop a mobile application to help their users self-monitor and communicate with clinicians.

We appeared to have everything in our favour – keen clinicians, willing patients and even a budget to build the mobile app. But like so many well-intentioned projects, it never saw the light of day. We spent all our time focusing on development, and it didn't even occur to us to consider either how it would be used in practice or what adaptive changes might be required.

Over the course of the project, which took much longer than we anticipated, clinicians were provided with smartphones for the first time. The desktop admin system we had created suddenly seemed outdated, and they didn't want to login to via their desktop computer. When I caught up with the lead clinician some years later, she told me they had ditched the app for the much more intuitive and simple off-the-shelf communication platform. It didn't have all the features of the app we had developed, but it did a good enough job and so they settled with that. It sort of made sense.

Thinking about Design

It is tempting for technologists to simply defer to a patient or a clinician's domain expertise in understanding the problem to be solved. But each on their own will not have the depth and breadth of the context in which the solution must operate to

Context Is King ■ 97

have the intended effect. The healthcare context is often described in technocratic terms using an engineering metaphor – moving parts that need to be fixed and so on – with specialist experts holding the knowledge. That is not to say their domain expertise is not of critical importance. But it only paints part of the picture.

What if the context is complex and emergent, not only about systems and processes but also values, beliefs and professional identity? There are multiple stakeholders in a system, from the administrator at one end to the commissioner at the other. A system may well combine more than one team and several organisations, all of whom have a stake in an existing process or pathway. Digital technology in a complex system, like a pebble skimmed across the surface of a lake, will create ripples that displace the status quo in imprecise and unpredictable ways. Put another way, I once sat on a conference panel with a GP who wearily opined: "Every time I am sold a technology I am told it will save me time; and it always adds extra work." Technology simply plonked on top of a system or process will invariably add more grind and more complexity.

Enter stage right, human-centred design. "Do we really understand what our users want? How do we make sensible, sustainable, financial decisions?" asks Imogen. "We are spending public money and if we really want to put it in the right places, having a user centred mindset is going to enable you to do that." Imogen Levey is one of the first user-centred designers to be employed by an NHS trust. She believes taking a human or user-centred design approach is a moral imperative when it comes to designing good services. "We shouldn't be led by what is the latest shiny thing … or because it's the clinician's latest fad or idea," she argues. Our conversation takes place over Hangouts along with Carolyn Manuel-Barkin who has a public health background and has worked in leading digital design agencies. "It is about making good investment decisions, full stop," agrees Carolyn.

Design with and for people who are going to use your product or service seems like common sense. It was human-centred design that most attracted me to the sphere of digital health. I had spent years in the NHS involving patients, and sometimes the public, in giving feedback on, as well as helping shape, healthcare services. Carolyn paints a cruel caricature of patient and public involvement in the NHS:

> It's like we're going to reorganise this whole thing and then we're going to have a community meeting to tell you about it, and you can be super disappointed about it and tell us none of it's going to work for you, but we've already made this decision and we're just going to write some colourful communications about why we're going to do this anyway.

She may be harsh, but she isn't completely off the mark.

Patient and public feedback most often takes the shape of a multiple-choice survey or a feedback form to be posted in the cardboard box on the reception desk.

98 ■ *Towards a Digital Ecology*

There are any number of committees and forums that have a patient representative invited to share their views; interviews and focus groups are sometimes used when evaluating services or undertaking research. These are all entirely appropriate and standard methods. But they lack oomph.

Design processes used in developing software are qualitatively different. They involve understanding users, not by asking them what they want, but finding out what problems they have, how they are solving them, and how technology might enable them to solve them in a better way. Finding these things out entails spending time with people, seeking to develop deep empathy and understanding of what matters to them. To have a real impact, design processes must engage with research, evidence and analysis as well as the wider policy context in which people live their lives.

Creating an engaging and intuitive user interface (UI) and an appealing user experience (UX) is the nucleus of a design process. Human-centred design approaches tend to be co-creative that is designing with and for the people who are going to use them. The discipline of *user-centred design* is about (re)designing services through generating deep empathy and understanding of the context in which technology will have to operate within. It's also about everything in between. "The blank space between a patient seeing their GP and seeing the consultant for the first time, that is part of a clinical journey, for the user that's part of the clinical journey, so [the opportunity is] what can you do in that blank space," says Carolyn. I was and am beguiled by this approach.

Discovery is jargon for making sure you understand the problem you are trying to solve before you design, build or buy a digital product. "We need to pioneer discovery," proclaims Imogen: "People do patient involvement, but nobody does discovery, and it's that idea of really understanding what problems we're trying to solve, people don't delve enough into that." Discovery is qualitatively different to asking people what they want. Carolyn is direct in her assessment of why people often find it hard to invest in discovery:

> It's hard for people to understand a process where they're not going to get a [product] at the end. So we're going to go through a process and we're still not going to have a thing … and the lack of certainty … it's really hard to take people on that journey and say this is what's going to create value.

User research is at the core of discovery practices, which is essentially understanding the needs, pain points, goals and aspirations of your users. Users may be anyone from patients, citizens, carers, clinicians or hospital porters. They exist outside the clinic or the hospital ward, so it is important to understand their lives in the round One research tool is *ethnography* that basically involves purposefully spending time in and observing the context in which technology will need to find its place. It is about being in a space but also disconnected from it, observing and learning.

Ethnography in a human-centred design process is a valuable tool in eliciting not only the explicit rules but the implicit culture and the context in which digital technology will need to find its place. At the very least, technology will need to fit within existing routines and practices and at best reshape and improve them.

Participatory workshops facilitate users to co-design products and services through creative and engaging activities, *making and doing* rather than simply talking. Designers test their products by watching people interact with them and observing what works and what doesn't. This highly immersive, kinaesthetic and empathic approach engages all the senses and is more impactful than the cognitive abstracted conversations of a committee or focus group. They are a great leveller when being undertaken with clinicians. Name badges are left at the door, and everyone sits together around a flip chart and post-it notes. The process of developing a digital product is highly iterative, showing people new versions of the application for feedback on a constant basis. This approach with short bursts of development followed by user testing means waste can be quickly eliminated and the most important features prioritised.

Design thinking is more than creating something that people want to use, is useful within a system and acceptable to an organisation, although each of those things is vitally important. Participatory design creates provenance for a digital product and builds advocacy throughout its development. The story of a product is almost as important as the product itself. The fact an asthma self-management tool was built with people affected by that respiratory condition and their clinicians, means that the asthma service in the next town or city is more likely to be warmly inclined towards it. Those patients and professionals who were involved in its development become its greatest advocates along the way. A clinician will be much more receptive to another clinician telling them something is great than an enthusiastic software developer.

The role of human-centred design is beginning to gain momentum in healthcare, with specialist consultancies emerging to support healthcare organisations in the design, development and implementation process. The NHS *Service Design Standards* conceptualise service design as the total experience of someone's interactions with an NHS service. Its mantra is "put people at the heart of everything you do."[5] This approach has been inspired by and adapted from the Government Digital Service which has transformed how we interact with transactional services such as filing for divorce or applying for road tax online. I can't help thinking that many of these government services are comparatively straightforward and linear compared to the complexities of healthcare. There are now designers in NHS Digital but very few operating in teams at a local NHS trust level. In fact, Imogen is a true pioneer. She believes that she is one of the first designers working in a local NHS trust and possibly the only one. And even then: "The trust didn't recruit a design thinker, they got a design thinker," she explains with a smile.

"When I started introducing the idea of user-centred design, clinicians really struggled with it," explains Imogen, "because I think they felt I was saying clinicians

100 ■ *Towards a Digital Ecology*

didn't matter, it's all about the [patient]." Imogen describes the challenge of balancing clinicians' priorities with those of patients. "The beauty of user-centred design and balancing that with clinical informatics is where the real power can be at a local trust," explains Imogen,

> It is finding the middle ground between different perspectives, needs and wants and [clinicians] letting go of some of their assumptions ... there's a lot of clinicians who say to me we see patients every day therefore we know what they need.

Our conversation reminded me of a human-centred design project for an app to help people remember to take their medication. During our co-creation activities, it became apparent that peer support, that is advice and encouragement from people in similar circumstances was an important factor in motivation to keep to a medication regime. In complete contrast, our co-creation activities with GPs determined that the one thing that would prohibit them from using or promoting the app would be the incorporation of a peer support feature. Patients' desire for peer support was seen by the GPs through the prism of clinical risk; what if patients gave each other inaccurate information? Where would the duty of care lie? In this instance, risk aversion won out, and patients did not get the feature that our user research suggested would have had the most impact.

Design thinking has a way to go before it is a common practice in the NHS. "Normally you get thrown into a meeting with a technology supplier who is demoing you their latest thing," groans Imogen. A self-professed troublemaker, she is carving out a pragmatic path in her organisation where she can hold the vision for digital services and try to avoid staff getting sidetracked by a shiny thing that they are desperate to buy. Imogen wants NHS trusts to start to think about websites and applications as services in their own right and move away from digital being the preserve of either the IT department or the communication and marketing function in a Trust. Her vision is for design practices to be integrated into improvement and innovation initiatives as standard practice.

Human-centred design is a practice common in the digital technology sector but that can be applied in any context. NHS trusts often have quality or service improvement teams, and there is a strong case for them to bring user-centred designers into their fold. The best technologies sit in the background, barely noticeable, but elegantly meeting a need or solving a problem. Spotify enables me to listen to any artist whenever and wherever I want with a few clicks. My banking app enables me to check my balance and move money about easily. I don't think about technology because it enables me to meet a need. Achieving the same in healthcare is so much more problematic, but the opportunity to build powerful experiences of patients, citizens and clinicians are there to be harnessed. Like drops of rain in an arid garden, human-centred design is an indispensable part of a digital ecology.

What Happens in the Margins

To illustrate why human-centred design is so important, we need to shift our gaze to what happens at the margins.

"One of the problems is that a large proportion of [nursing] activity that is done in any one place is completely bespoke and completely different." Anne tells me something I had not previously understood:

> Clinical practice is not a standard thing; the way the doctors, the nurses, the physios, the speech and language therapists do their work is nuanced to the environment they're working in and the patients they are working with; so we don't have standard operating procedures for some things that we do in clinical practice.

A recent commentary on evidence-based medicine reinforces not only the importance of context in the work of healthcare practitioners but also the strength of the relationship with a patient, how they are themselves feeling and even how they are incentivised in the form of targets they are required to meet.[6]

When Anne Cooper joined NHS Digital as Chief Nurse, her role was to bring a nursing perspective to technology projects as well as advocate for the role of technology to nurses, who happen to be the largest profession in the NHS. I ask Anne to explain to me why context matters so much in digital technology projects.

She tells me that if this variety of clinical practice is not surfaced and made visible through the design and development process, then technology projects that endeavour to codify and create systems to help clinical staff will inevitably miss the mark. It is also a big challenge for technologists because they need to be able to adapt their products to different contexts: "You need the technology to be an enabler to clinical practice," says Anne: "not something where we've got to translate and find ways to workaround." This codification process as a shared endeavour can be powerful, bringing to the surface what is implicitly understood, and meaningfully transforming practice. However, more often than not it is reductive in nature and easily rejected by the people who have to utilise those technologies in practice.

There is a normative view that technology is a progressive force and to resist it is to be guilty of intransigence. And whilst Anne is a technology advocate, she is concerned that without human-centred design between technologists and clinicians, we risk missing the important aspects of clinical practice that happen at the margins: "Think about when a nurse is assessing a patient," Anne explains: "in the olden days we would have had a form, and you'd go to the drawer and get the form out and you'd go through a series of questions that gives you a structure with which to assess somebody." When you've got a piece of paper and a pen in your hand, you can always write in the margins, you can always write extra things down, there are no restrictions. So if Gladys has come in and she has a cat at home and she's worried about the cat … you can always find a way, a space in the margins [to record it]."

102 ■ *Towards a Digital Ecology*

Anne is describing a sometimes reductive characteristic of digital technologies that cause frustration to clinicians:

> As soon as you go down into the world of drop down boxes and you try and codify everything, you lose the ability to bring the human being into the centre of that assessment. Free text is frowned upon because it's difficult to analyse, it's difficult to report on, it's difficult to use for decision support ... so there is a tendency to drive towards codified data collection.

Words scribbled in the paper margins get lost and forgotten with no value beyond the immediate. In electronic records the data lasts, it is persistent, it can have value beyond the individual encounter when it is combined into big datasets for planning and service improvement. Whilst emerging technologies such as artificial intelligence may be able to shape a fresher more personalised experience, clinicians are mostly interacting with the legacy systems of the past in their everyday work. No wonder they often feel frustrated.

In his 2016 report for the government on the future of health IT, American physician Bob Wachter recommends that *usability* be a core feature of any technology design and implementation. With a specific focus on electronic health records, his argument holds true for all types of digital technologies: "poorly designed or implemented EHRs [electronic health records] that do not support the way clinicians work also result in increased frustration, increased workload, and workarounds." He goes on to make the case that: "while there may be short-term gains from education of end-users, in general education and training cannot compensate for poor usability."[7] Elegantly designed products are not frivolous, they are a critical factor in determining whether clinicians and patients are prepared to use them in practice.

Human-centred design is a relatively new and somewhat alien concept within most of the NHS, despite the fact that a lack of appreciation of users' needs is cited as an important reason why innovation fails to be adopted within the healthcare system. Too often the focus is on the product and the supplier at the expense of facilitating NHS organisations to understand their challenges and find solutions to them. A digital ecology must nurture the soil of human-centred design if it is to create a habitat that enables clinicians to do their jobs well.

Culture Eats Digital for Breakfast

One of the more intangible factors identified within the NASSS framework that influences technology adoption, is an organisation's capacity to innovate. Trish and her team make the prosaic but salient point that innovation is hard work, and the effort required is almost always underestimated. Organisations need to have the bandwidth, the orientation, the expertise and the resources to do it well. According to Richard, an ex-CIO of a large acute trust and now employed by a large pharmacy "the [NHS] centre is good at giving us [vendors] plenty of work to do."

If an organisation does not have sufficient headspace to try something new, if it is crushed by targets, if it is a political football, where things that go wrong end up in the *Daily Mail*; if it has too little money and too many targets, any innovation it does muster is pretty damn impressive and almost entirely against the grain.

I worked in the NHS for over 20 years and its culture and constraints gently sucked me into its surf, enveloping me in its tides and pulling me deep within its waters. Innovation is typically regarded as a luxury rather than a necessity to survival.[8] It was only in a conversation with Frankie about her NHS initiation that those latent recollections were refreshed in my mind.

Frankie is not the actual name of the person I interviewed, she was happy to be open but she was worried about compromising her position as an innovation lead in an acute NHS trust. She is well respected and gets stuff done. I know because I have worked with her. I wanted her to not hold back on sharing the challenges as she has experienced. Her candour may be uncomfortable, but I am confident what she describes will be at least in part familiar to anyone who has worked in healthcare.

Frankie's background is not at all NHS. Working in a start-up in the early days of the iPhone, she was previously employed by a small company developing mobile apps for pop stars, airlines and high-end car brands. Frankie describes how, after a fairly spectacular fall out with her boss, she decided to initiate a *life laundry*, move cities and take a career break. She was introduced to a CIO who was looking for someone with an atypical NHS skillset: "he wanted someone with direct experience of working with mobile apps, [who understood] the process of rapid ideation, prototyping, development processes, delivery and metrics," explains Frankie. She took the leap and joined the Trust.

I was curious about Frankie's first impressions of her new organisation, having arrived from such a different working world. "Day one and I get this verbatim comment from my colleague 'God you're really optimistic, that won't last.' That stuck in my memory," she says with a wry smile. I could relate. I was similarly bamboozled by my initiation to the mental health NHS trust that constituted my first exposure to the NHS. In the early days, I thought seriously about leaving but ended by staying long enough for NHS culture to become familiar, whilst staying detached enough for it to always intrigue me.

The NHS is a heady mix of professional hierarchy, overlaid with managerial rankings, underpinned by jargon and acronyms that create an obfuscation that is barely penetrable to any newbie. It is bursting with people who want to make a difference. But they often find themselves wading through a thick soup of committees, reports and compliance. The NHS may not be one organisation, but its cultural characteristics are pervasive. This is important to know if you have an inclination to work with the NHS, either as an innovator from the outside or indeed you are an innovator like Frankie who wants to work in the NHS.

104 ◾ *Towards a Digital Ecology*

Frankie expands further on her experience of those beneath the surface traits:

> The culture is defeatist, stuff doesn't get finished, it doesn't get closed, there is an inability to accept failure and yet everything fails … morale is appalling, they start off on something and everyone assumes, they know it's going to be bad, they know it's going to be an uphill struggle, all the time, on everything, and that just wears people down.

Much of the NHS is running on empty, with too little gas in its engine to get to the destination it has been told it needs to reach. Everyone knows it isn't possible to get there, but they rev the engine and set off anyway. There is no other choice.

With never enough resources and always under too much pressure, Frankie's impressions resonate with my memories of trying to initiate change with the NHS trusts for whom I worked. Unless there is a policy drive or directive from the centre, it takes a superhuman effort to galvanise change: "People are there to maintain the status quo … it [the system] is totally opposed to change wherever possible … it will stimey innovation at every step, it will smother it in its crib, it doesn't want things to change, they are the guardians of orthodoxy, they are there to stop things from happening," says Frankie as she warms to her subject.

Whilst Frankie's views may seem hyperbolic, her words brought to mind a surgeon who I saw speak at a conference many years ago. He described how everything he did in his clinical practice was about looking back to the past, to his training, to established methods, to protocols, to avoiding harm and to elevating safety. Having developed one of the very first mobile applications used in emergency care, he was appointed into an innovation role in his NHS trust. He recounted the volte-face he had to perform – the blank page of novelty and emergence stood in sharp contrast to everything he had absorbed from his education and practice. His story exemplifies a profound tension between a true desire to do things better and an imperative to keep things the same.

This orientation towards prudence is manifested in NHS decision-making whereby the avoidance of exposure to criticism or risk trumps all. Frankie explains:

> The decision making matrices are a mess, delegating responsibility at lower levels has a tendency to default back up the chain when there's a difficult decision … or the risk gets mitigated to a committee so the committee makes the decision as opposed to an individual.

It is fiercely hard to navigate byzantine processes of decision-making to get new things off the ground. And when they do get off the ground, it is usually with too little resource, accompanied by the heavy weight of overbearing project management processes.

The adage, it's a feature not a bug, is apposite in this context. This is how the system is designed. Frankie explains: "I completely understand why, these are people who have got far too much work on and they haven't got proper agreements on what the priorities are." I have learnt this fact the hard way over the years. I have had a number of great conversations with dedicated clinicians who have thrown their heart and soul into an initiative that never quite happens because decisions never quite get made, or the money doesn't materialise, or priorities change.

Power counts too. And not in ways that you might expect. I recall working with a community team that cared for recovering patients who had been stepped-down from hospital treatment. The community staff explained to me that the hospital consultant had been successfully lobbied by a pharmaceutical company to recommend a self-management app as he discharged his patients to the community team. There was no discussion or debate with the community clinicians and they were not happy. Their patients arrived with the app and the clinicians were expected to incorporate it into their practice. The staff decided they didn't like it, not because it was good or bad, but because of how it had been foisted upon them. So they simply didn't comply with the consultant's wishes. The app was dead in the water.

I was struck by the extent to which Frankie and Trish have very similar things to say, albeit from different vantage points. In Trish's nomenclature: "The industry impetus of agile, rapid-iteration technology development and the 'fail early, fail often' principle typically followed for software products contrasts with the risk-averse, highly regulated, and randomized trial-dominated context of much biomedical innovation." Frankie's version goes like this:

> Agile, iterative working practices are the antithesis to the way the public sector works, pre-set, pre-agreed, fully planned, waterfall management; you're going from A to B, you know exactly where you're starting and exactly where you're ending up, despite the fact that is never how it works in practice.

Thinking Systems

So far this chapter has confirmed that ideas are cheap, but the realisation of those ideas in complex systems is to be cherished. How can we better nurture innovation and even better, spread it so that as many people as possible can benefit? The standardisation and efficiency of the Taylorist factory floor may have their place, but can they help us solve the challenges that lie ahead of us?

There are many different ways to achieve a goal. The most obvious means to an end isn't always the best. Many years ago, I set up an arts and mental health project. Our highlight of the year was a visual art exhibition in a fancy shopping centre. As I arrived early to the launch event, I couldn't help but be moved by the high-quality art on the walls. I noticed a young man, standing in front of a picture visibly

106 ■ *Towards a Digital Ecology*

trembling, so I went up to see if he was ok. It turned out he was standing in awe as he looked upon one of his artworks. Julian explained to me that not only was this the first time he had exhibited, it was the first time he had got a bus into the city centre in ten years. I felt incredibly moved. An occupational therapist might work with a person like Julian to help him build his confidence to use public transport using conventional methods. But for Julian, it was his new-found identity as an artist that created the breakthrough.

A creative and adaptive approach helps us solve problems and challenges in novel ways. When Bob Wachter, in his highly influential book The Digital Doctor (2017) called technology in health "the master of all adaptive challenges" he was spot on. We treat digital health as a technology project to be delivered by IT teams. But is it mostly a social process that depends on galvanising patients, clinicians, administrators and managers towards a common goal, in order to make an improvement which is enabled by technology. This is harder than it might seem.

Andy Evans, a regional chief information officer, makes the point well:

> You often successfully deliver the digital piece; not always, but it can happen; but the actual release of the benefit is tied to the change in the clinical behaviours, the way people work … and you've got this very slow return on investment because you actually need the sort of need the adaptive behaviour from the clinical community to go alongside it.

Perhaps it is because digital technologies are still comparatively so novel in healthcare that we put them at the centre of what are essentially improvement projects. The edification of technology above context is *one* of the reasons why technology projects so often fail.

Consultant radiologist, Rizwan, brings a clinical perspective to the theme of context and culture: "Almost the most important bit … what is so far a big inhibitor to digital innovation, is behaviours." He understands that dedicating time and effort to helping the people who are to use technology, incorporate it into both their formal and informal processes is invaluable:

> People don't see the pounds, shillings and pence of change management … you've just spent years of your life and a fortune buying this shiny new product which you know can be brilliant, but you have not bothered to give your colleagues the time, or they haven't been given the time to learn how to do it.

Through his observations, Rizwan is introducing another aspect of the adoption of innovation, which is sometimes seen as the territory of *organisational development* or *quality improvement* teams in the NHS. Both have a role in working with clinical teams to support them to improve their services. Rizwan mimics a disgruntled clinician: "'you know what mate, for ten years I've been clicking that box over there and I ain't changing for you' and then two months later 'you know, this thing you've bought is rubbish.'" Entrenched ways of working cannot be undone in an instant. Lasting change is built on relationships and trust. Rizwan sees this as a major inhibitor to innovation "because you've not got the bang for your buck for [the technology]."

An approach informed by systems theory, with an emphasis on patterns of relationships, values, culture and beliefs, presents a more helpful way to conceptualise digital health. I have heard clinicians derided on numerous occasions by digital health advocates for being resistant to technology. I am always left wondering if it would not be more valuable to seek to understand and develop empathy with their concerns about technology, to understand how that technology could be improved, to create space for them to work out how they might incorporate it into their practice and to decide that it might take more than it gives and decide to no longer use it.

Systems theory seeks to understand how systems function. Rachel Dunscombe, chief information officer and a fan of this approach describes it like Russian dolls: "it's systems within systems, so a department is a system in an organisation which is a system within a locality and on you go." She distinguishes between the standardisation required of technology systems and the personalisation of people: "variation in human biology is warranted [because] we are biologically different, we have different needs, communities have different needs." A systems theory approach understands how we lean into human needs, motivations and goals.

At this point, I'd like to introduce you to Andy, co-author of *Beyond the Fog*, a study into the future of NHS healthcare, commissioned by the Royal Free NHS Foundation Trust Charity. Having worked in a variety of innovation and strategy roles in many sectors, Andy has set up a think tank to create a platform to share what he has learnt. He begins by setting out the imperative, why we need to take digital innovation seriously.

"Healthcare is still largely an analogue process with some IT in the background," says Andy. "Health itself is going to be increasingly on a digital sub-strait. [Digital] will underpin almost everything to do with medicine and healthcare – the information that [healthcare practitioners] draw upon, the decision support systems that they use, the diagnostics, the treatment management – so in some sense, a healthcare system of the 21st Century is going to be a digital healthcare system."

Our conversation, a Zoom call in the summer of 2020, starts at a fairly abstracted level. Andy wants us to completely re-conceptualise how we think about our healthcare system: "It's somewhat ironic isn't it," he says, "that medicine is ultimately about biology, but we don't use a biological metaphor for our own healthcare system … we think of ourselves as a factory and we use engineering [as a metaphor]."

108 ■ *Towards a Digital Ecology*

This has not always been the case. It was in the early 1980s that the notion of managerialism began to creep into NHS operations.[9] Predicated on the idea that the health sector should operate more like a business, managers were introduced to the system, the language of efficiency, effectiveness and targets that we see today, became pervasive. "The healthcare system has borrowed from business, an industrial language of efficiency," explains Andy, "creating silos and division of labour, and then setting up targets that measure transactional performance." So why might this be bad for innovation? Surely, an efficient and effective healthcare service isn't a bad thing.

Our societal drift towards a digital substratum that increasingly underpins every aspect of our existence has similarly borrowed its nomenclature from industry. No doubt you will be familiar with the idea that the digital age, as it is often called, is the *fourth industrial revolution*. In a fascinating article, the Leading Edge Forum argues that we are in fact experiencing a *counter-industrial revolution* in which physical assets of the combustion engine are being superseded by *intangible assets* of software, data, brands and trust. The NHS is part of this incremental drift, systematically shedding its physical assets, in the shape of buildings and IT department servers, for intangible assets such as software and cloud hosting. How we might re-conceptualise healthcare is part of a wider societal metamorphosis that is less industrial and more ecological in its nature.[10]

Let's face it, our healthcare system has always dealt with the most important intangible asset of them all – *relationships* and *trust*. Andy believes an industrial metaphor is corrosive; it leads us to a narrow and reductive conceptualisation of innovation that fails to appreciate profound societal shifts we are experiencing: "health care can't be fully captured in transactional targets," he says: "what leads to good care isn't just the transaction that occurs; you can make a clinic very efficient by reducing the time a patient is seen from twelve minutes to ten minutes and it would hit all the targets and people would say that is much more efficiently run," Andy says, "but if people don't have time to express what their issues are, don't have time to ask questions, don't fully understand what the doctor is saying, then they go away less able to care for themselves." A ruthless focus on efficiency can inadvertently increase costs by completely missing the elaborateness of our humanity. Perhaps it would be better to lean into nuance rather than resist it.

What if we used a biological metaphor to think about the NHS – elevating ideas such as emergence, adaptiveness and yes, complexity? Andy believes this might unlock the door to more imaginative and creative approaches to the opportunities digital offers, in enabling a step-change to improving the healthcare system for all of us. For me, this way of thinking about healthcare could blow open our thinking, enabling us to radically re-conceptualise the sorts of expertise and ideas we value.

As well as the lived experience of patients and carers being at the heart of our orientation, we would venerate artists, philosophers, social scientists and historians for what they could bring to our re-imaging of healthcare. This may sound whacky, but it is when you involve diverse professions and perspectives, as we are starting to do with human-centred design, that we start to see things in different ways. I wonder if we should lean into those intangible assets that may facilitate a step change, rather than just create a digital version of what we did in our analogue existence. Maybe it is imagination that will save the NHS.

Nurturing a Habitat

My baptism into digital was characterised by failure in the face of complexity. As I groped towards an understanding of this experience, I coined the metaphor of a *habitat* to articulate the combinatorial factors that influence successful innovation. Borrowing from biology, a habitat is the array of resources present in an area that allows survival and reproduction. I recall searching for a concept that had an organic and earthy feel to it, attempting to counter the dominant industrial narrative or the sterile language of ecosystems. mHabitat was the name of the first digital project that I established, which still thrives to this day, having been on its own evolutionary journey over the years. The name is an expression of the ecological nature of healthcare systems that are metamorphosing from the analogue to the digital.

Without realising that there was a body of theory and literature behind this, an ecological approach in which people, organisations and the wider system around them began to fascinate me.[11] In the NASSS framework, Trish codifies this complexity of multiple-moving and interdependent parts in seven domains of condition, technology, value proposition, adopter, organisation, wider system, embedding and adapting over time. Andy's thinking steps us up a conceptual level to consider the extent to which how we think about innovation may influence our approach to it in practice. Frankie has a more practical take on how innovation may be enacted in an NHS context. These are all different lenses for the same challenge of culture and complexity.

When I ask Frankie if she thinks innovation is possible from within the NHS, she is emphatic. "Yes!" but quick to qualify: "on a small scale, generally in isolation, often as shadow IT, generally being led by individual clinicians doing their own thing." There is no shortage of good ideas simmering in every service but she sees those innovators as "coming up with brilliant ideas for innovation that organisations aren't willing or able to support."

Frankie's perspective resonates with my own experience. There are many examples of local innovations championed by bright entrepreneurial clinicians, of whom there is an abundance. But wider adoption is challenging in a fragmented NHS that is running on empty. Even the 15 Academic Health Science Networks, charged with supporting wider adoption in regions, have comparatively small budgets and teams to support these efforts.

110 ■ *Towards a Digital Ecology*

It is often the case that clinicians and managers are suspicious of the motives of the private sector and unfamiliar with how companies operate.[12] This leads to attempts to develop technologies in-house, often without an appreciation of the effort required to sustain them and naive ideas about how they might be sustained or even monetised. I can say this because I've been there myself. Having worked in a medium-sized digital health business, I look back and realise how naive I was thinking we could develop technologies in the NHS and sell them to our NHS colleagues. I didn't appreciate or understand everything that goes with running a successful company, marketing, sales and all the other things necessary to take a product to market. It can be done and sometimes is done. But it's a hard slog.

For Frankie, there needs to be a space, possibly separate to the mainstream operations of an NHS trust, where experimentation and imagination are permitted: "Unless you create a track within NHS organisations at a local level that can channel, direct and support that innovative thinking then it's already lost before it gets to the level of any serious thought." We need a more sophisticated approach that emphasises creativity and lateral thinking. Those are in short supply in a hard-pressed system.

I ask Frankie to describe what she thinks would help foster innovative thinking in an NHS organisation:

> It's a low governance environment. It's about iteration, it's about pace, it's about understanding that not everything will work. Give us a budget and we will give you an overall return on investment, like a stock portfolio. Some stuff will work, some stuff will fail. But demanding that everything works means you can never innovate. Spread bets on what will work on the basis of it being a benefit in the future. … there needs to be effectively a fund within an organisation.

Frankie is describing a permissive environment that allows the sort of creativity and off-centre thinking from which innovation can spring. But this requires the precious gift of *time* and headspace from the hurly-burly of operational services.

Anne Cooper thinks about *time* a lot. In an article, she wrote for the *Nursing Times*,[13] she makes a plea for nurses to have more time to think. Perplexed by this seemingly simple idea of creating *time and space* as a necessary condition for new ideas to flow, Anne immersed herself in the literature on healthcare innovation: "At first, I wondered if I had missed something … most of the things I read concerned doing more in the time available." Anne was perplexed, "There was plenty about how to fit in more tasks and how to be more productive, but there seems to be little about making time to think." I don't know about you, but I do my best thinking when I'm walking the dog. Just think what we could achieve when clinical staff have time combined with a permissive culture to *think* and exposure to different expertise and knowledge.

There are super examples of dedicated spaces created within and by NHS trusts to do just that. Salford Royal NHS Foundation Trust has a Living Lab and Experience Design Centres where clinicians and industry work together to solve problems collaboratively. Great Ormond Street Hospital has a dedicated space called DRIVE in which data and research projects flourish. The Health Foundry is a digital health co-working space that is owned by Guys and St Thomas' NHS Foundation Trust. I set up Co>Space North, a similar venue in central Leeds. Often funded from an NHS trust's charitable funds, we not only need more of these spaces, but we need to ramp up the diversity and the breadth of who we invite into them, whilst reaching out to non-NHS environments and developing relationships with them too.

To extend the biology metaphor, the NHS needs to become more of an amoeba, with the ability to stretch and adapt, a permeable membrane that allows for ideas and possibilities to move freely. People find ways to create these spaces but it is often against the tide and hidden in recesses. Time and space for people to convene is characteristic of a flourishing digital ecology.

Put a Dictator in Charge

There is a meme doing the rounds on social media. It goes like this: "Who led the digital transformation of your company? [A] CEO? [B] CTO? [C] COVID-19?" (MIT Sloan Management Review tweet, 19 November 2020)

As with many memes, there is some truth at the core. The pandemic did blow through the barriers of context and culture for a short period of time. "In times of crisis you appoint a dictator and get on with it," explains Frankie, "Covid became the dictator and we have achieved more this year that we have in the last three."

However, the heavy hand of the dictatorial rule is not without its challenges: "It's a double edged sword," says Frankie,

> it created the pathway in order to do stuff quickly, but it enabled a pathway to do stuff that was understood and tactically would fix problems that had been going round in circles for a very long time, tying up lots of time in committees.

The consequence of not making a decision suddenly became worse than making a decision.

Frankie observes that the pandemic forced adoption of what for the most part were well-understood technologies:

> The remedial stuff, that had taken three years, in fact it had taken longer than three years, at [name of Trust] we had tried doing video consultations using three or four different solutions for the three years I had been here, plus for a couple of years before I arrived, and it took us days to do it once it became a mandate.

112 ■ *Towards a Digital Ecology*

The pandemic forced a shift. It was the dictator that made the NHS introduce technologies that in reality, it should have probably done before. It stopped equivocation dead in its tracks. The danger we now face is a lack of imagination; a lack of appreciation of the seismic societal shift going on around our healthcare system; a tendency to simply replace an analogue process with a digital one. The NHS can begin to flourish again if we nurture and nourish it with time, resources and a permissive habitat to imagine a new future that can emerge from the best of what we already have. These are political and policy decisions, but they are also about mindset and orientation.

Giving birth is a transformative process. A mother's body has to heal and maybe even be repaired. Life is changed forever, in the most profound ways that are not even apparent or knowable to that small lump of life and its shell-shocked parents.

It is an everyday knowable story that is repeated minute by minute across the globe. But it is simultaneously the most personal and intimate experience for each of us. I will never forget Lesley, the community midwife who guided me through each of my three pregnancies. A sea of calm in the bewildering chaos of those first postpartum days, she helped me learn, adapt, adjust and incorporate in equal measure.

If we are to re-conceptualise digital transformation as a generative rather than technocratic process, then perhaps we may realise the benefits that we suspect are possible to achieve but which too often elude us. We would balance the repeatable with the unknowable and technocratic with the social. Context is king. We need to re-conceptualise a digital ecology and nurture it to grow.

Notes

1 https://www.nuffieldtrust.org.uk/files/2017-12/1513183510_nt-innovation-briefing-scc-web-2.pdf
2 https://www.nuffieldtrust.org.uk/files/2017-12/1513183510_nt-innovation-briefing-scc-web-2.pdf
3 https://www.rand.org/pubs/research_reports/RR2711.html
4 https://www.health.org.uk/publications/the-spread-challenge
5 https://service-manual.nhs.uk/
6 https://www.jscimedcentral.com/CommunityMedicine/communitymedicine-6-1047.pdf
7 https://assets.publishing.service.gov.uk/government/uploads/system/uploads/attachment_data/file/550866/Wachter_Review_Accessible.pdf
8 https://www.nuffieldtrust.org.uk/files/2017-12/1513183510_nt-innovation-briefing-scc-web-2.pdf
9 https://kar.kent.ac.uk/71495/1/64VidCalovskiThesis.pdf
10 https://leadingedgeforum.com/insights/the-counter-industrial-revolution/
11 https://www.sciencedirect.com/science/article/pii/S1532046403000844?via%3Dihub
12 https://bmchealthservres.biomedcentral.com/articles/10.1186/s12913-019-4790-x
13 https://www.nursingtimes.net/roles/nurse-managers/without-time-to-think-the-fire-of-innovation-dies-out-29-06-2012/

Chapter 7

The Social Determinants of Digital

The messaging from the NHS says 'go online'. Universal Credit is online, shopping is online…this means many people are excluded from the services they need to survive the crisis.

Evidence from Rich Denyer-Bewick, Citizens Online.[1]

The Wellness Myth

There is a common feature in the straplines and marketing materials of many digital health products that, I have to confess, irks me. I know that sounds a bit extra but it's true. *Empowering you to live a happy, healthier life! Helping you make lifestyle changes for a better you! So you can take responsibility for your own health!* It is as if all I have to do is make a few tweaks to my lifestyle choices and suddenly I will be the optimised, responsible, productive member of society that public health officials would like me to be. *Fitter, happier, more productive* as The Radiohead single goes.

An article in *The New Statesman* neatly captures the distaste that those lifestyle digital health products invoke in me, whenever I come across them:

The modern cult of wellness promotes pseudo-science, entrenches health inequalities and co-opts political terms such as "self-love" and "empowerment" into something you can buy. It encodes a rampant individualism: the idea that you alone are responsible for your well-being.[2]

DOI: 10.1201/9781032198798-7

113

114 ■ *Towards a Digital Ecology*

The stark reality is that not everyone finds themselves with the opportunity, motivation or circumstances to lead the healthy lifestyle that those mobile apps compel us to aspire to. Their straplines represent a sharp dissonance between the promise of digital health and the reality for the people who both have the most to gain and are the least likely to benefit. The 1997 number one Radiohead album *OK Computer* is a prescient exploration of consumerism, alienation and political malaise, throwing shade on our modern obsession with productivity.[3] *Comfortable, not drinking too much. Regular exercise at the gym three days a week.* You get the picture.

In order to understand the challenge of inequality in digital health, we need to turn our attention to social determinants that are the social, economic and political factors that shape our health and well-being. Whether we have a job, the conditions in which we live and the education we receive are by far and away the most important predictors of good health and well-being. These predictors are systemic factors of employment, housing and community which, despite the hyperbolic straplines, a mobile app is not going to readily solve.

Over the last 35 years, Michael Marmot has led rock star research highlighting the pernicious effects of social inequality. In an interview for the think tank NESTA, he argues that it is virtually impossible for people living in poverty to make healthy choices, even if they want to. "If people in the bottom ten percent of household income were to follow Public Health England's healthy eating advice," explains Marmot, "they would spend 74 per cent of their income on food." Healthy choices are literally out of reach for the poorest people in our society.

Marmot argues that,

> instead of asking how we can persuade people to make healthy choices, we should be asking how we can improve people's income so they can afford to eat, and how can we make it less prohibitive economically to eat healthily.[4]

I have this nagging worry that by pinning our hopes on mobile apps and digital platforms to persuade and nudge people to improve their health, we are obfuscating this unpalatable societal dilemma, which is the underbelly of our modern healthcare system.

What is the scale of the problem? Around four and a half million of us live in deep poverty and it is getting worse rather than getting better. Black and minority ethnic (BAME) families are between two and three times as likely to be in persistent poverty than white households; families with children are more likely to live in poverty, as are families who include a disabled person.[5] Many people were already living precarious lives before the pandemic. COVID-19 treated them with the most vicious blow of all.

The Social Determinants of Digital ■ 115

To make things worse, over the last decade, the Government has shifted spending away from services that help people stay healthy (public health) and instead focused on taxpayers' money on addressing the problems that could have been avoided in the first place (acute and emergency services).[6] This has a certain circularity that is hard to interrupt without a concerted effort and substantial reallocation of resources and effort.

In the face of these intransigent conditions, you can see why the questions we ask and the solutions we search for are never more important. Digital health tools and services could be the right answer to the wrong question. They could assist or they could obfuscate. We must pay sufficient attention to the root causes of the problems we are trying to solve if we have a hope of truly making things better. We must be on high alert for the plague of tech solutionism rearing its ugly head.

Hello Inequality, Let Me Introduce You to COVID-19

The pandemic has distributed the burden of its destruction in unfair and callous ways.

The startling intersectional impacts of ethnicity, alongside social and economic status, have become apparent as the virus has taken its devastating course. For the more fortunate, it meant an unexpected opportunity to bake sourdough, spend quality time with family and maybe take up a new hobby. For others, it meant enforced isolation along with a radical reduction in income, not to mention boredom and loneliness. For many, it was somewhere in between.

Halima is a Somalian woman who has found herself living in inner-city Birmingham, a single parent with five children aged between two and eleven. Although she is now a UK citizen, she entered the country as a refugee and is fortunate to have support from a local refugee charity. I know about Halima (not her real name) because a friend of mine volunteers for the charity and has been supporting her to learn English over the last year or more. Rebecca tells me that Halima lives in a high-rise flat in a deprived area of the city. She is scared of other people and worried for her children's safety. During the first lockdown, Halima did not leave her flat at all for fear she might catch the virus. Imagine staying in your flat with five young children for six whole months.

Halima is private about her health but admits to Rebecca that she takes medication for headaches. The physical and emotional weight of her situation would be hard for most of us to bear. Whilst in easier pre-lockdown times, Rebecca visited Halima in her tiny flat to practice spoken and written English. The pandemic put a sharp stop to that. "I send her an email with exercises on," says Rebecca, "she opens it and we talk via WhatsApp." Halima has one laptop for the family which doesn't have a webcam, and so she can't use it for video chat. "Her children

116 ■ *Towards a Digital Ecology*

help her with technology, but their knowledge is limited," explains Rebecca, "it's impossible to explain [reading and writing exercises] over the phone. I'm trying to find another laptop so we can do Zoom." Halima and Rebecca's story speaks to the daunting challenges faced by people whose existence is impregnated with the peril of poverty.

It is clear that the pandemic has thrown an unforgiving fluorescent beam on the haves and have-nots. In an opinion piece, entitled *Normality is now a luxury only the rich can afford,*[7] journalist Mark O'Connell lambasts what he dubs the "near hallucinogenically poor taste" exhibited by reality star Kim Kardashian when she informed the world of a birthday trip to a private island with friends: "where we could pretend things were normal just for a brief moment in time." Whilst this grotesque parade of wealth and privilege may be an outlier, it illuminates how differently the pandemic was experienced by those of us with money and resources, compared to those of us without.

Despite the *we're all in it together* mantra favoured by bureaucrats and health officials, it is evident that this couldn't be further from the truth. Rather than being a leveller, the risk of COVID-19 related death is more than four times as high for people of black ethnicity than for those of white ethnicity, after adjusting for age.[8] People who live in the richest areas of the country are half as likely to die of this nasty virus than those who live in the poorest. Disabled people have been amongst the hardest hit, and young people are twice as likely to lose their jobs.[9]

These confounding factors became apparent, not just in everyday life, but in the hospitals and on the wards of the NHS. The fact that black and minority health and care workers are more likely to be affected by the virus can, in part, be explained by their disproportionate employment in lower-paid key worker roles where they are more likely to work in either high exposure care environments or are less able to implement safe social distancing.[10]

A report from Public Health England, published in the early summer of 2020, suggested that historic racism, along with previously poor experiences of healthcare and racism in the workplace, means that those of us from BAME groups are less likely to seek help when needed, NHS staff are less likely to speak up when they have concerns about things that concern them.[11] This is the perfect storm of virus meets inequality, meets institutional racism.

There is a range of factors at play that speak to systemic societal inequality which was merely exacerbated by the sweep of the pandemic. None of these problems is new. People from BAME communities are overrepresented in lower socio-economic groups; overcrowded households increase the risk of infection; people are more likely to have worse outcomes from the virus when combined with pre-existing conditions such as Type 2 diabetes, which affect people from lower socio-economic backgrounds disproportionately.

These are unpalatable truths that the pandemic has served up on a plate and put squarely on the dinner table. Hello pandemic, let me introduce you to inequality, I think you'll get along well.

The Drum of Progress

The term *Luddite* has become synonymous with those who would stop progress. The word is bandied about to cast scorn on people who resist change and innovation, in particular developments in the technology sphere.

This now pejorative term has its roots in the 19th Century movement of English textile workers whose livelihoods were upended by the invention of industrial machinery. Eventually suppressed by the ruling class of the day, those workers had very real and legitimate concerns. It wasn't just automation that was destroying their highly skilled craft, it was the exploitative managerial practices that went with them.

I want to reclaim the word *Luddite* in the true sense of what I understand to be the meaning behind that movement centuries ago. This chapter does not argue against innovation. Digital has and can improve our lives in immeasurable ways. By the same token, it is not always a force for good. The advent of digital in the context of austerity and inequality, along with an underlying culture of individualism and consumerism, has a tendency to pump out certain types of solutions that amplify the differences between us rather than those which bind us together.

During the pandemic, we have seen a blank cheque for digital health, but has that money benefitted or further disadvantaged people already at the sharp end of the pandemic? One can only speculate that the money pumped into the system may have diverted constrained health resources to technology projects that only benefit those with the sharpest elbows and the loudest voices.

By holding a light to the social conditions in which digital innovation is grounded, we can start to ask critical questions and more importantly, we can start to re-imagine alternative futures and possibilities. It may move slowly, but the NHS is in a constant state of flux and reinvention. The question we should be asking is, are we creating the healthcare system that we want to have for ourselves, our families and our communities into the future?

To help me piece together the tiles in this mosaic, I interview experts whose experience and thinking I deeply admire. At the coalface, there is local authority digital inclusion officer, Rachel Benn; Emma Stone is a director for the leading digital inclusion charity, The Good Thinking Foundation and has a long-standing pedigree in the policy sector; Roz Davies is a social activist and managing director of an NHS social change team working in the field of inclusive digital transformation. As someone living with Type 1 diabetes, she combines professional expertise with personal insights into the role of technology in managing her condition. Sam Shah is a clinician and public health specialist who isn't afraid to speak out about discrimination within the NHS. Between them, they help me traverse the uneven landscape of digital and social inequality.

This chapter may expose the underbelly of digital that we do not want to see, but it is nevertheless fiercely optimistic. I muse over how we make sure we build digital tools and services for everyone, how we ensure the data we capture for policy and research tells the whole story and avoids casting shadows that exclude the experience

118 ■ *Towards a Digital Ecology*

of the most vulnerable and how we might create a digital workforce that thrives in its diversity. By shining a torch on it, we create the opportunity to change our course and steer in a fresh direction.

One Condition. Two Tales

Before we go further, I want to share two tales. They are both told by Roz, and they elucidate the stratospheric distance between the haves and have-nots in digital health. Over to Roz, in her own words:

"There are a few things that have improved the quality of my life and my successful management of Type 1 diabetes. The first was getting insulin. Without insulin you die. The second was doing a training course [on self management] which absolutely transformed how in control I was, how much I understood about diabetes and it gave me more power in my relationship with the [health] system as well.

And the third thing that happened was digital. I had learnt about the power of community and peer support through my NHS work on health champions, but then I discovered Twitter and I wondered what would happen if you blended this face-to-face stuff with digital. And I discovered the diabetes community online and I started to meet really interesting people. I couldn't believe how much I was learning and how expert and empathic people were. There's nothing like peer support in health, nothing. And through that I was learning about technology you could use to manage your diabetes. I found the sensor I've been using ever since, way before the NHS was using it, through that community. And it was life changing."

"A moment I had that was so stark, it was some freelance research I did on Type 2 diabetes in the South Asian community. And it has never left me. I will never forget going to this community group, it was an evening workshop, and I talked to the women first and then the men. There was this woman, and she was very sad. She had been diagnosed with depression, and she had Type 2 diabetes that she managed with insulin. She told me all her GP appointments were in the daytime when her husband was at work, and she had to go to the surgery to see the GP who she didn't understand and they never got an interpreter in. She didn't have a clue how to manage her diabetes and she was using insulin and I remember thinking that was pretty dangerous.

All of [the group] had technology at home but none of them were using it to manage their health. None of them had heard of Diabetes UK [the leading charity] and probably most of them wouldn't have been able to use it anyway as at that time because there was no translation into different languages. They were excluded in so many ways. The diabetes support wasn't culturally appropriate. I went looking online for anything I could find and I think I found two or three recipes and that was about it. It was terrible. This is a community in which diabetes is prevalent and they are completely excluded, both offline and online."

Pay-as-You-Go

All is not as it might seem. Whilst the majority of us have a smartphone, 25 million of us living with constrained income or on benefits cannot afford a monthly contract. Having to rely on pay-as-you-go is more expensive than broadband and can mean having to make choices between putting food on the table or letting your children get on a Zoom call for homeschooling.[12] The choices are stark.

With two and a half million new applications for Universal Credit made between the beginning of lockdown and the end of May, finances have been squeezed for many, like never before.[13] Pay-as-you-go means hitting data limits that stop you from doing basic things that others take for granted. This is what digital poverty looks like in one of the most affluent countries in the world. Whatever our views about digital, most of us don't have much of a choice about using it. In the next five years, it has been estimated that 90% of jobs will require digital skills. The internet has become as integral to our modern lives as running water and electricity.

I have been to countless digital health conferences over the years where tech start-ups with their pitch decks claim smartphone use is ubiquitous. It is a compelling narrative if you want the NHS to buy your product. However, such claims turn out to be untrue. It remains the case that 9% of UK adults do not use the internet, and just under a quarter have limited digital skills. Six million people cannot turn on a device, and over 7 million cannot open an app. The reality is more complicated than it might first appear.

Over the course of the pandemic, there has been a seismic shift in perceptions of digital exclusion. Just as we've not been able to hide from the unequal impacts of the virus on disadvantaged communities, the stark digital divide has punched us in the face. Whereas once we used to blithely refer to young people as digital natives, now we are seeing pupils can't homeschool because they don't have laptops. Things are no longer as clear as we once imagined.

Put simply, all these figures that I've just thrown at you point to the reality that there is a sizable chunk of the population who cannot or will not positively benefit from the momentum towards a digitised NHS. During the lockdown, digital suddenly became an essential component of being able to continue with our lives. Whether it was education, employment, social support or accessing health and welfare services, most things had to be done online.

Rather than being static, digital exclusion is complex, shifting and with many interdependent factors. A young person may use Snapchat and Instagram throughout the day but is completely floored when it comes to completing a job application online. A healthcare practitioner may be comfortable with online banking and shopping, but when it comes to an electronic patient record they lose their nerve. An older person may have once been online but with increasingly poor eyesight and failing dexterity, they have given up switching on their desktop computer. A single mother who was caught out by an email scam may have decided she no longer

120 ■ *Towards a Digital Ecology*

trusts the internet. A young professional may break their wrist and be temporarily impaired and unable to use their smartphone.

It is not enough to be digitally confident; we also need to be assured when it comes to making decisions about our own health and well-being. *Health literacy* is the phrase used to describe the: skills, motivation and ability to access, understand and use information to keep healthy.[14] When we have good health literacy we are more likely to stay well and have better health outcomes when we get ill.[15] As the world of health information has increasingly gone online, so our digital skills have become important to our health. All sorts of factors come into play, including how motivated we are, how interested we are, how easy we find it to search and find good quality information, and our ability to make sense of the information we find. Sometimes called eHealth literacy, digital and literacy have become inexorably conjoined.[16]

One Hundred Percent Digital

It was on a mid-May evening when I interviewed Rachel, digital inclusion coordinator for the libraries service in Leeds. Her team's mission is to reach the 15% of people in Leeds who do not use the internet via charities, community organisations and groups, with whom they are in contact. The team do this through a tablet lending scheme, through which they loan out 450 4G-enabled smart devices to people in poverty and through projects to build confidence and skills in those who lack them.

I am curious about the main reasons why people don't go online. Rachel tells me it can be a whole host of things but skills, motivation and access are the main factors. In her team's research, they have found poverty, deprivation and lack of employment are all mixed up with digital exclusion, and they focus their efforts on the parts of Leeds where these issues are most prevalent.

"A lot of people tell me they don't need to be online, they haven't been online their whole lives," says Rachel, "they tell me 'I lead a happy life, why do I need to be?'" For Rachel, this isn't about thrusting digital onto people, but it is about everyone having the opportunity to go online if they want to, helping them understand what the benefits might be. For some people, it might be when they might have to apply for universal credit or want to apply for a job and the employer requires them to submit their CV online, but Rachel wants to help people see about how people can use the internet more generally in their lives.

Rachel differentiates between the *hook*, the thing that might motivate people to go online and the *need* which might be about transacting with a government or health service. The team creates *hooks* by having devices available at luncheon clubs and other community activities where people can explore the internet and search for websites and resources that relate to their hobbies or other things that interest them. "Then further down the line they might need to order a prescription or something like that," says Rachel, "and then they already are familiar with navigating a website and find it less intimidating."

I'm ambivalent about the city's strapline of *100% Digital Leeds* – it seems both unobtainable and also a bit Orwellian at the same time. Rachel calls it "a lovely ideal" but explains that in reality, it captures an ambition which would see "everyone in Leeds having the opportunity and an informed choice about whether they go online." Rachel describes the city's holistic approach to digital inclusion:

> There's an assumption that if you're digitally excluded you can't turn a device on, but we class being digitally included is someone who has everything they need to use digital to improve their health and wellbeing and quality of life and access the opportunities they need.

This is an inexorable internet drift that is leaving people who don't use digital stranded on an analogue island. People who hold the purse strings of the NHS and other public services want people to go online because that is how they hope they can drive efficiencies, meeting increasing demand with dwindling resources. They hope and perhaps believe that *digital first* is good for everyone. But this orientation can lead to a compulsion to big-up the good things technology has to offer whilst downplaying the downsides.

The digital mantra beats the drum that it is good to be online. But maybe the reality is actually that it simply is increasingly hard to get things done in a world where everything from claiming universal credit, searching for a job and booking a holiday takes place on the internet. The majority of us have some concerns, with 81% of 12–15-year-olds and 62% of adults report having had a harmful experience online. That is a lot of people. We are mostly worried about the content we see and our interactions with others that may cause disquiet or distress.[17] Over half of adults and young people are worried about our privacy and how our data is used. Our relationship with digital technologies is not a straightforward one.

"It's not going back," remarks Emma, when I ask her about the downsides of digital inclusion. "Digital isn't going to stop here." Emma describes something surprising she learnt when reviewing the evidence on the relationship between online harms and digital inclusion. "There can be really bad and damaging consequences from the really bad behaviors that go on [online] as well as frauds and scams," she tells me, "but as with anything … people build their resilience and learn about what is safe and what isn't, through doing it." During her research, Emma came to the realisation that digital inclusion is about supporting people to navigate the harms as well as the positives that being online presents.

The Law of Inverse Care

> You are always balancing the things that digital can enable you to do which are wonderful and amazing and which can help to create a more level playing field, and which can help to reduce inequalities, and which can help to motivate people or support them, and help them feel connected and improve quality of life, and amplify community action.

122 ■ *Towards a Digital Ecology*

Emma sets out the digital inclusion dilemma: "But exactly at the same point, you've got to work hard to make sure that it doesn't also end up compounding and contributing to further inequalities and further injustices."

The inverse care law was coined by Julian Tudor Hart in a 1971 paper for *The Lancet*, in which he suggested a perverse relationship between the need for healthcare services and their actual utilisation. Put another way, the people who least need healthcare are the most likely to access it, whilst those who are in most need are least likely to receive it.

It is also the case that how we access and make use of services is radically different depending on our social and economic circumstances. A consistent theme of this book is the fragmented nature of our NHS, its bold three-letter acronym masking many different services, all organised by their own internal logic and need to sustain themselves. The consequence of this complexity is that the poorest people are the most likely to end up at the sharp end of services when all the preventative and early intervention stuff has not touched the sides. To put it in bleak terms, figures from NHS Digital show that people in the most deprived parts of England are more than twice as likely to show up at A&E than people in more affluent parts of the country.

It turns out that the exact same people who have the most to gain from using digital health technologies are the ones who are the least likely to use them. We are yet again benefitting the educated and the affluent at the expense of the vulnerable and excluded. There is a real and present danger that we re-purpose the inverse care law in a digital guise. Digital has become a social determinant of health.

Chronic health conditions, such as Type 2 diabetes, are more than twice as common in the least well-off and well-educated segments of society than the most affluent and well-educated. If we combine these stark facts with digital exclusion, that is less access to broadband and lower digital literacy, then we can see how disadvantage is easily compounded in the sphere of digital health. Silicon Valley tech bros are often the subject of ridicule for designing products for their white, male, affluent and educated counterparts. But what if we are falling into the same trap in digital health.

Digital exclusion is a double whammy – it not only limits access to digital-first health services, it can also impact the wider determinants of health such as the ability to get a job or secure good quality housing. Combined with health literacy, digital literacy is about more than being able to download an app. It's also about trust, motivation and a belief in your abilities and a sense of self-efficacy and worth. All those things are more likely to be knocked if you are lower down life's pecking order.

There is a double bind, in which poorer people are increasingly compelled to go online to get the support they need from the government. Applying for jobs, housing and even universal credit, have all shifted from analogue to digital. Rachel tells me, "We've got younger people, 18, 19, 20 years old, that can use a smartphone but when it comes to applying for Universal Credit, they don't have the skills to do that."

To illustrate her point, Rachel describes working with a group of young mothers experiencing poverty, all of whom had a smartphone or a tablet. They told Rachel that they could all use email,

The Social Determinants of Digital ■ 123

> but as the session went on, we realised they all had email addresses, somewhere down the line someone had set one up for them … but many didn't know how to navigate their inbox, they'd never sent an email, they'd never attached a picture or a document or a CV. They all use their smartphone to call friends and family … but they can't do lots of other things.

Public services need people to go online because that is how they have to deliver services in increasingly constrained times. So whilst many of us might associate the internet with freedom and limitless possibility, for others, it's about finding a job and getting access to benefits. "We knew that it wasn't just about delivering skills sessions, and putting on 'how to use an iPad' or 'how to use a computer,'" explains Rachel. The team uses impressively creative methods to entice people to try out the internet. With an iPad lending scheme, charities running luncheon clubs for older people show guests how to use the devices to find content that relates to their interests and hobbies. "Further down the line, they might use the NHS App to order prescriptions," says Rachel.

I ask Emma if efforts to help people get online to access NHS services are really just a sticking plaster that covers over more profound inequalities. If digital inequality is merely a symptom, then treating it on its own fails to get to the root cause. "I don't think it's a sticking plaster but I don't think it's the solution alone." I ask Emma to explain: "Digital inclusion for health only, would be a sticking plaster but actually we need to be joining the dots and embedding digital inclusion in all aspects of people's lives." When thinking broadly about all the factors that contribute to our health and well-being, then digital inclusion will help people to improve their circumstances and contribute to making their lives easier.

Designing for Everyone

Digital inclusion is both a consequence of improved social conditions and a means of people being able to improve their lot. Digital technologies must be part of the solution rather than a distraction from the material realities experienced by a significant proportion of the population. I don't buy the argument that I've heard many times that if we give digital technologies to the more affluent and capable then we free up services for the most vulnerable. My inclination tells me that in a context of ever constrained resources, that sort of thinking opens the backdoor to a two-tier health system. It obscures the attention we must pay to the wider social determinants of health.

There are two competing approaches to how issues of digital exclusion are thought about in the NHS. I have heard many people assert that if we give digital tools to the people who can use them, this will free up space and time for people who can't use them to access face-to-face services. We effectively create a

124 ■ *Towards a Digital Ecology*

two-track system. Another argument is that we focus on digital inclusion efforts so that everyone is able to use them, and choices about how to access digital or face-to-face services are open to everyone. This approach recognises that not everyone will want or be prepared to use digital technologies, but they should have the option.

Emma believes that the apparently common-sense two-track approach is deeply problematic:

> it doesn't at all speak to user experience, which is that even the most digitally enabled person may at times want to have a non-digital experience and interaction ... [binary thinking] takes you to a point where you are designing a *digital* service rather than a *health* service.

By designing with and for people who are most able, you are not testing those products and services to be usable and inclusive. People's abilities and circumstances change over time. They are not static.

We need to avoid thinking about [digital exclusion] in really binary terms," says Emma, "where we have a digital track for those who can and a non-digital track for those who can't." She explains why she believes this is fundamentally the wrong approach:

> you've got to move away from thinking about digital inclusion in relation to a [clinical] service pathway ... it's digital inclusion in relation to health outcomes, services and pathways but also the wider determinants of health. Digital inclusion is not only important so someone can access that particular cancer pathway that happens to be digital enabled, it's also important for everything else in people's lives now, education and employment, all those things that can make life easier and make you connected to the world we live in now.

For Emma, we need a health service that is flexible enough for people to choose the channels that work best for them in the circumstances they are in and which are able to adapt to their changing needs, preferences and abilities. Digital should not be the lobster pot in which you get caught up, never to find your way out. Everyone wins from inclusivity – people who will benefit the most get the access and you get upstream benefits when people are able to improve their lives and well-being in other ways, preventing ill health and enabling people to thrive. "The pandemic has been interesting, because loads of people have had to do it, they haven't had an option ... sometimes when you have to do something then it's won over people who might have been more sceptical. And that's always been the fascinating thing about digital health, we're actually starting from a pretty low base even those of us who were capable of using platforms such as Zoom and

WhatsApp or even electronic prescriptions, weren't using them because we didn't have to."

For Emma, the big question is, who is responsible for digital inclusion? "What is the responsibility of the NHS to invest in the support for that wider digital inclusion, rather than going for a sink or swim, and we'll just pick up the ones who sink?" Emma describes Good Thinking's experience of developing local *digital health hubs* to promote digital inclusion in the everyday places that people go to in towns and cities across the country. In an evaluation, they found that the ones based in GP surgeries tended to focus in a transactional way on specific activities such as ordering a prescription, whereas community-focused ones in libraries tended to think about inclusion more broadly and holistically. The NHS needs to be part of the answer, but it is a bigger question that needs to be answered across government departments, driven by the political will to make a difference.

Data Shadows

As my weekday morning conversation with Emma continues, I try to discreetly eat my breakfast whilst throwing a ball for a bored dog with my left arm out of camera view, hoping none of these are posing too much of a distraction. Emma moves on to the topic of data, sharing her thoughts about what digital exclusion means for the data that mobile apps and platforms amass in huge quantities. "Given that we are now relying on digital footprints to plan [health services] then you have a massive data planning gap around the people who are already least represented," explains Emma, "You're compounding all of those biases in terms of planning and resource allocation."

Here are some facts about data. Around 30% of the entire world's stored data is generated and captured in health systems, each one of us typically generates around 80 megabytes of health system data a year from medical imaging and electronic patient record, a typical hospital stay involves a collection of several hundred individual items of data and our GP record incorporates every record of every consultation going back over decades. The healthcare system is swimming in the data that we generate from our interactions with its services. But whose data is in and whose data never gets captured or codified in the first place?[18]

To find the answer to the question, we need to enter the sphere of data bias. It was a surprising and pleasant surprise to see her on the speaker list. Digital health conferences have a tendency to focus on NHS, industry and academic themes, but rarely do they facilitate critical thinking about the wider societal implications of our trajectory towards a digital-first NHS. So keynote speaker, Caroline Criado Perez, author of *Invisible Women: Exposing Data Bias in a World Designed for Men* (2019) was a welcome intrusion into a panoply of suited (mostly) men selling digital gadgets and gizmos with promises of system transformation.

126 ■ *Towards a Digital Ecology*

Whilst Perez focuses primarily on gender discrimination in her analysis of how data reinforces a world orientated towards men, her work nods to broader issues of inequality and their systemic effects. Going back to the ancient Greeks, Perez illuminates how the male body has been the default norm, to the detriment of women throughout the history of healthcare and clinical research.

Because women have been largely absent from medical research, she argues, data specific to women has been systematically excluded from medical education. Gender bias is perpetuated because the data we generate is derived from the default male body. A rather stunning example given by Perez relates to the female *Viagra* that when released in 2015 was found to potentially interact negatively with alcohol. When the manufacturer quite rightly ran a clinical trial, they recruited 25 participants, of which only two were women, and they did not sex-disaggregate the data in their analysis.[19]

The researchers had investigated the contraindications of a female drug on mostly male bodies, even when it is well known that alcohol impacts female and male bodies very differently. As a layperson, this story seems bizarre. But in fact, this example is only one of the many described by Perez, which between them point to a systematic bias in which data renders women's bodies and women's health less visible.

I was struck by a fiercely contemporary example of this type of bias in the use of personal protective equipment (PPE) during the pandemic, which has been widely reported to be in short supply, putting NHS and other key worker staff at risk of infection. A BBC news article[20] highlights the limitation of one-size-fits-all PPE which is ill-fitting and uncomfortable for many women. This is not a new issue; a TUC report in 2017[21] found that:

> most PPE is based on the sizes and characteristics of male populations from certain countries in Europe and the United States. As a result, most women, and also many men, experience problems finding suitable and comfortable PPE because they do not conform to this standard male worker model.

So why are gender and other forms of difference and inequality salient to digital health? The simple answer is that digital technologies are primarily interfaces for collecting and presenting data. Medical technologies are increasingly combining digital technologies and real-world data to inform clinical research. With a bias towards male bodies as the norm, the increasing amounts of data we are gathering are further amplifying this bias. The notion of *health data poverty* has been coined as the inability of individuals, groups or populations to benefit from discovery or innovation due to insufficient data that are adequately representative.[22] If we are collecting data with gaps and shadows, and we use this for determining priorities and investment in healthcare, then we have a problem.

And our biggest problem lies in the field of Artificial Intelligence (AI), which has developed a bad reputation over recent times, for amplifying bias. Nowhere in the sphere of digital health hype is there more hyperbole than when it comes to AI, with any number of start-ups claiming that they can disrupt the healthcare system with intelligent systems that can outperform doctors in the detection of disease or automate back-office functions. AI can be described as a set of advanced technologies that enable machines to carry out highly complex tasks that require intelligence if a person were to perform them; intelligence can be defined as *problem-solving* and *an intelligent system* as one which takes the best possible action in a given situation[23].

We have reason to be cautious. The hype of AI is counterbalanced by discordant voices pointing out its limitations in real-world settings. Relying on large datasets to train its algorithms, time and again AI has been shown to spew out the bias and stereotypes that are embedded within the data that is shovelled into them.

AI has started to gain steady traction in the field of X-rays and scans which are collectively known as medical imaging. Trained on large datasets, algorithms can start to be used for identifying disease and provide decision support for clinicians. Ophthalmology is a speciality that has begun to use AI because of the crucial role of imaging in detecting diseases such as diabetic retinopathy, age-related macular degeneration, glaucoma and cataracts.

A group of researchers undertook a global review of all publicly available ophthalmology datasets to ascertain their quality and completeness. Through their investigation, they found 94 unique open datasets that are cited over and again by multiple studies. Between them, those datasets comprise over 500,000 images from around 100,000 patients. The researchers uncovered a problem. The data quality was highly variable with ethnicity as the least routinely captured datapoint, closely followed by gender. Training algorithms on these datasets, which according to the researchers is commonplace, will obscure any differences there may be for men and women, along with people from different ethnic backgrounds.[24]

In an editorial for *The Lancet* entitled *Challenging racism in the use of health data* (2021), the authors explore how data is infused with inequality from design through to input, analysis and application. The design of the research questions that get asked in the first place is permeated with underrepresentation from people from BAME communities; the data is less likely to include ethnic minority people who are less well-represented in research, recording of ethnicity is routinely patchy so differences are overlooked. A more insidious effect is the analytical decisions that get made which can interpret racial inequalities in the underlying data as biological facts rather than a reflection of the societal effects of racism. When those algorithms get applied in real-world clinical settings, all these gaps and shadows are compounded into a further reinforcement to make the experience of people from BAME backgrounds marginalised or completely invisible.[25]

Professor Brian Cantwell Smith[26] is an expert in philosophy and computer science at the University of Toronto. He makes a distinction between *reckoning* and *judgement*[27] whereby reckoning is the ability to manipulate data and recognise patterns, and judgement is the process of deliberative thought "grounded in ethical commitment and responsible action, appropriate to the situation in which it is deployed."

128 ■ *Towards a Digital Ecology*

He argues that the measurement of individual health data contains an implicit and toxic assumption that each of us is responsible for managing our own health. This normative elevation of the responsible patient and upstanding citizen neutralises the social determinants of health and renders inequality invisible. The responsibility shifts from governments and decision makers, and obligations are distributed amongst the very individuals who are the least able to act on them. AI just amplifies this bias more.[28]

We have a lot of work to do in order to generate good quality data, at scale, which avoids encoding the discrimination and bias that permeates our everyday societal realities. The fact that we are becoming conscious of this is a start. We need diversity at every level if we are going to properly shift the dial on this endemic problem.

Who Leads Digital Health Matters

"If you're serving a diverse set of population needs, which you are in the NHS, then you need a diversity of thought which by definition means you need diverse teams," Indi Singh explains as we chat over Zoom one afternoon. "We recognise we have a diverse population of needs, but we don't take the next set of steps."

What if one way to develop data-driven technologies that meet divergent needs is to have more diverse people designing and developing them? Having worked in charity and NHS settings, which tend to be fairly female-dominated, switching to the digital world literally gave me a headache. I recall going to one event at which I was the only female speaker out of the seven on the stage and the only woman on the invite list of over 50. When I complained to the organisers, it not only caused consternation, but sometime later I found myself called up with an invitation to attend an event because they told me they needed a woman there. I had inadvertently become the token woman. It didn't feel too comfortable to be in that position.

The lack of gender and ethnic diversity self-perpetuates itself. I chaired the first meetup in Leeds of One HealthTech, a volunteer-led group promoting diversity in technology. During the session, a couple of women in their 20s who worked at NHS Digital stood up and told the group how difficult they found it being the only women in a technology team. One described how she had been asked by one of her male peers to make the tea, mistaking her for a secretary. They were seriously thinking about leaving.

Sam Shah thinks about the issue of inequality in respect of the NHS workforce and the start-up community a lot. Voted in the top 100 UK Tech Asian Stars in 2020[29] and the fourth most influential BAME Tech Leader in the *Financial Times* in 2019,[30] he has an impressive pedigree and a public platform for his views to be heard. In an article for Health IT News entitled *Is that a glass ceiling I can see through?*, he argues: "Diverse people inevitably bring diverse views. If we reflect diversity in decision-making, then, in turn, we can achieve decisions that are more reflective of society."[31]

The Social Determinants of Digital ■ 129

I interview Sam at the end of a long working week of what felt like never-ending Zoom calls. The initial appeal of remote working has long since faded, as I realise how much I pine for a handshake or hug from my friends and colleagues. We begin our conversation idly planning a get-together once the pandemic zombies have receded and life can return to some sort of normal.

On to the topic in hand and Sam tells me that even as a senior director at NHS England and NHSX, he experienced discrimination: "When I look across the national organisations, at one point I was one of the very few directors who was non-white." He recalls how he has been overlooked for jobs for which he was more than qualified and how he has been excluded from decision-making with his peers: "And I think, if it happens at that level, what chance does anyone else have lower down in the system."

"Inequalities exist in every part of the system, they've existed for the last thousand years and they will exist for the next thousand years," says Sam, "it's how we respond to them that counts." He recalls members of his team approaching him because colleagues would routinely call them by the names of other non-white colleagues saying "oh you look so similar to the other person, that's why I got confused." This didn't just happen once. It happened again and again. Sam remembers how he raised it with his senior peers "and nobody wanted to do anything about it. It was literally swept under the carpet and ignored."

Whilst Sam's experience has been more positive at a regional and local level, he worries about how remote national leaders are from the realities of prejudice and inequality: "We've got a mismatch between the decision makers having no connection with the people for whom we're trying to solve problems across the NHS," he argues. For Sam, this has to start at the top: "If we are a system trying to solve [healthcare] problems for society and we can't even get it right in our own organisation, what hope do we have of solving these problems?"

In October 2019, the issue of discrimination reared its head under the headline: *NHSX removes job advert amid criticism it excludes BAME applicants* in Digital Health's industry news. The article reported that an advertisement for a chief nursing information officer (CNIO) was removed after two days when some people on Twitter pointed out that the advert effectively excluded BAME individuals. The role stated that applications must have "proven and significant experience at director level," which would automatically narrow the field to less than eight black and minority nurses who hold director positions in the NHS. Bias is not always overt, or even conscious, but it has material consequences.

Diversity isn't just a challenge for the NHS. It is also a challenge for start-ups, SMEs and companies building technologies for healthcare. "Imagine those startups, and the founders, and the people in them," says Sam, "if we don't have [diverse teams] we lose that diversity of thought, we lose that inclusivity in our process." Diversity is about building better products that meet people's needs: "We all come with our biases, and I do too, but if we all come with our biases, we get that melting pot, we will at least mitigate some of those biases, we will be able to modify some of them."

130 ■ *Towards a Digital Ecology*

The Shuri Network has a mission to promote diversity within the health technology sector and advocate for BAME women, promoting leadership and career development. Speaking at a digital health conference, Heather Caudle and Ijeoma Azodo from the Shuri Network argue that without a diverse and inclusive team, "unconscious bias" can be built into technology, ultimately putting patients at risk.[32]

Sometimes called the "triple threat" of low income, increased health needs and challenges with textual, technical and health literacy, it turns out that people whose needs and ability differ from the norm are often forgotten about and so further disadvantaged.

This disadvantage is threaded throughout the system, tightly sewn into the fabric of the digital health sector: "We know that it's more difficult for ethnic minority founders to get finances and funding, it's a known phenomenon when you look at who gets funded," explains Sam, "We know that in terms of who gets a seat at the table when dealing with the NHS, it's very polar, it's very uniform."

A 2020 report from McKinsey entitled *Diversity wins: how inclusion matters* sets out a clear data-informed business case for diversity, which shows that companies with more women and ethnic minority employees perform better and are more profitable than their less diverse counterparts. Having tracked 1,000 companies in 15 countries over five years, trends show that the higher the representation, the higher the likelihood of outperformance. However, hiring diverse talent isn't sufficient in itself, it is the experience people have in the workplace that shapes whether they remain and thrive. The report advocates not only diverse representation in leadership roles but also tackling the sorts of discrimination that Sam recounts to me, assertively and head-on.[33]

According to the McKinsey report, companies whose leaders welcome diverse talents and include multiple perspectives are likely to emerge from the pandemic crisis stronger. It is clear that diversity wins, now more than ever, the report concludes.[34] So back to the pandemic. What have we learnt about digital inequality and how to tackle it?

Just as Vital as a Food Parcel

It took a pandemic to make us realise we can't live without the internet. It has literally become the lifeline that can drag us out of the swamp of loneliness and isolation whilst connecting us to the things we depend on every day for our survival. During the pandemic, the internet was as vital as a food parcel to those of us who felt its impact the most.

Digital exclusion is experienced through daily omissions and indignities. Take for example, the letter sent by the NHS to those at highest risk of COVID-19 complications. Its various links to online information and support, for which the most part there was no offline equivalent, would have been largely irrelevant to the 175,000 or so non-internet users who received that letter.[35]

The Social Determinants of Digital ■ 131

"It's hard to look at Covid as a positive," says Rachel, when I ask her how it has affected her 100% Digital team. "Lots of services are behaving very reactively … doors are shut, so how do we reach those service users who are in need? Harder to reach now is even harder to reach." The need and demand for the team's support had increased exponentially, and the team was busier than ever.

Rachel tells me that all of their 450 4G-enabled iPads are out on loan to charities with lots waiting and a funding bid in the pipeline to get more. As we speak over the summer pandemic months, the team has been building the capacity of charities to help get people online through information, advice and webinars.

Rachel describes a spike in demand from organisations who come to her team saying "before we didn't really see a massive need for digital, but it's all we can offer our service users right now, so please can you help us." Rachel says her team is struggling to meet demand and she is worried that people already in need are now even more socially isolated and lonely.

"There's lots of amazing work going on in the city to get food parcels, prescriptions and all of that [out to vulnerable people] and we are just very keen to get digital aligned with that," Rachel explains, "because staying connected, being aware of all of that advice and guidance which is online, is just as vital as a food parcel." Rachel worries about people who can only afford small data plans and can no longer access the free Wi-Fi zones in the city "so that data that they have got has to last all day."

I was curious about how Rachel's team actually supports a charity that urgently needs to shift its activities online:

> Organisations were saying [to us] I used to run five sessions a week for people, we've got 1200 members, and now they're not going anywhere, they're literally not accessing anything, how do we get these activities online? How do we create a virtual offer other than welfare calls?

Those phone calls are massively time-consuming for these small organisations, Rachel was convinced there had to be a better way, "It would have more effect having a virtual session where someone's engaging in something interactive and it's social … the difference between a voice call and a video call is massive."

Rachel and her team trialled their COVID-19 response with one charity in the first week of lockdown to work out how they could best provide support. "They identified three service users who had a digital device … we offered them support to get onto the Zoom platform, so they did one-to-one calls talking that service user through how to use Zoom." But that was not as straightforward as it might seem, "we instantly found challenges that every service user has a different device, and trying to explain it over the phone, you can't physically see what you're trying to explain."

The team created a toolkit for how to use Zoom for each separate device so now the support can be tailored, and staff can email instructions to them if they have an email address. Workers have even found themselves going to people's houses and

132 ■ *Towards a Digital Ecology*

talking through the window or standing at the garden fence to explain things to people in person:

> We trialled a virtual coffee morning, which was great, and we do a round-robin, how's everyone doing, a real mental wellbeing check-in … and they all got so much out of it, people were saying 'I had a reason to get up in the morning' 'I had a reason to put my lipstick on' that real sense that people have something to look forward to.

Once they had developed a model that works, they engaged volunteers to do the call to get people set up with Zoom. In a stroke of genius, they also encouraged people who had got online to help their friends and families to do it too, "if I can do it, you can do it." They started to scale the approach across the city. "As the weeks have gone on, more [organisations] have been able to do it, a variety of things, history talks, life coaching sessions, mindfulness, managing anxiety, quizzes, coffee mornings, exercise sessions." Even people in a Breathe Easy group were getting their pulmonary rehabilitation support online.

I ask Rachel how they are supporting people who don't have a device in the first place, so can't benefit from the support they have developed. She tells me that in addition to the tablet lending scheme, they are working with a new initiative called DevicesDotNow,

> that's obviously a national programme, but we are signposting organisations to that to get devices that have got data built in, and we support funding bids as well, so to help organisations get the funding to get their own devices that they can give to service users.

The team has become genius at unearthing funding opportunities from benevolent companies that are willing to share reserves of cash to help them have a wider impact.

As with other aspects of the pandemic, charities and civil society responded at pace to the ravaging effects of the virus on the people Rachel describes to me. It happened in the very early days of that pandemic when we were still adjusting to the self-enforced isolation required to suture the pernicious viral spread. Realising the desperate nature of the situation, charities such as The Good Thinking Foundation and FutureDotNow came together to raise funds for devices and data to be distributed to people most in need, in an initiative called DevicesDotNow. They provided 10,000 of the most vulnerable people with devices, data and support.

Even though not having access to a device is a barrier "confidence is still the biggest," says Rachel,

> the amount of people who did have a device, but it was just in a box, or not being used, or just [people] not wanting to engage … and in those

first weeks it was 'yeah I won't bother because we'll be back in the coffee mornings next month, not realising the impact of Covid.

For Rachel, it's about motivating people, building their confidence, "people whose first language is not English are facing a big barrier, so giving instructions over the phone is challenging," she tells me.

An investigation by the Health Service Journal in early June revealed an inequality crack in the government's COVID-19 online test and trace system. The process included completing an online form on the NHS.UK website to order a test kit. Instructions are given to take a swab of the inside of your nose and the back of your throat, using a long cotton bud, via a kit delivered to your home. The HSJ found out that behind the scenes, the online application process was administered by a credit check company that used their rating system to verify the identity of people requesting the kit.

Whilst it was not a credit check and did not affect people's credit score, what it did do was exclude people who do not transact online and do not have online transactions that can be measured by a credit check company. The fact that you need an email address and that you asked for your national insurance number (not mandatory) are all steps in the process likely to exclude vulnerable and excluded groups such as migrants and travellers and people without a stable address.

The HSJ reported that if people refuse permission to access the TransUnion database, or if they refuse it, then they have to choose the drive-through option. This could be an impossible option for someone without a car or access to transport. Inequalities creep in through the cracks when the people designing systems are oblivious to them.

Beyond the Stats

"Make it person centred!"

This is the response from Rachel when I ask her what her hopes are for a post-pandemic digitally inclusive future. She advocates that "we stop, think and reflect about what changes we need to make going forward, so we are *never* in this position again."

Rachel recognises that this is a collaborative effort between different parts of government, civil society and the third sector. She wants her city to be a place where "people *do* have access to the internet, a device, the skills and support," and there is the capacity to reach out to everyone and offer them the help they need to get online. "If you're not on the ground working [in digital inclusion] it's easy to lose sight of what the problem is because you're so far removed from it," she tells me. Rachel sees the issue and its effects, upfront and personal every working day, and she wants things to change.

The fact that digital exclusion touches so many aspects of people's lives means it also touches on the responsibilities of many parts of government, from the

134 ■ *Towards a Digital Ecology*

Department of Health and Care, the Department of Culture Media and Sport to the Department of Work and Pensions. According to Emma, digital exclusion is everyone's and yet nobody's responsibility: "It's almost like there's much greater recognition of digital exclusion of patients and carers and citizens, but actually there's still not much clarity about what's the responsibility of the NHS itself."

Whilst the NHS is being told it needs to go digital, the consequences for those of us living in digital poverty run the risk of going unnoticed. "It just feels like everyone notices it now more," says Emma, "but whose responsibility is it to lead and coordinate and take action around this [issue]?" Emma believes we need to ask the right questions to have a hope of taking the right approach:

> who is driving digital inclusion and what is the real goal of it? And how far is the goal person-centred and about what that individual needs more broadly and holistically, as opposed to this is digital inclusion because the NHS needs it?

A letter from Simon Stevens, the chief executive of the NHS, on 31 July 2020, provided instructions to NHS organisations about how they should restore operations and prepare for a third phase pandemic response. All these communications are published on NHS England's website. The emphasis of the briefing is on inequality, with an urgent directive to support those people most affected by the pandemic.

Buried in the letter is an instruction to: "develop digitally enabled care pathways in ways which increase inclusion, including reviewing who is using new primary, outpatient and mental health digitally enabled care pathways by 31 March." Roz tells me that regions understand there is a problem but they are looking for more direction from the centre to do more to improve digital inclusion. "If you understand the NHS, it's very centrally driven, and that phase three letter has had a really powerful effect actually, just that one line has had a powerful effect," Roz tells me.

Roz describes a sense of urgency across the regions:

> Most [integrated care systems] are recognising digital inclusion as a priority but it's early days. There are a handful that really get, and then there's a load who get it but haven't got very far, and then there's a few who are not even bothered about it yet.

Roz counters my scepticism with enthusiasm; she is optimistic about the future:

> We can't move for people wanting to talk to us about this, CIOs and CCIOs included. Those people would not have been talking about digital inclusion a couple of years ago, so they're ready, they understand it's an issue, but they don't know what to do.

She explains that they have clocked on to the fact that "If we carry on with this digital by default regardless, then there's a big flaw in the plan."

Roz believes that because the NHS is so large, is such a big employer and has so many volunteers, it can leverage its resources and its might to make things better. Roz believes this is essentially an issue of social change: "and social change doesn't come from government, it comes from civil society." As large organisations and employers within local communities, NHS organisations can actively contribute to improving social and economic conditions through how they employ people, purchase goods and services, use buildings and spaces and work in partnership;

> The NHS is a movement in itself and we've really seen that in the last year. It's really come into its own. The NHS was created from social change and I think people in the NHS, and remember the NHS is people, have been incredible over covid, they've come together, they've challenged, they've taken a scientific approach [to the pandemic] and sometimes in opposition to this government's philosophy.

The notion of NHS organisations as *anchor institutions* whereby they choose to make a positive difference in their communities is gaining currency and is one way in which they might consider their contribution to evening out inequality.[36] It could be anything from lending a community space to a digital inclusion project or giving used laptops to a charity. With a bit of creative thinking, the NHS can continue its tradition and momentum towards social change.

Digital exclusion is just one of the consequences of systemic inequality that casts a heavy persistent shadow over society at large. As the intersection of so many other socio-economic factors, there is no quick fix, despite the fact those in charge would like you to believe it is the case. Systemic challenges call for systemic changes. And those have to be wanted, voted for and enacted by governments, fought for by ordinary people.

I am alert to the fact that these systemic barriers may feel remote for start-ups and SMEs developing digital products and services for the NHS. I ask Emma that beyond inclusive design practices, what should any good company be considering? "It's about understanding that your market is not simply divided into those who have access and those who don't. Actually there are those issues about skills and confidence and how much data you can afford."

Emma implores start-ups to think carefully about the demographics of who will be using their product and avoiding making assumptions about their access, confidence and capability:

> People can get the 'I don't have a device' and they can get 'I cant afford home broadband' …. What isn't visible is 'well I have a device but I can really only use it to do these [small number of] things and anything else is too complicated, or I'm not interested, or it feels really dangerous to me.

136 ◼ *Towards a Digital Ecology*

In a digital inclusion review, The Kings' Fund identifies factors that increase the likelihood that digital technology will actually get used by people who are least digitally included. I was particularly struck by the need to tailor digital services to people's contexts, understanding how they live their lives day-to-day when they are not in the GP surgery or the clinic. Making sure that information is not only relevant but credible to people is another factor – do I look at a mobile app and think this is something that I can relate to, feel happy using, and says something about my life?

Some good news to accompany Roz's enthusiasm is that the All-Party Parliamentary Group on Social Integration produced a report[37] during the pandemic that makes the case for expanding and developing the sorts of initiatives that Rachel is involved in. They conclude: "The COVID-19 crisis has exposed a huge digital divide in this country" and state that "it is essential that, when the current crisis period ends, there is long-term commitment from the Government, educational institutions, employers and civil society to reduce digital exclusion."[38] This appears to be a topic that has risen up the agenda that maybe the Government can no longer ignore.

It is clear that digital exclusion is a symptom of deep inequality and lack of opportunity experienced by the very people the NHS most needs to reach out and support. A modern NHS must meet their needs first and foremost. How do we help our 70-year-old NHS keep those core founding principles at its core – meeting the needs of everyone, free at the point of delivery, based on clinical need, not ability to pay? Rachel is proud to work in a city whose stated ambition is that people who are the poorest improve their health the fastest. This is a call to arms to all of us whether we be mobile app developers, AI experts, policymakers or everyday patients and citizens. Let's harness the inexorable push towards digital technology that creates an ecology that works for everyone.

Notes

1 https://socialintegrationappg.org.uk/wp-content/uploads/2020/06/Social-Connection-in-the-COVID-19-Crisis.pdf
2 https://www.newstatesman.com/politics/health/2020/06/dark-side-wellness-industry
3 https://en.wikipedia.org/wiki/OK_Computer
4 https://www.nesta.org.uk/feature/health-design/we-dont-want-normal-we-want-better/?utm_source=Nesta+Weekly+Newsletter&utm_campaign=3e44a1c66c-EMAIL_CAMPAIGN_2020_05_26_11_41_COPY_03&utm_medium=email&utm_term=0_d17364114d-3e44a1c66c-182283923
5 https://socialmetricscommission.org.uk/
6 https://www.health.org.uk/publications/long-reads/will-covid-19-be-a-watershed-moment-for-health-inequalities?utm_campaign=11582911_COVID-19%20and%20health%20inequalities%20%2011%20June%202020%20%20WARM&utm_medium=email&utm_source=The%20Health%20Foundation&dm_i=4Y2,6W9FJ,18YGUJ,RP6OU,1

The Social Determinants of Digital ■ 137

7 https://www.theguardian.com/commentisfree/2020/nov/09/normality-luxury-wealthy-covid-pandemic-kim-kardashian

8 https://www.health.org.uk/news-and-comment/charts-and-infographics/emerging-findings-on-the-impact-of-covid-19-on-black-and-min?utm_campaign=11582911_COVID-19%20and%20health%20inequalities%20%2011%20June%202020%20%20WARM&utm_medium=email&utm_source=The%20Health%20Foundation&dm_i=4Y2,6W9FJ,18YGUJ,RP6OU,1

9 https://www.health.org.uk/news-and-comment/charts-and-infographics/same-pandemic-unequal-impacts

10 https://www.cebm.net/wp-content/uploads/2020/05/BAME-COVID-Rapid-Data-Evidence-Review-Final-Hidden-in-Plain-Sight-compressed.pdf

11 https://assets.publishing.service.gov.uk/government/uploads/system/uploads/attachment_data/file/892376/COVID_stakeholder_engagement_synthesis_beyond_the_data.pdf

12 https://phw.nhs.wales/publications/publications1/digital-technology-and-health-inequalities-a-scoping-review/

13 https://www.goodthingsfoundation.org/sites/default/files/research-publications/good_things_foundation_covid19_response_report_march_june_2020.pdf

14 https://diabetes.jmir.org/2018/4/e10925/pdf

15 https://www.acpjournals.org/doi/pdf/10.7326/0003-4819-155-2-201107190-00005

16 https://www.goodthingsfoundation.org/sites/default/files/research-publications/digital_inclusion_in_health_and_care-_lessons_learned_from_the_nhs_widening_digital_participation_programme_2017-2020__0.pdf

17 https://www.ofcom.org.uk/__data/assets/pdf_file/0027/196407/online-nation-2020-report.pdf (p.29)

18 https://www.health.org.uk/sites/default/files/upload/publications/2019/Untapped%20potential.pdf

19 Perez, 2019, p.207

20 https://www.bbc.co.uk/news/health-52454741

21 https://www.tuc.org.uk/sites/default/files/PPEandwomenguidance.pdf

22 https://www.thelancet.com/journals/landig/article/PIIS2589-7500(20)30317-4/fulltext?mc_cid=5c9789452b&mc_eid=ada8f378ea

23 http://ai.ahsnnetwork.com/about/ai-in-health-and-care/

24 https://www.thelancet.com/journals/landig/article/PIIS2589-7500(20)30240-5/fulltext

25 https://www.thelancet.com/journals/landig/article/PIIS2589-7500(21)00019-4/fulltext

26 https://ischool.utoronto.ca/profile/brian-cantwell-smith/

27 https://www.theguardian.com/commentisfree/2020/may/16/for-all-its-sophistication-ai-isnt-fit-to-make-life-or-death-decisions-for-us

28 https://www.adalovelaceinstitute.org/wp-content/uploads/2020/11/The-data-will-see-you-now-Ada-Lovelace-Institute-Oct-2020.pdf

29 https://asiansintech.com/top-100-asian-stars-in-uk-tech-2020/

30 https://amp.ft.com/content/43f7cece-0086-11ea-be59-e49b2a136b8d

31 https://www.healthcareitnews.com/blog/emea/glass-ceiling-i-can-see-through

32 https://www.digitalhealth.net/2019/10/diversity-in-digital-health-is-a-matter-of-patient-safety/

33 https://www.mckinsey.com/~/media/McKinsey/Featured%20Insights/Diversity%20and%20Inclusion/Diversity%20wins%20How%20inclusion%20matters/Diversity-wins-How-inclusion-matters-vF.pdf

138 ■ Towards a Digital Ecology

34 https://www.mckinsey.com/~/media/McKinsey/Featured%20Insights/Diversity%20 and%20Inclusion/Diversity%20wins%20How%20inclusion%20matters/Diversity-wins-How-inclusion-matters-vF.pdf
35 https://www.goodthingsfoundation.org/sites/default/files/research-publications/good_things_foundation_covid19_response_report_march_june_2020.pdf
36 https://www.health.org.uk/publications/long-reads/anchors-in-a-storm?utm_campaign=12186513_HALN%20launch%20%2023%20Feb%202021%20%20COLD%20audiences&utm_medium=email&utm_source=The%20Health%20Foundation&dm_i=4Y2,79769,18YGUJ,TEVLV,1
37 https://socialintegrationappg.org.uk/wp-content/uploads/2020/06/Social-Connection-in-the-COVID-19-Crisis.pdf
38 https://socialintegrationappg.org.uk/wp-content/uploads/2020/06/Social-Connection-in-the-COVID-19-Crisis.pdf

Chapter 8

The Jeopardy of Trust

> Data is not, and has never been, neutral. Data practices have social practices 'baked in', so when we talk about data we are also talking about the socio technical structures around its capture. How data has been gathered, interpreted and used reflects accepted social norms. We are always in the process of constructing data, and our relationship with it is dynamic and often unequal. Choices society makes about the production and use of data reflects the distribution of power and is conditioned by power asymmetries.[1]

Interoperability is the technical challenge of systems being able to seamlessly share data between them. But there is a human challenge too. That is the challenge of trust. It is not just the spectre of NPfIT that looms over efforts to digitise the NHS. There are a number of high-profile data debacles that cast a long shadow over endeavours to use data for what is known as *secondary purposes* that is to improve care, for research and to develop new products and services for healthcare.

Health data is valuable. Despite the fragmentation of the NHS, our healthcare system remains the single largest integrated healthcare provider in the world, with primary care patient records covering the entire population from birth through to death.[2] Electronic patient record systems in hospitals are less well-established but nevertheless house around 23 million secondary episodic patient records. A 2019 report by global consultancy, EY, estimated that the 55 million GP records held by the NHS have an indicative market value of several billion pounds. The data stakes are high.

There are a number of reasons why data is so valuable. It begins with the personal. Data helps clinicians diagnose and treat us. Our data tells a deeply personal story about who we are, where we have come from, what conditions we may experience in the future and what might be preventable. Tools such as predictive risk

DOI: 10.1201/9781032198798-8

139

140 ■ *Towards a Digital Ecology*

algorithms use data from electronic records to predict the possibility of an individual developing an illness or needing emergency treatment; they can support and enhance clinical decision-making by analysing data in a way that it would be hard for an individual clinician to do. Data is interwoven into the tapestry of our healthcare system, threads that combine together to create deeply rich woven fabric.

Once that data is combined with millions of other similar datasets, it enables analysts to see patterns and develop insights at a population level. These insights can be used to find new ways to predict or diagnose illness and improve care. This data can also be used to innovate – helping find new solutions to intransigent healthcare issues. But it is not just the NHS that has a role in innovating, so do universities, pharmaceutical companies and increasingly technology companies. And things are moving fast. Developments in technology are not only outpacing policy and regulation but also racing ahead of public attitudes and tolerances to how data is kept safe, used and accounted for.[3]

The promise of data to innovate and improve health is significant. Not only do we need public trust but we need that data to be usable. If we get our act together to standardise and codify data, then we can use it to treat the things about us that are not standard and codified. But at the moment we have the reverse. Because data is not routinely standardised, clean, comprehensive and consistent, it can't be used to create insight that would enable care to be better personalised to our personal needs. Unstandardised data equals standardised care. You get what you are given.

The Boundaries of Health Data

Let us pause for a moment to consider what constitutes health data. It is no longer just the information that is captured in our clinical record. Clues to our health are also rendered through the smartphones that many of us carry in our pockets. With advances in data science, everyday data that we spew out as we go about our daily lives can and is used to infer how healthy (or not) we are. What we search for online, our supermarket loyalty card, the widget on our smartphone that records the steps we take, the words and phrases we use on social media platforms, even *how* we use our smartphone; all of these are data points that can be used as proxies for our health.[4] This is where it starts to become fiendishly complicated.

Data only becomes really valuable when it is aggregated, processed and linked to create a longitudinal dataset, showing patterns over time. However, as we have seen in previous chapters, lack of interoperability and standardisation means that there are significant costs in curating, processing and analysing patient data.[5] The NHS has not been great at nurturing data analytics capability, that is experts who can make sense of the data we do collect, in order that we can do good things with it.[6] Much of this data remains fragmented, siloed and unanalysed. Even now, more patient data than we might imagine sits in paper records, stored in massive filing cabinets and moved around on trolleys by porters. Try and think back to your last

The Jeopardy of Trust ■ 141

inpatient encounter or outpatient appointment, recall how much was written down with paper and pen.

Fatima's most recent outpatient hospital visit was to have a suspicious lump in her breast examined. Having had previous mammograms, this was not the first time she had visited that particular hospital clinic. Fatima idly flicked through ragged copies of *OK!* magazine with the familiar dread in her stomach as she waited to be called in for her appointment. As she entered the consultation room, she observed the consultant rifling through her paper notes, held together with metal tags. Perplexed, her doctor couldn't locate details of her previous visit some years earlier. It was left to Sarah to dredge her memory in order to recall and recount what she hoped were the most salient facts.

Some weeks later, when she got a call back from a nurse to tell her that her mammogram was clear, she exhaled with relief. The doctor had given her the all-clear during her appointment, but it was good to know her test results confirmed the clinical assessment. However that was not the end of the story. Somewhat embarrassed, the nurse told Fatima that the doctor had either not written up her notes or she had failed to press record on her dictaphone. Either way, there was no record of the consultation. Fatima had to go back and repeat the consultation just so that part of her longitudinal record was correct in case of a future encounter. She couldn't help but imagine what this mistake had cost the NHS trust (never mind the personal inconvenience and time taken out of work) and what it would add up to if multiplied across appointments at a regional or even national scale.

Through our publicly funded, free at the point of demand NHS, we are collectively bound in a social contract that binds citizens, professionals and institutions together in equitable healthcare for all. But these firm foundations were established when our data was captured in handwritten notes on paper, bound together and stored on shelves and in filing cabinets. We have work to do in order to make sense of what this social contract means when it comes to the gallons of data we produce between us as patients, citizens and professionals each and every day.

However, a debate about information that operates in a closed loop between patients and clinicians is just one part of the story. It was no surprise to me to discover that the global *quantified self-movement*, where self-tracking and health monitoring are everything, has its origins in the Californian tech scene.[7] Whether it be steps, calories or vital signs, everything is quantified for an optimised health-fulfilled existence.

The tools that were once the domain of health professionals are now embedded in the hardware of our smartphone or smartwatch. We have become our own physicians and created our own personal surveillance systems. As the ethos of quantification, which used to be the preserve of geeks, has seeped into our everyday existence, virtuosity has become intrinsically linked to a willingness to quantify our lives. The information in our health records is now just a fraction of the data we produce and is used for all sorts of purposes we may not appreciate or fully understand.

142 ■ *Towards a Digital Ecology*

The Data That Didn't Care

Back in 2006, Clive Humby, American scientist and inventor of the Tesco Clubcard, coined the phrase *data is the new oil*, and if data is oil then healthcare data is rocket fuel, as NHS England learnt to their cost back in 2013. Recognising the value of data for *secondary purposes* of planning services and medical research, the national care.data programme set out to take data from GP practices and put it into a central database for use by planners, researchers and industry.

Not only would the anonymised data be used by the NHS, it would also be used by research and even commercial organisations. The public were informed by letter that this process would happen automatically unless they opted out by informing their GP. This did not go down well. Headlines such as *care.data: how did it all go so wrong?* from the BBC[8] reflect the massive outcry that ensued, both from clinicians and the public. A concerted campaign soon thwarted what many believed was essentially a reasonable programme with laudable aims. So how *did* it all go so wrong?

The project was abandoned just a year after it began, after widespread criticism, including a damning report from The Major Projects Authority, which concluded there were "major issues with project definition, schedule, budget, quality and/or benefits delivery, which … do not appear to be manageable or resolvable."[9] With uncanny echoes of the previously doomed NPfIT programme which had finally limped to a sorry end just a year earlier, this was a centrally led project that attempted to move at pace. As is so often the case, the project failed to win support from key stakeholders and fell into a chasm of ill-defined scope, uncertain achievability and incompetent implementation.

Around the same time care.data was abandoned, another uncomfortable and embarrassing data mess-up was under scrutiny. Sir Nick Partridge, a non-executive director of the Health and Social Care Information Centre (HSCIC), was asked to lead a review of data[10] that had been released by the NHS Information Centre (a predecessor organisation). Partridge concludes that: "It disappoints me to report that the review has discovered lapses in the strict arrangements that were supposed to be in place to ensure that people's personal data would never be used improperly."

The report determines that despite the fact there was no evidence of harm arising from this gaff "It does not excuse errors that … still would create concerns for the public about the controls that are in place." He concludes that this is as much about trust and confidence as it is about security. There are a number of what the report determines are "grave lapses" that it uncovered in tight controls on our data. This left a heavy question hanging over the NHS – is our healthcare system competent to be trusted with keeping our data safe and secure?

There are few people better placed to reflect on NHS data lapses such as care. data and its ramifications for the present day, than Dr Natalie Banner. As the lead for Understanding Patient Data (UPD), an initiative hosted at the Wellcome Trust, Natalie has a formidable background. She has a PhD in philosophy and has held policy roles in ethics and the governance of genetic and genomic data as well as advocating

The Jeopardy of Trust ■ 143

on behalf of the research sector's on the introduction of GDPR. It is fair to speculate that what she doesn't know about patient data probably isn't worth knowing.

My conversation with Natalie takes place in early June, over a now customary video call. The early evening sun pouring into my makeshift office meant I had to adjust my laptop to see the screen. The warmth of the fading day seemed to reflect an emerging optimism as the first lockdown was beginning to ease and the curve of the pandemic appeared to be descending. At that point, the death toll globally was 365,105 globally and 38,243 in the UK according to the Johns Hopkins dashboard. Little did we know, we were only experiencing a brief reprieve in the pandemic ordeal.

Coronavirus was dominating the news, and in particular, the story of the prime minister's aide Dominic Cummings and his 240-mile trip from London to Durham in the early days of the lockdown. This story was pertinent to my conversation with Natalie because talk of data inevitably turns to talk of public trust in our institutions and those who govern them.

Even though she maintains the motivation behind care.data was ostensibly a sound one, Natalie describes how its execution in practice was disastrous. Not only did the NHS make it difficult for people to opt out of sharing their data: "if you registered for certain opt outs you wouldn't get invited for screening services, so it would actually impact on your care."

The badly thought through technical implementation was compounded by what Natalie described as an old-fashioned and paternalistic attitude on the part of NHS bureaucrats:

> It was like 'we can tell people what's happening if we have to' but there wasn't a sense that actually, hello, this is data that's come from people, it matters to them, they have a right to be informed, they have a right to express a view or a choice.

NHS bosses failed to understand the impact of what they were trying to achieve: "It was all dismissed because the data was so important and it was valuable and all you have to do is educate people and they will understand how much it matters."

Whilst care.data may be less present in the general public's memory, it weighs heavily in the memories of those who work in healthcare: "It's created a real culture of risk aversion, of anything to do with data," says Natalie, as she describes an atmosphere of "absolute terror" when it comes to data: "If we get this wrong, we are going to be in it, we will have The Daily Mail down our throats." As digital technologies generating vast swathes of data become more present in the NHS, the fear of getting it wrong with data is ever more heightened.

A Cautionary Tale

There is another story that runs deep in recent digital health history, which illuminates tensions between public and private interests. In 2016, the Royal Free London

144 ■ *Towards a Digital Ecology*

NHS Foundation Trust announced a partnership with DeepMind to develop Streams, an app that improves the detection of acute kidney injury by immediately reviewing blood test results for signs of deterioration and sending an alert with the results to the most appropriate clinician via a dedicated handheld device.

In April 2016, The *New Scientist* first ran the damning story.[11] The Royal Free had provided personal data of around 1.6 million patients, without explicit consent, as part of this trial to test an alert, diagnosis and detection system for acute kidney injury. The data included highly personal and sensitive details such as whether patients had been diagnosed with HIV, experienced depression or even if they had ever undergone an abortion.

What turbocharged this into a public interest story was the fact that the start-up had been acquired by Google. DeepMind was now owned by one of the big four global technology companies, whose business model is predicated on monetising personal data – that is the data that you and I produce every time we do a search using their internet engine. The case created profound questions about a private organisation's access to large publicly generated health datasets on which they could build products and services. Indeed, a memorandum of understanding between the two parties released under a Freedom of Information Request[12] sets out DeepMind's ambitions for the partnership: "a clinical and operational test-bed, a strategic steer in product development and, most of all, for data for machine learning research." It is evident that data was at the heart of their digital health ambitions.

The big four global conglomerates (Google, Apple, Facebook and Amazon) all have an interest in digital health.[13] DeepMind achieved what many a start-up dreams of – they were acquired by one of the most powerful private companies in the world – creating wealth for themselves and their investors. Companies such as Google who buy out start-ups are invariably interested not only in the innovation itself but in the data that it gives them access to. Health data is massively valuable. And a small number of powerful companies with monopolistic control of large health datasets should raise alarm bells. Large amounts of data in the hands of a small number of private operators has the potential to inhibit innovation – putting others off even attempting to enter the field.

In their critique of the case, Powels and Hodson[14] call this incident "a prism of the future" of digital health where private interests collide with public health priorities and where the stakes are high. They argue that, with access to large datasets, companies such as Google could obtain a monopolistic position over health analytics not just in the UK but internationally. Data transferred into private hands take them out of democratic control, public scrutiny and accountability. It turns out that Google knows a lot about us but we know little about them – a one-way mirror.

This particular incident raised an interesting conundrum that we will come back to later – how might we rethink our data assets as a public resource that is held in the commons rather than by private organisations. This is both a challenge and an opportunity for our National Health Service. But it needs the expertise and the nouse to leverage its power and realise the value of the data for which it is custodian and keeper.

WannaCry

If you happen to mention the word *WannaCry* to a friend or colleague who was working in IT back in 2017 then you're likely to see a visible shudder. I recall an urgent call from our head of the IT department the day after the events which started on Friday 12 May, asking me to come to the office and have my laptop updated with the latest software patches. It was the day the NHS got held to ransom.

Stephen was an NHS chief information officer at the time and remembers it all too well: "I think I was sitting in my office and everyone was like, quick look at the news, I think it was BBC, and then also text messages from a number of CIOs saying, hey something's going on." Even though his Trust was reasonably well prepared, this wasn't the case for everyone:

> Some [Trusts] got hit badly, there were stories of people, when they got hit, they shut everything down, they shut down all the accesses to the outside world, but then when the switch to kill [the virus] was discovered, you could only get it if you were accessing the outside world, so people were like oh shit I've just shut everything down.

WannaCry was a significant global cyber security event that happened to particularly affect the NHS. The WannaCry ransomware encrypted data and files on 230, 000 computers in 150 countries. Whilst it wasn't specifically aimed at the NHS, it blocked key systems, preventing staff from accessing patient data and critical services such as MRI scanners. The attack affected 236 hospitals and 595 GP practices, resulting in the cancellation of 20,000 appointments and cost the NHS around £92 million in service disruption and emergency IT upgrades.

The disruption to clinical services brought into startling relief just how dependent the NHS is on IT systems. Out of date infrastructure makes systems massively vulnerable to attacks, running old computers that aren't actively supported by operating systems. Stephen is scathing, "I don't care what they say the reasons are" [old systems and PCs],

> they just shouldn't be doing it, it's as simple as that. The security risks [are huge] and if it's a hassle to renew the application, or modernise it, or something, there is always a way round it, you can do something, for me it's like, get it out of there, get it out of there, it's not on.

In a retrospective analysis of WannaCry in the science journal *Nature*, the authors conclude that healthcare is one of the most vulnerable sectors to cyberattacks. This is simply because our healthcare system is running too many out-of-date systems. Whilst the incident has resulted in an increase in cybersecurity investment, the authors argue that there still remains a need for an increase in IT budgets "to ensure that current systems can be sustained securely and that healthcare systems are resilient in the face of attacks."

146 ■ *Towards a Digital Ecology*

Cybercrime is on the up, and this is a particular worry for the NHS for reasons that won't surprise you. According to *The Lancet*: "health-care organisations also take substantially longer than other industries to contain data breaches because of a lack of resources, both financial resources and trained personnel, and inefficient infrastructure." Cyberattacks are for the most part opportunistic and target those organisations that are the least prepared. The NHS is a sitting duck.

The most common type of data breach in healthcare is known as misdelivery which covers for example, sending an email and addresses to the wrong distribution list, sometimes with a file containing sensitive data. Human error is alive and well. The second most common data breach is an attack through web applications. As more organisations create mobile applications to interact with patients: "they create additional lucrative attack surfaces." As digital technologies embed themselves into the fabric of healthcare, these sorts of risks do too.

Despite their best efforts, *The Lancet* reports that they were unable to find evidence of a catalogue that systematically lists all software and hardware deployed within the NHS. They conclude that the NHS is ill-prepared for a future attack and that the NHS is at risk of: "substantial reputational and financial loss, and, most importantly, risk to patients' safety." WannaCry showed how dependent we already are on digital technology to deliver NHS services. With massive efforts to digitise the NHS, this will only increase. We need to get our security sorted.

Cybersecurity issues remain a real threat. In the first two months of the pandemic panic, the NHS received almost 30,000 malicious emails. It turns out that it is not just the virus that has spread across the globe, it has been closely tailed by an increase in cybercrime. Enterprising criminals played on people's pandemic fears by sending malicious emails about the virus, asking people to click on a document that took them to a fake webpage which then harvested login details. We might think we're wise to this stuff, but it's easy to get caught out when our minds are busy and we're wading through an overbearing inbox.

The wholesale pandemic shift to homeworking increased security risks and resulted in NHS Digital issuing guidance to staff, which included imploring people to not click on suspicious links or open any suspicious attachments, change the admin/default password on the home broadband router and make sure they are running all the latest versions of software on all their devices. With cybersecurity, the responsibility of individual GP practices and NHS trusts, NHS Digital even has a *Keep I.T. Confidential* campaign in an attempt to build awareness of good local security practices.

Cybersecurity is not just about IT systems, it's also about the minutiae of how many of us manage our personal health through mobile apps and devices. For those of us with elderly parents, the allure of wearable devices or sensors in homes to keep a check on their well-being is powerful. With busy lives and long distances keeping us apart, why wouldn't we use technology to keep us connected? The benefits seem clear and the risks negligible.

Security consultancy Pen Test Partners, who have a reputation for ethical hacking to winkle out security weaknesses, found a worrying problem with a smartwatch that can trigger reminders to the wearer to take their medication. What they found was scary: "Like every smart tracker watch we've looked at, anyone with some basic hacking skills could track the wearer, audio bug them using the watch, or perhaps worst, could trigger the medication alert as often as they want." The team speculates that for an older person with memory problems who is perhaps taking multiple medications, an overdose is not inconceivable. Whilst they contacted the company involved, and the vulnerability was quickly secured, it highlights the risks that security gaps can provide. These are real-world problems not obvious to the casual observer.

Andy Evans, a regional chief information officer in the Midlands, is a concerned man. He is seriously worried about online attacks, combined with what he sees as a laissez-faire attitude towards cybersecurity. He puts down this complacency, in part, to cognitive overload on the part of clinicians and managers. During the pandemic he found that there was only so much people could cope with managing. "I had several conversations with doctors where they said to me 'If you don't do this someone will die' and I said you know if you get this wrong and we have a WannaCry then thousands will die."

It might not be uppermost in many people's minds, but for Andy cybersecurity is a persistent nagging headache that won't go away. Keen to persuade me that he's not being dramatic, Andy implores me to look at the National Cyber Security Centre website. The first headline I encounter proudly proclaims that the organisation defended us from 700 cyberattacks during the first pandemic wave.[15] This is clearly a real and present challenge that we should take seriously.

"The next time we have a WannaCry they'll take all the data," says Andy: "We got collateral damage, [from WannaCry] we accidentally got caught in the target" but the sophistication of cybercrime has moved on, and Andy believes in the NHS we're struggling to keep up. An impassioned advocate for cybersecurity, Andy finishes up by reminding us the stakes are high: "We know if we get [cybersecurity] wrong then it's game over, the public will never trust us again."

Amazonian Challenges

One data problem in healthcare is an asymmetric relationship between the NHS and big tech giants. When the NHS is collaborating with massive profit-making companies over the data it stewards on behalf of the public, it starts to get messy. When the NHS starts to monetise the very data it is acting as a steward for, the lines become increasingly blurred. Under the headline "Amazon ready to cash in on free access to NHS data" on 8 December,[16] *The Times* broke a story arguing that Amazon has been given access to vast swathes of data that it could then use to develop commercial products without any benefit back to the NHS.

148 ■ *Towards a Digital Ecology*

The Ada Lovelace Institute pick up the story in a post[17] in which they explain that although the deal was struck between Amazon and the NHS in December 2018, it wasn't announced until six months later and the contract was only put in the public domain[18] after a freedom of information request by a campaign group, Privacy International. On the surface, the deal seems a reasonable one. Amazon's Alexa can access NHS website data to give reliable health information to its users.

However, digging into the heavily redacted contract, Ada Lovelace highlights what they call some significant asymmetries of power, in which they argue Amazon get a significantly better deal than the NHS:

> It permits Amazon to access 'all healthcare information' including 'symptoms, causes and definitions' and 'other materials' held by the Secretary of State for Health and Social Care. Under this contract, Amazon is free to use the data to make, advertise and sell 'new products, applications, cloud-based services and/or distributed software' and can share the information with affiliates and third parties. The license applies around the world and cannot be withdrawn, giving Amazon free access to this data in perpetuity.

They make the case that the government is relatively under-resourced to strike decent deals with massive companies and is in a weak position to make deals that benefit the public and which maintain trust.

Even more disturbing, the contract gives Amazon the right to vet all publicity from the Department of Health and Social Care and that it can't issue any press releases or other publicity without their prior written consent. This is a clear tension between public bodies with democratic accountability and private companies in whose interests it is to control and contain the message, this cannot be good for democracy. And it can't be good for innovation.

The Internet of Health

The social contract which I cited at the beginning of this chapter is relatively easy to define when it involves citizens and the state. However, it starts to fray when private organisations enter the field. These are the big tech companies and the digital health start-ups that capture and analyse and feedback our health status to us. Sometimes we are active agents and sometimes we are passive know-nothings. Sometimes we can harness that data to improve our health. On other occasions, it can have unforeseen and unwanted consequences. Often we don't have much choice.

The traces we often unwittingly leave behind us as we conduct our online lives have been given the fancy name of *digital phenotyping*. The idea is that these crumbs of activity are harvested through algorithms that start to paint an inferred picture of our health. In 2017, Facebook hit the headlines when it created an algorithm to

The Jeopardy of Trust ■ 149

detect when people might be suicidal by analysing the content of their posts.[19] *The New York Times* reported that one person had been visited by police after posting on Facebook and was taken to hospital against their will for a mental health assessment.[20] This example raises all sorts of confounding questions about the role of technology companies in public health as well as how they use our data and the real-world actions they may take as a result. Not only are the lines between health data and non-health data blurred, we are gently slipping into a world of veiled surveillance.

Facebook may have had good intentions in their attempts to prevent suicide. At the very least they will have wanted to find ways to minimise the negative press associated with a spate of people taking their own lives whilst live streaming on the platform. But what about when companies exploit the data leaking from our online clicks to not only predict but to monetise our health. Knowing we are overweight or sad, eating too many takeaways, or not doing enough exercise, are all opportunities to sell us pills, diets and exercise apps. It is not a huge leap into a more dystopian future where our application for life insurance or a loan is turned down because we've eaten one too many doughnuts. This is the Orwellian reality we may find ourselves sleepwalking into, one small slumbering step at a time.

I recall a conference where an enthusiastic start-up presented their occupational health solution that they were already selling in the US and hoping to bring to the UK. It has seared itself in my mind because it so disturbed me. They showed an organisational dashboard that gave an overview of their employee's health and well-being. Managers could see at a glance how much sleep an employee had had the night before and even what their hydration levels were like. I don't know about you, but I don't believe my employer has a right to know how many beers I glugged the night before or that I stayed up later than I would have liked binging on a box set. Both Fitbit and Jawbone have developed enterprise solutions, including trackers and dashboards to help employers assess workplace wellness and chivvy staff to improve their health.[21] This is a future of ubiquitous quantification and management by an algorithm. It's not a future that appeals to me.

One London

> I would assume also that the information that they have at the GP, the hospital can see it too. I'm not sure, because sometimes when you go to the hospital, they ask so many questions, but you think, how can you not know? Don't you have all my information? It is exhausting because you're in so much pain and still need to explain it.
>
> One London Citizens' Summit participant[22]

I wonder where this backdrop of mistrust and concern leaves us today. Almost half of us are not happy for companies to collect and use our personal information under any circumstances. This is an upward trend.[23] There was a time when Facebook and

150 ■ *Towards a Digital Ecology*

Instagram were seen as the good guys, disrupting us all with their novel platforms, seducing us into a world of convenience and connectivity. They may still have us in their grasp, but the honeymoon period is over. We have become wiser to their obfuscated business models. It is increasingly apparent that our pact with these digital ogres gets us free stuff in return for our time, attention and data.

This decline in public trust bestows a murky backdrop for our attitudes towards health data. Within this landscape of equivocal trust, big tech giants at the forefront of the canvas and debacles like care.data and WannaCry at the back, what hope does the NHS have of building public confidence. Well, it turns out there is a seed of hope in a London project which has attempted a more mature conversation with the public on this ever-fraught issue.

"It was quite a personal journey," says Amy Darlington as I interview her from my sitting room on a sunny midsummer day. I feel see the sun streaming in through the French windows as I transcribe our conversation. I first met Amy when she was designing an ambitious public participation exercise around the use of data in the capital city. As a communications expert and executive director at Imperial College Health Partners, Amy has worked in the field of public engagement for more years than she cares to remember.

"I didn't really understand public deliberation," explains Amy: "I didn't understand the power of it. And I am now the strongest advocate. When there are complex problems, it's a really good methodology to get very considered and informed public opinion to help inform decision making and policy." Amy is the force behind an ambitious undertaking that sought to dig deep into public attitudes towards health and care data amongst residents of London. It's an interesting case study on how to meaningfully involve lay people in a purposeful debate on an important topic.

"We have to do more to build public trust in the uses of health and care data. Huge mistakes have been made in the past, it's a hugely complicated area, and it's rife with confusion." This was the drive for Amy and her team when health and care organisations in London came together as One London to apply to be one of the shared care record sites under the Local Health and Care Record Exemplar (LCHRE) programme back in 2018. With a 15-million-pound prize, London was one of five regions that won bids to connect the myriad of separate health and care records together so that information could be shared for individual care, planning services and research.

Amy was certain that, if they were going to get this right, they had to involve London residents. She describes a high level of anxiety amongst the team who knew this was a complicated topic: "people just expect that their personal data is shared for treatment and care already; NHS providers are anxious about what they can and can't do; clinicians are unclear about what their patients do and don't want; privacy campaigners are concerned about the role of commercial organisations "and on and on it goes," sighs Amy.

The Jeopardy of Trust ▪ 151

"The fact that there is a legal basis for sharing data … we felt didn't provide us with the level of legitimacy that was needed for a programme such as One London to have longevity." Amy and the team quickly recognised that one of the key risks to that programme was "a lack of public trust and confidence in realising the many benefits that are there when joining up health and care information."

"So we said, we really need to invest in a meaningful conversation with Londoners," and when the One London team was successful in their bid, it was down to Amy to lead this daunting part of the project. Having that conversation with the 9 million London residents, who between them speak 300 languages was going to be no small challenge.[24]

"All our premise for engagement was, we need to have a strong understanding of what people's expectations are with the use of health and care data" but more importantly that "what their expectations are, rooted in how a health and care system operates." This is the approach that makes the One London stand out from more common attempts to get out onto the streets or compose a questionnaire or any other approach that simply asks people for their views.

> Historic engagement had tended to either focus on perceived benefits or perceived concerns but it hadn't got into a conversation with the public about how they weight up those benefits and concerns. What benefits are you willing to give up to address your concerns, what matters most, what is most important in the context of reality [of how services work.

The team wanted to explore public views in the *context* of the day-to-day realities, constraints and limitations of how the healthcare system actually operates. This called for a much more sophisticated approach than simply asking a member of the public for an opinion in a survey or focus group. Most of us harbour general warm feelings towards the NHS and some sense of trust that our information is used for good purposes. That is even if we think about that sort of stuff at all. So any view we might be asked for is likely to be fairly ill-informed. There's no nice way of putting it.

Amy smiles as she explains,

> whenever you talk to the public there is a very strong expectation that their information is shared with the clinicians who need to see it to support their direct care and they're really annoyed and frustrated when they hear that that isn't happening across the board.

Amy knew she wanted a deliberative exercise that brought Londoners together to think deeply about these issues. But she was less sure about what was already known on this subject. The initial phase of the project concentrated on drawing together insights from research and participation work that had already been done about public attitudes to data sharing. Amy's team commissioned market research

152 ■ *Towards a Digital Ecology*

company, Ipsos Mori, conduct interviews with 169 Londoners from less frequently heard groups to plug the gap in intelligence on their views and experiences.

This research confirmed what people in the field already know. Whilst people expect their data to be shared for their direct care, they are less happy with it being used for what is referred to as *secondary purposes* that are for research or commercial purposes such as the development of new drugs, technologies or treatments. We are generally vague and uneasy about our data used in ways that seem remote and unclear. Where has it gone? How will it be used? How long will it be kept for? Is it in my best interests? And how will I ever know?

Amy realised that she needed to find a way of introducing real-world scenarios, constraints and limitations that health and care systems operate within.

It was for this reason she decided upon a Citizens' Summit, a four-day participation process with 100 Londoners who were recruited to reflect the diversity of the city. The planning was forensic. Participants were chosen based on demographic characteristics such as gender, age, socio-economic group, ethnicity, and health status reflective of London's population. People were even recruited to reflect a range of attitudes towards data sharing:

> I've worked in engagement for a long time and I've never been in a room with such a diverse group of people, recruited off the streets, across thirty boroughs of London …. they came from all walks of life and had very different perspectives.

Starting with the end goal and then working backwards meant that the conversations were rooted in a wider context. "The reasoning of this was really important," says Amy. "We wanted to understand from Londoners, what would make something more or less trustworthy, more or less acceptable, where were the red lines, where were the grey areas, and why did people feel that way."

The One London team were in luck, the deliberative exercise took place just weeks before the pandemic struck, where people could freely shake hands, chat and sit huddled around a table:

> We had four full days with these one hundred Londoners to really get into the depths of the trade-offs. Our whole design was not asking people whether we should or should not share data, it was 'this is happening so how do we do it in a trustworthy way?' but by the way, when you're thinking about that, here are all the constraints and you have to tell us what is acceptable within these constraints.

Experts in the field gave evidence over the course of each day to help inform people's thinking, and everything was recorded and curated online for the sake of transparency.[25]

Amy and the One London team weren't always able to anticipate the points of view of those 100 Londoners. A particular surprise came through discussion about

The Jeopardy of Trust ■ 153

proactive care, or in other words, using data to screen and approach people who may be at risk of a particular disease. "They were like 'get on with population health management," recounts Amy, "why aren't you doing it? This makes complete sense, we want to have a preventative health service.'" But when it came to the notion of being contacted by a health professional out of the blue because they were at risk of a disease was a different matter:

> the biggest bone of contention was 'if I was in that cohort and I was proactively contacted, I don't know how I'd feel about that, and I think there might need to be some sort of consent model about whether someone can contact me to tell me I might be at risk of something.

Amy explains what happens next:

> We [policy makers] can take those recommendations and that can shape our commercial model and shape our governance and shape how we grant data access, or not, and to whom, because we now understand at a very granular level what matters to people and what's important.

I ask Amy if we should be taking more of this approach to working out answers to intransigent challenges in the NHS. "It was really amazing to see one hundred people debate these issues, it was just phenomenal," says Amy,

> it could be seen as the silver bullet … but it's not. It's a really good methodology to inform public policy … but it is not grassroots community engagement, it's depth, it's not breadth, in deliberation terms it's big but it's not big when you're talking about nine million people.

Amy is an advocate for deliberation as part of a mixed bag: "There is a place for deliberation but alongside other forms of engagement."

As we wrap up our conversation, I ask Amy to reflect on care.data and the extent to which the work of One London had to be done as a consequence. "We absolutely did not want to repeat the mistakes of the past," says Amy, "the ambition [of care.data] was probably the right one, but the execution was absolutely not."

Amy tells me that it was fear of another care.data that tipped the balance when it came to securing cash for the Citizens' Summit. Like me, she spent many years in healthcare advocating for meaningful patient and public involvement: "[I] got very frustrated with the response of 'let's just get someone sitting on a board' this tick box, tokenistic approach." With a command-and-control culture driving a knife through the core of our healthcare service, it can be scary asking people for views and opinions which might not accord with those of decision-makers. But whilst health bosses were sceptical, she tells me they are now the biggest champions.

For Amy, this process has shown what can be done in terms of public engagement on complex topics when it is properly invested in: "We shouldn/t shy away

154 ■ *Towards a Digital Ecology*

… we should invite [the public] into the complexity, because when we do amazing things can happen," she concludes:

> I think we've won the argument in London at a regional level but I think there's still quite a lot of work to do at a national level to understand what it takes to build trust with the public. And I think there's a lot of talk about the need for public trust, but I think they equate that to privacy, if we've got privacy rules and good governance then we've got people's trust, and it is absolutely not the same thing. Privacy is important and all those rules are important, but we learnt it is so much more than that.

The big takeaway for me from the One London experiment is that it is abundantly clear that most of us are pretty clueless about how the data we leak as we go about our everyday lives is stored and exploited for either commercial or social or healthcare ends. It's clear that we mostly expect our personal health data to be shared between healthcare professionals who are providing us with care. We are pretty shocked when we find out this often isn't the case.

The idea that our data might be used to plan services or for research is for the part something that we don't often consider. Many are nervous about our data being shared with non-healthcare organisations, and in particular, we don't like it being shared with commercial companies. And finally, the greater clarity, and the more we have an opportunity to understand how it all works, the more positive we are and the more we would rather like to have access to our own data as well as everyone else.[26]

The Controversies Continue

As I write this chapter, there is a privacy debate blowing in the wind. Amidst a flurry of media, many of us are ditching WhatsApp for messaging platforms such as Signal and Telegraph after criticism of their privacy credentials and concerns over future monetisation plans from their parent Facebook. Privacy matters.

A recent study in *The Lancet* indicates a shift in public opinion towards being less willing to share our data with commercial organisations and with tech organisations.[27] We know this is a problem for innovation because technologies like AI rely on massive data sets to train their algorithms. It is a problem because population health approaches require large datasets to plan health services across a region. We have seen how important data is during the pandemic to create insights on trends and spikes in a contagion that enable governments to manage lockdown measures.

Who has access to our data, and how they use it matters. And the work that Amy and her team did to build trust on data sharing in London is easily blown to

The Jeopardy of Trust ■ 155

the wind unless adopted consistently across healthcare. Over the seemingly endless pandemic months, Palantir and Faculty were just the two of many private technology firms brought in to help the NHS deliver the COVID-19 data store. This store pulls in health data from a variety of sources to help authorities gain insights into the pandemic. Official information about the store explains that the data processed in the store is either pseudonymised, anonymised or aggregated and therefore does not identify any individual. [28]

However, both appointments were controversial. Palantir is mired in controversy through its work in the US associated with deporting undocumented migrants; Faculty was previously associated with Dominic Cumming's leave campaign that took the UK out of Europe. After challenges from legal experts and civil society organisations, such as Open Democracy and Amnesty, along with the inevitable media storm, the contracts with both companies were put into the public domain.[29] It is transparency that is unwillingly given and only when wrenched out of those in power. I wonder how the One London participants, who spent four long days carefully deliberating about how health and care use our data, might have felt when they opened their newspapers or scrolled their Twitter feed to see these stories in the headlines.

The simple message here is that the NHS and government must be wilfully transparent about how they use our data and who they bring in to do this, if they are to retain public trust. The relationship between private companies and public organisations dealing with the data that emerges from our lives must be transparent and accountable. Even for those of us less interested in the ins-and-outs of public sector contracts, the mood music played out in the steady stream of tweets, articles and media chatter lay toxic foundations of suspicion and concern. And these niggling concerns are set amongst a broader backdrop of worries about how technology companies use our data in other parts of our lives.

Phil Booth has dedicated his life's work to holding those in power to account for how they use our data. After a protracted battle with the government on his NO2ID campaign with strapline *stop the database state*,[30] Phil set up medConfidential in 2013 after he was approached by a group of medics who were concerned about data sharing in the NHS. On a customary Zoom call on a Friday evening after a long working day, I ask Phil to set out his manifesto for a principled and sound approach to data use in the NHS. Unsurprisingly, he has given this quite a bit of thought. He begins with the meta-question that has informed medConfidential's approach: "Ok so what are the essential data characteristics that would make data use within the NHS useful and sustainable for the long haul?"

Phil and his small team have developed a simple set of principles for data that assert that it must be *consensual, safe* and *transparent*. This is the lens through which they assess every data-related initiative that comes up in our public healthcare system, using a scorecard which they publish on their website.[31] Phil's mission is to "fight [each] battle in order to make progress towards the thing that we think is going to be the long term solution."

156 ■ *Towards a Digital Ecology*

Phil is an advocate of what he calls *data usage reports*, statements of how our data is used that create a channel between us as individuals and the institutions that make use of our data. Think of your bank statement which you may get sent through the post, or if you are like me, check out on your banking app and download it as a PDF if you so wish. This is the ultimate in transparency and accountability: "if there is a data breach for example, you can know whose data was affected and what mitigations you're taking … and you can tell people definitively that they weren't affected," explains Phil, "and so a lot of fear and worry evaporates."

"We're not talking transparency just for the sheer hell of it," says Phil, "it is absolutely functional, operationally really desirable to open up that channel and make good use of it as well." He argues that this is not only the way to build public confidence and willingness to share their data for secondary users but also to generate enthusiasm for such endeavours:

> when someone wins a nobel prize [for health research] you can ping everyone and say, guess what, your and your families data was involved in the research that won a nobel prize! There's a whole bunch of good news to be fed that there's no way to do at the moment.

As a member of the oversight group for the One London citizen summit, I ask Phil for his view about this and initiatives like it. "It was certainly a well designed process," he tells me. But he is concerned that endeavours at a local level run the risk of creating lots of local frameworks that lose a coherent national picture that is easy for the public to understand "[we need] a coherent singular framework that every integrated care system [can use]," he asserts.

According to Phil, public engagement activities on the use of data are "utterly pointless if there isn't an output and [could even be] corrosive." He is impatient to see impact and results: "this stuff has to feed into the actual machinery that is actually going to do something about it." Phil concludes our conversation by refocusing on what he believes matters most in the ongoing debate about data:

> Everyone wants the data for research and innovation … [but] unless you focus on doing the care bit first and get that absolutely right, I mean the data will still be there, it will be available, but the primary focus has to be on delivering care … any deviation from that because hey we want to do research or whatever, erodes trust and actually screws you up.

Phil's mantra is simple:

> focus on patient safety and quality of care, that's it, and we're going to use all of our information systems and make sure they work across the piece, and I guarantee you we will have wonderful, lovely rich data for other purposes as well.

A Social Contract

The more healthcare professionals have access to our data, the more we want to have access to it as well. This is an important theme in the evidence review conducted by One London. However, it is balanced by concern from some that by having access to their data, they may also have responsibility pushed to them that they do not want or cannot cope with.[32]

So why can't we be custodians of our own data? There are some who advocate taking our paternalistic healthcare system and flipping it upside down in which the interoperability that eludes public services resides in us as patients and citizens.

In addition to working as a digital technology specialist, Rachel Dunscombe lives with Type 1 diabetes. She sees the value in what she calls *citizen science* and peer communities coming together to learn about their condition through shared data. She believes we are working towards a time when we will regard access to our data as a human right. Sir Tim Berners-Lee, inventor of the World Wide Web, has a plan for what he refers to as "mid course correction" for the problem of proprietary data silos that we cannot influence or control across all aspects of our online transactions.

His answer is *Solid*, an interoperable and open standards initiative that allows citizens to bring our data together into a decentralised data store called a *Pod*. His website describes it as "like a personal Web server for your data" in which you control the data in your pod and "you can share slices of your data with the people, organizations, and applications you choose, and you can revoke that access at any time."[33] This momentum towards citizens as custodians of our own data beginning to pick up pace but is not something on the immediate patient horizon. At the moment, I will have to make do with the patient portal provided by my GP's electronic patient record provider that is tethered to one system and gives me basic access to some information and some transactions. It's a start, but there is so much more possibility if only our dreams could be more desirous and venturesome.

I began this chapter by talking about the social contract that our healthcare system binds us together in, whether we are aware of it or not. Thinking more deeply about this social contract may hold the key to how we think about our healthcare data. In a public deliberation exercise, Genomics England, came up with a way of thinking about this social contract which may be helpful when considering how we might approach secondary data use.[34]

They identify three aspects of the social contract, which they define as *reciprocity, altruism* and *solidarity*. Those are all lovely words, but what do they mean in this context? *Reciprocity* is about how we transact with healthcare services – we expect to be provided with good quality healthcare services and in return, we turn up for our appointments and take our medicine. *Altruism* is based on the idea that we help others without immediate benefit; we show altruism every time we drive up to the curb to let an ambulance race by, when we donate blood or when we participate in healthcare research. Finally, *solidarity* is a shared recognition that good health for each of us as individuals enables us to prosper as a whole; each time we have a

158 ■ *Towards a Digital Ecology*

vaccination we are showing solidarity with others, and healthcare professionals show solidarity when they treat everyone equally and with respect.

There are some emerging approaches to data sharing that hold promise. A Data Trust is one model whereby an independent group or entity stewards data on behalf of a group of people with what is called a fiduciary duty which involves "stewarding data with impartiality, prudence, transparency and undivided loyalty."[35]

The UK Data Biobank[36] is a charity that hosts in-depth genetic and health information from half a million UK participants in a large-scale biomedical database that can be used for pioneering research.

DataKind is a global organisation that brings together data scientists to volunteer with charities and other social change organisations to help them make use of their data to make the world a better place. The team's impact includes inspiring projects such as the creation of a civic dashboard for Citizens Advice to help them identify emerging social issues from the data generated by its interactions with the 5,000 people who walk into its 3,000 bureaus each day.

A massive advocate for open data, the physician, writer and broadcaster Ben Goldacre has become a regular presence at digital health conferences. He argues for a collaborative approach to data science in the NHS that produces a shared *commons* of knowledge and insight that can be shared and built upon. He advocates that the NHS should use open software tools and create a public library of "tagged, edited and curated workbooks and 'how-to guides', with the patient data stripped out" that can be easily reused by others. He makes the case that we should insist that code that has been developed with public resources is put into the public domain by default.[37] This data commons overcomes the big problem of data in the vaults of commercial companies whose value is locked away. Suddenly, innovation is blown wide open.

In addition to new governance models and social purpose organisations popping up to help us address the data challenge, a set of tools are also emerging which help technologists design data-driven technologies with ethics in mind. Developed by the Open Data Institute, the Data Ethics Canvas is one such tool that has been designed to help health teams identify and manage ethical issues in data projects.[38] Another is The Consequence scanner, which is billed as "a way for organisations to consider the potential consequences of their product or service on people, communities and the planet." Developed by now-defunct charity DotEveryone, the scanner is one of the various tools which can be incorporated into projects where data is at the core.

When we think about making our data available for secondary uses as something which binds us together in a shared social contract, we may start to feel very differently about it. However, these perhaps lofty ideals may be easier to sign up to if you have the luxury of confidence in your public institutions. We need to experience that social contract to be able to believe and invest in it. And the reality is that decades of social inequality have insidiously undermined it, like a dog worrying at a wound until it becomes infected and sore. The institutions progressing this important agenda need to look and sound more like the people who have less confidence in them if they have any chance of winning their trust. And for the most part, they don't.

The Jeopardy of Trust ■ 159

COVID-19 has shown us, if we didn't already know it, that our health and even our lives are contingent upon the behaviours of others. If we are sensible, we will build on this moment of clarity to even out the inequalities and reinvigorate our social contract with each other. I can't help but conclude that a strengthened sense of mutual regard, shared responsibility and reinvigorated trust in our public institutions are preconditions to us being happy to share data for our collective good.

In their excellent critique *The Data Will See You Know*[39] the Ada Lovelace Institute poses a series of questions that aim to lay the foundations for future consideration about healthcare data. They ask questions about governance and the legal frameworks that underpin trustworthy use of data and they ask how we can bolster solidarity and societal well-being. They pose interesting challenges, such as how we might harness the affordances of technology to increase the ability for people to participate in and influence the structures that govern health and data. These are urgent questions which demand the attention of citizens, civil society, the healthcare system, corporates and government.

We may feel somewhat suffocated as we scrabble for answers to these insistent questions, overwhelmed by the steep gradient of the challenge that lies ahead of us. However, there may be reasons for optimism. I ask Natalie where she thinks we are now as we round up our call. Natalie is upbeat:

> It's definitely changed in the last few years, people are much more aware and much more respectful that this data has come from people and is about people, and they have a right to understand it, but also to express a choice … it's a step in the right direction.

I reflect on whether we will ever be able to get from under the cloud of care.data and move forwards. Natalie has a slightly different perspective: "I think perhaps without the shock of care.data, perhaps [the shift] might not have happened."

If we can reflect and harness what we have learnt as the pandemic subsides, as we learn from new models of data custodianship, and as we use deliberative processes and the influence of civil society to make sense of both the challenges and the opportunities, maybe we can fork the code towards a fairer data-rich future as part of a thriving digital ecology.

Notes

1 https://www.adalovelaceinstitute.org/report/rethinking-data-prospectus/

2 https://assets.ey.com/content/dam/ey-sites/ey-com/en_gl/topics/life-sciences/life-sciences-pdfs/ey-value-of-health-care-data-v20-final.pdf

3 https://understandingpatientdata.org.uk/sites/default/files/2020-03/Foundations%20of%20Fairness%20-%20Summary%20and%20Analysis.pdf

4 https://www.adalovelaceinstitute.org/blog/health-datafication-digital-phenotyping-and-the-internet-of-health/

160 ■ Towards a Digital Ecology

5 https://assets.ey.com/content/dam/ey-sites/ey-com/en_gl/topics/life-sciences/life-sci-ences-pdfs/ey-value-of-health-care-data-v20-final.pdf
6 https://www.health.org.uk/sites/default/files/upload/publications/2019/Untapped%20potential.pdf
7 https://journals.sagepub.com/doi/pdf/10.1177/2055207616689509
8 https://www.bbc.co.uk/news/health-26259101
9 https://www.theguardian.com/politics/2015/jun/26/nhs-patient-data-plans-unachievable-review-health
10 https://www.gov.uk/government/publications/review-of-data-releases-made-by-the-nhs-information-centre
11 https://www.newscientist.com/article/2086454-revealed-google-ai-has-access-to-huge-haul-of-nhs-patient-data/
12 https://link.springer.com/article/10.1007/s12553-017-0179-1
13 https://healthcareweekly.com/how-the-big-4-tech-companies-are-leading-healthcare-innovation/
14 https://link.springer.com/article/10.1007/s12553-017-0179-1
15 https://www.ncsc.gov.uk/news/ncsc-defends-uk-700-cyber-attack-national-pandemic
16 https://www.thetimes.co.uk/article/amazon-ready-to-cash-in-on-free-access-to-nhs-data-bbzp52n5m
17 https://www.adalovelaceinstitute.org/health-data-partnerships-adas-view/
18 https://www.contractsfinder.service.gov.uk/Notice/919533b2-4d46-4c72-bf2b-4e320cff572e
19 https://www.businessinsider.com/facebook-is-using-ai-to-try-to-predict-if-youre-suicidal-2018-12?r=US&IR=T
20 https://www.nytimes.com/2018/12/31/technology/facebook-suicide-screening-algo-rithm.html
21 https://www.adalovelaceinstitute.org/wp-content/uploads/2020/11/The-data-will-see-you-now-Ada-Lovelace-Institute-Oct-2020.pdf
22 https://www.onelondon.online/wp-content/uploads/2020/07/Public-deliberation-in-the-use-of-health-and-care-data.pdf p.26
23 https://www.ofcom.org.uk/__data/assets/pdf_file/0027/196407/online-nation-2020-re-port.pdf
24 https://en.wikipedia.org/wiki/London
25 https://onelondon.online/citizenssummit/
26 https://understandingpatientdata.org.uk/sites/default/files/2019-07/Understanding%20public%20expectations%20of%20the%20use%20of%20health%20and%20care%20data.pdf
27 https://www.thelancet.com/journals/landig/article/PIIS2589-7500(20)30161-8/fulltext
28 https://www.england.nhs.uk/contact-us/privacy-notice/how-we-use-your-information/covid-19-response/nhs-covid-19-data-store/
29 https://www.digitalhealth.net/2020/11/data-contracts-with-palantir-risk-undermining-core-values-of-nhs/
30 https://www.no2id.net/
31 https://medconfidential.org/for-patients/loopholes/
32 https://understandingpatientdata.org.uk/sites/default/files/2019-07/Understanding%20public%20expectations%20of%20the%20use%20of%20health%20and%20care%20data.pdf
33 https://solidproject.org/about

The Jeopardy of Trust ■ 161

34 https://www.ipsos.com/sites/default/files/ct/publication/documents/2019-04/public-dialogue-on-genomic-medicine-full-report.pdf
35 https://theodi.org/article/what-is-a-data-trust
36 https://www.ukbiobank.ac.uk/
37 https://journals.sagepub.com/doi/10.1177/0141076820930666
38 https://theodi.org/article/data-ethics-canvas/?__cf_chl_jschl_tk__=41c1e34775c8351ec2 60790f20339beċ09d1f837-1612210922-0-AY9ZbsDB4ajoBB5ljz6IQb6Qi-FInhmkuCJWzNftkgsQ2hWKzqE6WRDg595-75uVW7PKnpf8yglJxMyo4VENSZM-0KYsbF_KIQvX8WlLCNelzKgUm5Y9qdQY_H7jKXbnbTAhwux-BE_3WzTeT5xSDdi LpI9urxkC2oNUZrkbexvFNXJEut9ZVYvBWEQdLXzSqsNFJtVxXiilOQF3bTeV1LDiv TNfR6FssDMgwREff5rwNDJjsX-dar_qSVYKLDVLNUX5M8Rd1qggaquFqf1trCuo-Tiq5f02y7AlWzaGPeln3hPgTuFEmS-IhYSpOiXCszDH2KSpyqAw02U4JRd0fCmo1I
39 https://www.adalovelaceinstitute.org/wp-content/uploads/2020/11/The-data-will-see-you-now-Ada-Lovelace-Institute-Oct-2020.pdf

Chapter 9

Bending the Curve on Digital Mental Health

Introduction

The use of digital technologies for patient care was still in its infancy back in 2013. It felt like the wild west. My first tentative steps into the frontier were taken as an employee of an NHS trust which provides mental health services. At that time, digital wasn't such a commonly used term. Back then it was all about mobile apps and the common nomenclature was mobile health or mHealth. I coined *mHealthHabitat* (then shortened to mHabitat) as the name for the team I went on to establish, using an ecological metaphor for the many factors that digital health is contingent upon if it is to flourish. Right from the get-go, I was fascinated by the many combinatorial factors that can mean the success or failure of a digital technology intended for use by patients.

In this chapter, I shine the spotlight on secondary care therapy services as a case study for digital adoption. With the flora and fauna of comparatively mature digital services, I wonder what this subset of mental health services can tell us about the requisite factors that need to exist for digital adoption to prosper. Struck by the pervasiveness of private-sector provision in this ecology, I am troubled about what this might mean for the future of the NHS. It is clear to me that there is an imperative for NHS services to adapt to and nurture their digital habitat if they are going to save themselves. The question is how.

Like every other part of the NHS, mental health services were shaken by the pandemic, tripped into making rapid adjustments to how they were delivered, out of necessity rather than choice. It is apparent that some of these changes may have eased the way for therapy services to embrace technology more enthusiastically than

DOI: 10.1201/9781032198798-9

163

164 ■ *Towards a Digital Ecology*

they might have done before. If they can capitalise on the tactics they *had* to make and manoeuvre them into embedded practices, then maybe this could unlock their survival. The contested role of digital technologies in secondary care mental health services is the cornerstone of my inquiry over the course of this chapter.

However, before we delve into the digital habitat of mental health therapy, I want to step back and explore the extent to which the pandemic exacerbated pressure on mental health services. We need to understand what has changed in order to understand what this means for mental health and the provision of therapy services. It is evident that COVID-19 propelled us into a parallel pandemic of the mind and soul.

A Mental Health Pandemic

The pandemic ricocheted through our lives, wreaking havoc in everything that we know protects our mental health and well-being. Our jobs, our housing, our relationships and our social connections all came under unprecedented strain. The situation was grave, not only for our mental health but for the services that pertain to our emotional well-being.

The term *disaster mental health* has been coined for a strand of research that explores the impacts of disasters. Disasters affect millions of people around the world every year. To put it in perspective, there's at least one somewhere on the planet every single day. Disasters are events that threaten harm or death to a large group of people; they disrupt services and social networks; they have ripple effects in terms of physical and mental health.[1] Sound familiar? Yes, we have lived through a disaster of epic proportions. Whether it be boredom, loneliness or grief, the pandemic affected each and every one of us. With the largest enforced isolation in living history, even the most robust of us has felt the consequences of these most tumultuous times.[2]

Most people bounce back from a disaster and find a way to cope. However, that is not the case for everyone. During the first wave of the pandemic, the Royal College of Psychiatrists (RCPsych) reported an increase in urgent and emergency mental health cases, including people who were suicidal. This rise in demand was coupled with a significant drop in routine appointments, indicating a likely build-up of people needing, but not getting mental health support. The professional body for the psychiatry profession, registered its concerns about a tsunami of demand that could overpower mental health services, hurling them up and sucking them down into its deadly tide.[3]

Mental health charities and think tanks were quick to try and predict the impact so they could lobby the Government to do something about it. The Centre for Mental Health is one of those organisations having developed a model which forecasted that up to 20% of the population would need either new or additional mental health support as a direct consequence of the pandemic. This equates to 10 million people of whom one and a half million are children and young people under the age

Bending the Curve ■ 165

of 18. That is a tidal wave of distress and misery which would displace and engulf the already beleaguered services struggling to stay afloat.

Whilst the longer-term impacts are predicted and modelled, we do know what happened during the first wave and early lockdown because researchers have had an opportunity to find out. The COVID-19 Social Study[4] from University College London is one of those projects, producing reports on the basis of surveys from around 70,000 people around the UK, each sharing their experiences in a ten-minute online survey as well as in-depth interviews. It is often the case that research can seem lofty and out of reach, but this one chimes with the mood of viral immediacy, producing outputs each and every week to illuminate the riptides of this disaster of the body and the mind.

These weekly reports give a snapshot into the mood of the nation as we were swept up in the pandemic wave. In those very early days, it was somewhat bizarrely toilet paper that was uppermost on our minds, as supplies were stripped from the shelves by panicked customers. The week one study report shows public concern about getting food (and maybe also toilet paper) was actually far greater than any worries about actually contracting the virus. As the first swell of the pandemic subsided and lockdown restrictions began to ease, the study shows higher than average depression and anxiety but some indication they are on the decrease. With the persistent grip of social determinants always present, the mental health consequences of the pandemic were highest in young adults, people living alone, people with lower household income, those living with children and the many of us living in urban areas.[5]

None of this should be a surprise, many of the things that help us feel good about life, or at the very least help us cope when we don't feel so good, were ripped away from us. And to add insult to injury, the services that are there for us when we get to the point we drum up the courage to ask for help, were decimated. A quarter of us who reached out for help as we were sucked into those violent early pandemic days, found that there was none available.[6]

Before we consider how digital technologies played a role in the first wave of the pandemic, I want to take you back to the early days of digital mental health and set the scene for what was about to come.

A Salutary Lesson

The Samaritans Radar app weighs heavily in the history of digital technologies in mental health. The year was 2014 and I remember it well. It was in the early days of patient-facing digital services when every charity seemed to want a mobile app without much of an idea of what it might do or achieve. Mobile apps were cool and every on-point charity should have one. Radar has become a salutary lesson in how *not* to approach the use of technology in the sphere of mental health.

I happened to know some of the people involved in the debacle, and it became a pivotal case study in my postdoctoral thesis. I recall attending a workshop in the

166 ■ *Towards a Digital Ecology*

London Headquarters of Twitter, where the beleaguered suicide prevention charity gathered experts to help them reflect and regroup. I have to confess that my main recollection of that day is texting photos of Twitter HQ to my children, tickled by their Silicon Valley-esque table tennis table, free snacks and inevitable bean bags. But back to the matter in hand, how did the 70-year-old charity get it so wrong?

The Samaritans work through volunteers who provide listening support services over the telephone. One of those volunteers happened to work for a digital marketing agency who perhaps wanted to bring their skills to help The Samaritans do something cool with digital. Using an algorithm that was supposed to be able to spot words indicating mental distress, they launched an application that monitored the content of tweets. If you had signed up to the app, it would have automatically monitored the tweets of everyone you follow and sent you an alert if the algorithm spotted a tweet which it determined might indicate mental distress. The idea was that you could reach out and offer support to that person, an everyday Samaritan, choosing to stop and care when others might walk by.

But to become a volunteer with The Samaritans takes a certain predisposition along with training and supervision. Consider for a moment if you would have known what was the right thing to do or say if an alert had popped up in your inbox. Consider if you would have the confidence and skills to help someone you may hardly or not even know on the basis of a tweet. I'm not sure I would. These were just a few of the implications of the well-intentioned project that the charity completely failed to anticipate. There were more.

What if I have malicious intent, using the app to seek out vulnerable people? What if the algorithm fails to spot sarcasm? (Worst day at work EVER. Think I'll end it now.) What if the algorithm misses actual distress conveyed in such a way it fails to recognise the real meaning? What if I am actually distressed, but the last thing I want is one of my followers on Twitter getting in touch with me? These were just some of the concerns of mental health activists and privacy campaigners, who through a flurry of intense activity, managed to disgrace the charity in the media and get the app taken down within the space of two short weeks.

This mishap is a sobering lesson in how not to do digital. Taking technology and looking at how you can apply it in a certain context, often ends up in an innovation attempting to solve a problem that may not even be there. Failing to understand the attitudes, beliefs and behaviours of people the app is intended for, and not accounting for the privacy of those affected by the technology, is suspect. Developing a technology that turns out *not* to do what you intend it to do can be downright dangerous.

Perhaps the more profound point is that The Samaritans inadvertently reduced something complex, subtle and personal into an algorithm and application that wasn't sophisticated enough to do what they had hoped. This is the story of a charity trying to do a good thing that was way out of its depth. It is a classic case of tech-solutionism, the idea that technology is the key to solving any problem and where the algorithm reigns supreme.

Bending the Curve ■ 167

Other mental health services watched The Samaritans get burnt and made a pledge to think twice before they leapt into the confusing world of apps and algorithms. It set an uncomfortable path for digital mental health, whilst serving as an early warning for how things can so easily go wrong.

Cinderella Services

Despite the much-publicised Radar disaster, it is no surprise that so many people want to innovate in this sector. Mental health problems are all too common, and many entrepreneurs are motivated by their own experience or that of a close friend or family member. A cursory glance at the app stores shows any number of mobile apps with a mental health theme. But even though mental health services are notoriously underfunded, digital mental health is surprisingly one of the more mature sectors. To understand why this is the case, we need to travel back to 2006 and the work of an eminent economist.

Mental health services are often described as the Cinderella of health and care services because they have forever been under-considered and under-resourced. Mental health advocates argue that this underfunding is a false economy because good mental health is strongly associated with good physical health, it turns out you can't have one without the other.[7] Combined together, good mental and physical health is not just a good thing for each of us as individuals but for society as a whole. Good mental health is a societal asset that is not only good for ourselves but also good for our economy, we are more productive when we are happy.[8]

Under the Blair Labour Government, it was finally time for Cinderella to go to the ball. This sea change was instigated by the work of Professor Richard Layard, an economist at the London School of Economics, who produced The Depression Report.[9] This paper set out a clear connection between the scale of mental health difficulties in the UK and the cost to not only people's lives but to the economy, which at that time, Layard estimated to be some £12 billion a year. Suddenly, mental health services were re-conceptualised as an investment rather than a cost.

The argument he made was simple – mental health problems are common, one in six of us will experience depression or anxiety and one family in three is affected. There are inexpensive evidence-based psychological therapies that have a positive effect for at least half of people who use them, in the shape of cognitive behaviour therapy (CBT). But they weren't being routinely prescribed, with only one in four of those with anxiety or depression offered this form of therapy. With insufficient numbers of trained therapists, there was a problem in the system. Medication was often the only option prescribed by a GP, despite evidence suggesting that therapy has longer-lasting effects than drugs, as well as being more cost-effective.

Here is a boiled-down version of how Improving Access to Psychological Therapy (IAPT) works. The service offers a range of National Institute for Clinical Excellence (NICE) recommended psychological therapies, including cognitive behavioural therapies. CBT is a family of talking therapies, based on the idea that

168 ▪ *Towards a Digital Ecology*

thoughts, feelings, what we do and how our bodies feel are all connected. If we change one of these, we can alter all the others. When we're low or upset, we often fall into patterns of thinking and responding which can worsen how we feel. CBT works to help us notice and change problematic thinking styles or behaviour patterns so we can feel better.[10]

IAPT operates with what is called a stepped care model, which matches intensity and duration of the intervention with the severity of symptoms; low-intensity interventions (such as group education) are offered to people with mild to moderate symptoms and stepped-up intensity (one-to-one talking therapy) for those who are more severely affected. This means that the right resources are deployed in the best way, as cost-effectively as possible. Put simply, higher-intensity interventions cost more and so are only offered to the people who most need them.

Layard's report put the cost of recovery from mental health problems at £750 a person, an insignificant drop in the ocean compared to the economic costs of untreated mental misery. The maths was simple. Layard argued that the money which the government spent on training therapists would pay for itself. And so, Improving Access to Psychological Therapy (IAPT) Services were born just two years later, providing secondary care CBT at scale. GPs could now refer patients experiencing anxiety and depression to this new service. Cinderella had been rescued from the servants quarters by her baron economist and had finally arrived at the ball.

The Fruit That Hangs the Lowest

To understand why digital is comparatively mature in the 140 IAPT services across the country, we need to understand the conditions under which these services operate. They give us some clues as to why this may be the case and could hold the key to other health services beyond therapy services. It seems that there are a number of particular features to IAPT that have made it highly attractive to start-ups and amenable to digital technology adoption. Let me offer an explanation through the lens of what matters to a digital health start-up from a purely business perspective.

If I am creating a new digital health company, I want a large market, as do my investors. Mental health problems, such as depression and anxiety, are common which is bad news for society, but good news for a start-up that wants lots of users and an opportunity to scale their business. Around 900,000 people access IAPT services each year, which sounds like a lot but is still only a drop in the ocean (15%) of those of us who actually experience anxiety or depression.[11] The Government has plans to expand IAPT services, with an ambition for almost 2 million adults able to access treatment each year by 2024.[12]

Along with a large group of potential users, there is demand for IAPT from the public that services are routinely unable to meet. The fact that there are still not enough trained therapists is a headache for IAPT services. So, they are constantly looking for ways to reduce their waiting lists and see more patients. IAPT is highly target driven and measures everything in order to continually enable services to review and improve. The pressure to deliver waiting time targets is immense, with three-quarters of people referred to IAPT expected to enter treatment within six weeks and just under 100% within 18 weeks.[13] All of this means that IAPT services are looking for creative ways to manage demand so that they can meet the needs of their local population and don't miss their targets. This is a nicely defined customer problem to be solved which isn't often the case in health services.

The prescriptive nature of IAPT services means it is relatively easy to demonstrate how a (digital) intervention creates benefits. The IAPT service manual sets out clear characteristics of a well-run service, along with standard measures and reporting. It is target driven and patient outcomes are closely measured, with a requirement for a minimum 50% recovery rate for all individuals completing treatment. The clearly defined model means that an entrepreneur has a clear idea of what their innovation needs to deliver. There are few grey areas.

IAPT is one of the few parts of the NHS (other than GP practices) that has pretty much ubiquitous electronic patient record coverage. Even better, IAPT isn't plagued by the curse of non-interoperability which stimies innovation in so many parts of the NHS. IAPTUS, the leading electronic patient record provider, has an interoperability widget that enables other products and services to integrate with it. The fact that data can move seamlessly between the NHS and digital products or services, in theory at least, makes it easy for therapists to use them and for NHS trusts and commissioners to buy them. This seems like it could be game-changing.

All of this is an innovator's dream, a large market, a clearly defined problem to be solved, a well-defined service model that is consistent across the country and a mature underpinning technology infrastructure. Digitally enabled therapy is now included in the core IAPT manual alongside face-to-face interventions.[14] But there is even more. A common barrier to the take-up of digital products in the NHS is the paucity of evidence that it actually works. Clinicians, who have been trained to deliver evidence-based interventions, are easily put off by promises from a start-up that can't back up their claims. However, this is not the case in IAPT. In mid-2020, the leading open-access science journal, *Nature*, ran an article on a study that found that internet-based CBT is clinically and cost-effective when delivered as part of a stepped care model in IAPT services. There is a compelling clinical and cost-benefit case that has been made through any number of high-quality studies.[15] The case continues to stack up in favour of digital.

Finally, maybe there is something about the relative infancy of IAPT that has a part to play in its cultivated digital health ecosystem. At the tender age of 14, IAPT is the teen of mental health services. As a comparatively youthful service, it is perhaps more amenable than others to new ideas and different ways of working. The fact that its inception coincided with the genesis of Facebook, along with a real acceleration of digital and social media is worth noting. And whilst the two have no obvious relationship, IAPT has done its growing up in parallel with the emergence of digital technologies both in health and the wider world.

The Detractors

The IAPT model has transformed mental health care by making therapies available to many people who would have otherwise not received any help. However, it's not without its detractors and the lens of the start-up and the marketplace is not without its limitations. Digital technologies are for the part designed within and constrained by the normative paradigm within which they are conceived. As a result, digital technologies will often (although not inevitably) reinforce and perpetuate the dominant modality within which they have been conceived, developed and evaluated.

IAPT's foundations were laid within an economist mindset which accounted for value in terms of pounds and pence. The therapy service's origins have been closely tied with successive government's efforts to get people with mental health problems off benefits and back into work. There is a line of argument that this utilitarian approach to mental distress, tied to neoliberal notions of productivity and self-optimisation, fails to engage with the deeper and more profound existential aspects of what it is to be human.

There has been a small but consistent strand of criticism on the perceived reductive nature of IAPT's emphasis on CBT, which some argue gives primacy to adjusting thought patterns at the expense of helping people make sense of past experiences and to how their social and economic situations impact on their distress. The minutely prescribed and highly structured nature of IAPT is argued by some to be stressful and demoralising for the therapists who deliver it. Targets require high throughput of patients and can leave practitioners feel like a cog in an industrialised wheel.

Its managerial foundations fit well within the economic paradigm from which it originates, but perhaps not in one which searches more deeply into the human condition. Whilst this more existential challenge is not the primary subject of this chapter, the salient point for us to keep in mind is that digital technologies can facilitate the delivery of services within an existing system (broken or otherwise) or they can fundamentally reshape it. We may want to double down and reinforce a normative model or we may be inspired to completely rethink and reinvent it.

A Faster Horse

The next step in my case study of digital therapy is to delineate the sorts of products and services that start-ups and SMEs develop for people accessing IAPT services. To do so, I interview Chris from Mayden, the company behind the leading IAPT electronic patient record (EPR) provider. It is just before the Christmas of 2020 and as a turbulent year is drawing to a close, we are both in a reflective mood. Chris begins by recounting the genesis of IAPTUS, which has turned out to have created a firm foundation for a digital health ecosystem. It is a story of chance and serendipity.

"It was literally a random conversation on an exhibition stand at the NHS Confederation conference," he explains. The founder, another Chris, had set up

Bending the Curve ■ 171

Mayden as a consultancy back in the early 2000s. He was at the conference to promote a magazine that he had produced and his wife was there to help him. She ended up in a random conversation with a clinician who happened to be the clinical lead for one of the two initial IAPT pilot sites.

Given that the IAPT pilots asked for a lot of data to be reported, the clinician was looking for help to develop something that would capture them. "Over the course of the discussion [his wife said] said 'well we do healthcare web systems' and he went 'great let's have one of them.' So a couple of weeks later, Mayden was building the first version of IAPTUS." Chris reflects on this serendipitous moment that seeded a business and created a path for use of digital technologies in IAPT,

> We were like the little mouse scurrying around the elephant, they [big EPR vendors] didn't notice we were here, no one was interested in doing it anyway ... today would you build an EPR from scratch for a random thing? Probably not.

So what exactly is the ecosystem of digital products and services for which Chris and his company unwittingly created the foundations, as IAPT took its first baby pilot steps. The 20th Century motor car manufacturer, Henry Ford, is famously associated with the adage: "If I had asked people what they wanted they would have said faster horses." Digital IAPT services exemplify the spectrum between doing the same thing faster and creating a step change in the provision that marks a break with the norm.

Firstly, there are software products in the shape of video consultation platforms that enable clinicians to deliver therapy remotely; then there are mobile applications that act as an adjunct to care, enabling patients to do activities such as keeping a diary, recording steps towards goals, tracking thoughts and feelings and so on. These are discrete products that help clinicians do what they do differently or enhance the existing model of care, still delivered by NHS therapists. They represent faster horses, a useful adjunct to enhance the existing model of care.

The second group is arguably more game-changing and also somewhat more problematic insofar as they take the shape of services rather than products. Instead of licensing a product to be delivered by an NHS therapist, a number of companies provide a whole service, including employing the therapists themselves. SilverCloud and IESO are two of the leading private companies selling digital therapy services to the NHS. These services are supplementing rather than competing with NHS IAPT services, helping them reduce waiting lists and manage demand. However, private providers within NHS services is a political hot potato and one that evokes strong emotions. We will return to this later in the chapter.

SilverCloud was founded in 2012, around four years after the birth of IAPT. It is a digital service that offers 30 guided therapy programmes whereby the user works through a series of CBT topics at their own pace. A therapist checks in with the patient at regular intervals to review progress via asynchronous messaging,

172 ■ *Towards a Digital Ecology*

increasing the intensity to synchronous chat, telephone or video consultation for people with higher needs. The courses have features such as videos, activities, quizzes, audio guides and an online journal. Users have the option to share content with their supporters which gives the feel of a private social network. I wondered what makes this approach different to traditional face-to-face IAPT services.

During the summer months of the first pandemic wave, I interviewed Lloyd who, with an impressive pedigree in the digital health sector, runs SilverCloud sales across Europe. Lloyd believes that digital services have created a step change in the IAPT delivery model. "You have digital solutions which are still a one-to-one model [online consultations and messaging services]," he explains,

> you have the efficiencies in that the person doesn't have to come in and you can do it remotely, but you still have the problem of scheduling and availability. So if there's a surge on capacity, you can't meet that demand.

Put simply, the person to person model is not scalable because it relies on a synchronous interaction between two people.

In contrast, guided therapy services have a one-to-many model, whereby a therapist can support around six times as many people at any one time. The therapist guides their patients through self-help modules and provides asynchronous messaging for support. "You get huge efficiency savings … because you have flexibility," explains Lloyd, "you can prevent people coming into IAPT [through guided support] and can help with meeting demand in a service as well, so it has something to offer right across the continuum of delivery." Lloyd describes how digital platforms can also be used to step patients down from care at the point of discharge from an IAPT service.

Digital services, such as SilverCloud, represent an innovation in IAPT provision because they have a scalable model. They have created a platform, along with a set of CBT content, that can reach more patients with fewer therapists. Video and messaging services take therapy online, but they still require the patient and the therapist to be engaging with each other at the same time. However, guided therapy using asynchronous messaging entirely interrupts the episodic and synchronous model of care. Now one therapist can support multiple patients at the same time. The costs are reduced, more people can be reached, and profits for a private company are within reach.

However, not all benefits are planned or even expected, even by the companies who would regard themselves as the digital disruptors. An academic study of patients' experience of using SilverCloud threw up an unexpected result that intrigued me. It reminded me of when Twitter changed the *favourite* feature to a *heart* icon. The icon had originally been designed by Twitter to enable people to tag tweets that they wanted to curate in a *favourite* list that they could go back to. However, as we know humans have a pesky habit of using technologies in ways not imagined or intended by their creators. People began using the favourite button in the same way as a thumbs-up button on Facebook, to show others that they liked it. Catching on to this, Twitter changed the icon to the heart icon that we see at the bottom of our tweets today.

You may wonder how this story is relevant to the SilverCloud digital therapy platform. Well, its creators designed it to mirror traditional therapy, expecting patients to complete one module a week, taking around 40 minutes to do so. However, a research study found that many patients actually use it in a completely different way than they had imagined. Rather than visit the platform weekly, they were going to it for in-the-moment assistance at the point they felt they needed it, to find answers or seek help.[16]

Clinical services are for the most part designed on the basis of episodic care, organised around set appointment times and locations. But smartphones and laptops afford the opportunity for people to get what they need when they need it. The idea that you can get help at the moment that you need it has the fancy title of ecological momentary interventions. SilverCloud designed a faster horse, but their patients redesigned it into a motor car.

In Search of the Gold Standard

Of all the parts of the human condition that the NHS pokes and prods, treats and cares for, it seems to me that our minds are the most exquisitely personal and private. It is for this reason that mental health services are at their core about relationships. In my experience, the instinct of mental health practitioners is to recoil at the notion of digital technology as a medium to deliver care. They see a binary between the gold standard of face-to-face treatment and the relative paucity of that which is mediated by digital.

For many, technology conjures up everything that is the antithesis to human connection – remote, mechanical and impersonal. But how fair is this assessment, and what does the evidence tell us about the utility of digital technologies in mental IAPT? Maybe they can be as good, or even better, than the standard treatment. I wonder what happens to relationships between mental health practitioners and patients when digital is in the mix. It turns out there is a substantial body of evidence we can draw on to understand what works and what doesn't.

A ton of randomised control trials (RCTs) have been done on digital therapy services. Regarded in the NHS as the most robust standard for clinical research, a control group is given the existing intervention (or no intervention), and their results are compared to a similar group who has the intervention. The results are compared to see if the new intervention is equal to or better than the existing one. Such trials show that people often don't stay the course with purely online interventions, or to put it in NHS speak, these sorts of interventions suffer from high attrition and non-adherence. It is rather the case that online interventions are most effective when they are a blend of human support (delivered face-to-face, message, email or phone) and

174 ■ *Towards a Digital Ecology*

self-directed activities (such as educational modules). On the whole, the evidence suggests that we do not respond well to purely self-guided interventions. However, as technology matures and improves this may well change.

I am curious about the upsides and downsides of digital therapies. The abundance of research in this field throws up some common themes. For many, the convenience and flexibility of online therapy can reduce feelings of stress, and the onus on them to engage with the treatment can be a positive stimulus. On the downside, poor quality content that doesn't feel personal or tailored to the individual along with technical and usability issues can be a barrier. Lack of privacy and the amount of self-directed work required from the individual can also create frustration and ultimately have a negative impact on personal motivation. Online therapies aren't for everyone, and they are less likely to work for people with a learning disability and people with low literacy, along with a lack of digital skills. There would be a big issue of parity and equal access if the NHS were ever to go down a purely digital first route.

What about the cost of digital IAPT services compared to face-to-face services? The National Institute for Health and Care Excellence (NICE) is the body that provides national guidance and advice to improve health and social care. Back in 2018, they put together an expert panel to review particular technologies and produce briefings intended to inform the NHS of their effectiveness. The panel's review of SilverCloud's Space for Depression course concludes there is a "partial case for adoption based on a comparative review of its use in three IAPT services.[17] Whilst limited in scope, it is an attempt to understand the extent to which a digital therapy costs or saves the NHS money. Where it does work well, the briefing shows that the SilverCloud course has similar clinical outcomes and is generally less costly than standard care.

The most telling conclusion from the briefing is that digital therapy services are most effective when time is spent by the IAPT service planning and helping therapists to offer it as part of routine care. In my conversation with Lloyd, he raises the same issue:

> Everyone in the NHS, they don't have the time or the capacity to invest in new things that are going to layer on top. So the tension is that there are a lot of private suppliers that have fantastic solutions but being able to get the bandwidth for change is quite difficult to do.

This theme that occurs over and over again – ignore the adaptive nature of digital health at your peril. Its impact is only ever as good as the time and care spent working out how it fits into the everyday routines of clinicians and only implemented in practice insofar as clinicians are supporters and advocates. These are the human factors that make the difference between success and failure and should never be underestimated. Yet time and time again NHS organisations buy technology, apparently seduced by the product and with scant regard for conditions necessary for it to realise its true value.

RCTs and other forms of research-based evidence are costly and time-consuming. However, internet-enabled therapies offer the opportunity to collect real-time data which can be used to measure impact. From September 2020, IAPT services have been required to collect and report data on a new category, namely *Internet-Enabled Therapy*. NHS Digital, who analyse and report the data, define this sort of therapy as patients working through materials on the internet with a therapist inputting with encouragement, clarifications and feedback at key points.[18] Data on digital therapies are now part of the common reported dataset.

Scores taken from referrals having internet-enabled therapy are now incorporated into the calculation of patient outcomes alongside those from care contact-based referrals. Over time, this will enable a comparison of the efficacy of internet-enabled therapy with other forms of treatment. This is a massive move forward in embedding measurement and comparison of digital services and creates accountability and transparency which is very welcome and sets a path for other disciplines in which digital mediated care and treatment are becoming more commonplace.

A Digital Mental Health Pandemic

In those early spring pandemic days, IAPT experienced the same drop in activity as GP surgeries and hospital outpatient appointments. Flatlining referrals were accompanied by a big spike in antidepressant subscribing to 6 million people in England over the summer months.[19] The number of people diagnosed with depression doubled during the first wave of the pandemic.[20] The high tide of the pandemic tsunami was sweeping up its victims and sucking them into its watery depths.

I asked Chris to tell me what story the data collected in IAPTUS told us about how things changed in that first wave. With the platform covering two-thirds of IAPT providers, the data offers a good indication of overall IAPT activity. Chris describes a dramatic 70% fall in referrals in the first two weeks of lockdown along with a comparable drop in treatment as therapists adjusted to remote working.

However, from that point on, there was a gradual rise in both referrals and treatment, and it is clear that services did not collapse as some worried they might. "DNA [did not attend] rates fell, and recovery rates have increased," says Chris, speculating that more people completed treatment during the first wave because they were stuck at home with less of the competing demands that might otherwise mean they drop out.

As the ability to meet in person became impossible, so the remote consultation came into its own. It is a familiar story. "People weren't able to do their traditional ways of treatment," recalls Lloyd from SilverCloud, "and so digital had to replace your normal ways of working, it had to slot in, it happened over night, it had to." Suddenly NHS therapists, who were mostly used to delivering face-to-face services, found themselves either redeployed or working from their own homes to deliver therapy into the homes of their patients via video or phone.

176 ■ Towards a Digital Ecology

Whilst much of that shift was common sense, the national IAPT team promptly launched a weekly webinar series aimed at helping clinicians get used to exploiting features such as video screen share to help their clients engage in collaborative exercises that they would ordinarily do face to face. This was a backstage response to the pandemic that was not obvious to patients at the receiving end of treatment, but which sought to equip therapists who were experiencing a seismic shift to their usual practice. A total of 16 weekly webinars were recorded in the first wave of lockdown, proving wildly popular with therapists – one webinar on PTSD had 1,610 live viewers and 4,000 within the subsequent week.

All curated on a platform called NHS Futures, I watched the first video for therapists that came out in March, aimed at teaching therapists how to treat PTSD remotely using CBT. As well as showing pre-recorded videos with methods of intervention role played, the speakers provide self-care tips for therapists working from home. These include encouraging therapists to move around and do something pleasurable after remote sessions, keep workspace separate from their non-work space to delineate the two, marking the end of the working day. The webinar series was a valuable resource for therapists, giving guidance on adapting to new working practices and acclimatising to remote working. It is striking to see the sorts of things clinicians had to consider as they adapted to new working practices and accommodated the use of technologies.

I ask Chris what he thinks this reshaping of working practices will mean in the longer term for NHS IAPT services, along with their digital counterparts. What he goes on to say, probably reflects the most significant impact the pandemic had on IAPT services: "[They] wouldn't have planned to have a remote workforce, but one being forced upon them," explains Chris, "they are seeing the advantages of doing it, and it's kind of worked, recovery rates are high and satisfaction rates are pretty good." The pandemic tsunami may have wrecked our mental health, but it has forced a disruption to everyday practice that just might enable NHS IAPT services to save themselves. Let me explain.

There has been a steady drain of NHS trained therapists to the private sector and digital-first services over the years. "Loads [of therapists] would feel a moral obligation to work for the people who have trained them and the NHS, so why are they leaving?" Chris speculates:

> The workforce is predominantly female, it's predominantly young, and therefore there is quite a high churn for maternity leave and then when they're wanting to come back, what is a high priority for them is flexibility. Now a lot of the [digital companies] provide that flexibility, you can work the hours that you want to work and so they can fit it in in the evening when the kids are in bed.

However that flexibility has not been offered by 9 am to 5 pm NHS IAPT services up until now.

It is not just therapists who are dissatisfied with the status quo, it is patients also, explains Chris: "and actually if you ask patients when do they want to receive care, they typically want it in the evening too". I ask Chris why services haven't been adapted, but he doesn't have an answer. He is as bewildered as I am. "It doesn't make sense!" he tells me, rolling his eyes. A common theme in my many conversations with clinicians is one of inertia, whereby things have always been done a certain way and so they continue. The relative advantage of making a change in the ordinary state of things just doesn't stack up. However, all that changes when a disaster strikes.

In our conversation, Chris and I speculate about whether the pandemic might be the wake-up call NHS IAPT services need to redesign their working practices: "Now having been forced to do it in Covid and the wheels haven't fallen off," observes Chris:

> and in the areas difficult to recruit in … they're like, hey we don't have to recruit [there], I can recruit anywhere … so some providers are realising they don't have to deliver a service wholly by setting up local teams, they can do it by sharing a workforce over a wider area regardless of where the staff are going to be.

Suddenly, options and possibilities have opened up for NHS services, and if they are smart they won't need to rely on private services in quite the way they have done so before. Rather than buying in flexibility, they can own that flexibility for themselves.

Could this be the wake-up call the NHS needs to embrace the benefits of digital technologies in order to deliver flexible services that aren't entirely bound by location and appointment? What if they could redesign services so they meet the preferences of a significant cohort of patients at the same time as creating a thriving happy workforce. As importantly, what does it mean for NHS services if they don't take the opportunity to make this shift when digital-first private services are willing and able to do so? As the pandemic curve flattens, now is the time to bend the curve of digital mental health.

Bending the Curve on Digital Mental Health

In the very early spring days of the pandemic, Boston-based psychiatrist and prolific academic John Torous produced an editorial in the *Journal for Medical Internet Research*. In his paper, he argues that whilst governments around the world are attempting to flatten the curve of the spread of the virus, it is time to accelerate and bend the curve on digital mental health.

There is no doubt that John is the go-to expert for digital mental health, and I was fortunate to interview him in the early summer of 2020. In our conversation, John reflects on the shift to remote care: "We've seen that telehealth has really stepped up for mental health care and we've seen that mobile apps have a role too

178 ■ *Towards a Digital Ecology*

but it hasn't quite been the same role as telehealth." He observes that the groundwork in telehealth and the obvious advantage of remote interactions has resulted in wide adoption but: "when we can move to apps and wearables and monitoring, move towards digital programmes and therapies, then it becomes closer to asynchronous psychiatry." John believes that freed from temporal and geographical boundaries, we can bend the curve beyond synchronous care to reach more people within the limited resources at our disposal.

John's perspective is wider than the secondary care therapy services which we have largely explored in this chapter. His purview is not only technology but also the human factors in how digital can play a positive role in what is essentially a relational discipline. "The most pressing issue we have to consider," he tells me, "is are we going to increase access to care or are we going to increase a digital divide?" His team have instigated two very interesting innovations to address this concern.

It became apparent to John that many of his patients were not confident in technology:

> many people may have a smartphone but no one has shown them how to download an app … to use the alarm feature for when you want to track when to take a medication, how to use notes to keep track of important medical information.

In order to address this he has firstly created a short course for people to learn digital skills in a group environment: "digital literacy skills are very learnable," he explains: "it's not fancy, it's not machine learning, it's not a new app, it's not a new device, it's working with people and helping them become ready to use technology."

Secondly, his team has created a new *digital navigator* role which he likens to a radiologist having a technician to support them in routine scans. Rather than trying to persuade clinicians to change their practice: "we know it's very hard to implement change into healthcare, we have centuries, if not decades of evidence, and we know just giving people new technology is not going to fix everything." At the end of an appointment with his patient, he brings in the navigator to spend time with his patient to set up a sleep monitoring app or whatever they have determined between them might help. Before the subsequent appointment, the navigator downloads and prepares the data so John and his patient can review it together in their consultation. "Learning from decades of prior research and experience," says John: "hybrid solutions that offer a blend of face-to-face and online or app-based treatment will be the most effective solution." John has a simple prescription that could just work.

To Save the NHS Click Here

One of the more contested aspects of digital in the NHS is the extent to which some digital companies move health services from public to private hands. Private providers

Bending the Curve ■ 179

delivering healthcare is not particular to digital companies and has been increasingly a feature of the healthcare landscape since the Lansley reforms and primed through the introduction of an internal market back in the 80s. I am curious about whether the slow progress on digital adoption on the part of NHS provided IAPT services makes them vulnerable to losing contracts when they are re-tendered by commissioners. It is definitely the case that there are increasing numbers of what could be described as digital-first private IAPT providers competing with NHS IAPT services.

In an investigation into NHS spending, the Nuffield Institute found that NHS-provided mental health care has seen a fall in revenue whilst the independent sector has seen it rise. A decline in revenue raises worrying questions about the sustainability of NHS trusts insofar as each organisation needs to deliver a critical mass of services in order to be viable.[21] If an NHS trust loses a service such as IAPT to a private-sector provider, then its overall viability comes under threat. Private companies tend to go for the simplest and easiest services to be delivered where there is a profit to be made. Equally for NHS trusts, these less-complex services provide a counterbalance to more complex mental health services such as forensic units and assertive outreach teams. If they are left providing only the more complex and challenging services then they are more vulnerable to being destabilised. There is a ripple effect that, whilst not immediately obvious, displaces the balance of healthcare.

Further calculations by The Nuffield Trust indicate that over the last decade around 20% of annual public spending on health services in England has gone to private providers.[22] Recent data from NHS Digital tells a similar story, indicating that the vast bulk of IAPT provision is provided by NHS trusts, with just under 10% delivered by charities and another 10% delivered by private companies. The threat to NHS providers is still relatively small but is nevertheless present. A recent award to a digital-first private company of an 86 million pounds IAPT contract proved controversial when it ousted a not-for-profit provider.[23] There is a tension operating at the substratum of digital health that at the very least must be rendered visible if we are to determine the digital ecology we want to nurture.

As we have seen, NHS IAPT services routinely outsource patients to private companies when they can't meet demand. These companies appear to be doing well. SilverCloud recently raised $60 million in a Series B investment round and has a valuation of between 58–87 million euros. IESO has similarly raised a total of £18.7M in funding over five rounds of investment.[24] The role these companies play in NHS provision is still small but appears to be growing. In September 2020, NHS Digital started recording internet-enabled therapy which could be delivered by any provider, including in-house NHS developed products. Figures show that in September 2020 only 5% of services were delivered in this way but it grew dramatically to just over 27% in November.[25] The data has not been collected over a long enough period of time to show trends, but the fact that over a quarter of interventions are digital in the most recent figures, is startling.

It is not my intention in this chapter to deliberate extensively on the rights and wrongs of privately delivered NHS services. However, the shifts in the pandemic do

180 ■ *Towards a Digital Ecology*

highlight how previous working practices within IAPT appear to have neither met the needs of patients or the workforce and have resulted in outsourcing to meet demand and meant it is less competitive than its private counterparts. This shift provides an existential and a practical challenge for NHS organisations. If IAPT services can leverage and embed the changes they have been forced to make, then maybe this provides a promising approach that will secure their ability to thrive in the future.

If NHS providers fail to do this then they will end up with dwindling services which are the most difficult to deliver and succumb to a deficit that ultimately has to be picked up by the public purse.

An Open Future

My first ever single was Are Friends Electric by Gary Numan; I still have a photo of me holding the treasured vinyl seven-inch record in my grubby eight-year-old hands. My Adam and the Ants phase involved listening to scratchy mix-tapes my friend's older brother had made for us on a tape recorder. My first Walkman, along with the novelty of walking up my local town high street listening to Madness on my headphones, was like nothing else. My CD collection is now confined to a box in the attic, and I am now one of 232 million people who subscribe to Spotify.[26]

The music streaming platform has transformed how many of us consume music. Through one subscription we can access any artist, genre or playlist we might imagine. We trade convenience and accessibility with the joy of owning a single or album. Or we do both. Digital technologies mean that music can be shared in an instant, released from its vinyl prison and distributed in a click. The only thing preventing it from leaking out to the world in an instant is the copyright that protects it.

What could IAPT (and the wider NHS) learn from platforms such as Spotify when it comes to delivering services personalised to people's needs and preferences? I ask this question to illustrate how we might think creatively and laterally about enabling equitable access to a range of therapies and other clinical services through the affordances of platform technologies.

IAPT has in some ways always been a digital service. From those very early days when IAPTUS was conceived, its delivery has been underpinned by technology. A relatively mature ecosystem of digital products and services has grown around it. Those digital services are like the CDs of therapy; an IAPT service buys the CD in the form of a digital service and that is what therapists and clinicians have available to them, whether or not they like the artist or the album. It is a start, but you still get what you are given, even if it meets your needs and preferences less well than something else. What's more, just like copyright, the data is locked away in proprietary systems, apart from that which NHS Digital compels it to provide for reporting purposes.

Bending the Curve ▪ 181

Does the Spotify model hold the key to re-conceptualising how digital services are offered and licensed? We are already some of the way there. NHSX is busy creating frameworks for different categories of digital products and services, a bit like an online record store where you can peruse and download an album. They have done the background work to make sure the album meets all the right standards so you can play it from your smartphone or laptop without a problem. They could easily create a framework for digital IAPT services but that would only solve the purchasing problem.

What if the NHSs were to behave less like a record store and more like Spotify, creating not only the standards and governance for digital providers but also a delivery platform to which regional integrated care systems could subscribe. That fee may be calculated according to the size of the population and could be a balance of national retainer and local purchasing. The difference is that it wouldn't be a one-album purchase, it would be any number of tracks that meet the requisite standards to be used as required according to local needs.

This would mean that as an IAPT therapist I could log on and scroll through the range of digital therapy services approved for use via the open platform's front end. I could prescribe a self-guided depression course for one patient, a course of messaged-based CBT for another and an education class or mobile app for another. I could personalise the intervention to the specific requirements, circumstances and preferences of each of my patients. As a patient, my choice is expanded and my likelihood of sticking with intervention may be increased as a result. I am not limited by the one-off purchasing decision of the IAPT that provides the service in my local area. The role of a digital navigator seems to fit nicely within this approach, helping patients onboard and use the application prescribed to them.

There are wins for the NHS too. Spotify captures huge amounts of data, which when combined, start to generate insights at a population level about our music preferences and listening habits. The platform, with the right permissions, would curate the data and release it from proprietary applications. It could be used for real-world evaluation as well as improvement and research. In the interests of accountability and transparency, the data would be made available to inform what works and what doesn't, opening up insights for patients, commissioners and the public. With good quality insight, digital health companies could start to be reimbursed for the benefit (outcomes) they bring to patients, moving to a value-based payment model rather than paying for activity.

Healthcare data is generated by patients, administrators and clinicians and funded through the public purse. Releasing that data so that it can be used equally by a start-up, corporate or researcher could release new insight leading to innovation rather than it being monopolised by the private companies who currently hang on to it for their benefit alone.[27]

What's in it for the digital service providers? They have an active marketplace and an easy way to make their services available to the NHS. They will be able to get to market more quickly. This is not an entirely new concept. SilverCloud has

182 ■ *Towards a Digital Ecology*

already integrated its platform with the EPIC electronic patient platform, part of a proprietary walled garden called the *App Orchard*.[28] Rather than being led by another vendor, the approach I describe would be truly open and the standards and data remain within public hands.

This open platform model could add value to the research community too. As well as being highly prescriptive and target driven, digital IAPT products and services also attract a lot of interest from academic researchers. Driven by the desire to generate new knowledge, academics often create digital platforms through which they ask users to generate data for research purposes, or they develop digital interventions which they assess as to their efficacy as a novel mode of intervention. A good example of an open research platform is OpenSafely[29] which is a secure analytics platform for electronic health records in the NHS. It was created during the pandemic to analyse over 24 million pseudonymised primary care NHS records in order to answer clinical and public health questions. It was developed with cooperation from one of the largest primary care electronic patient record providers.

Sometimes researchers have an idea for a novel digital product or service that could add value to IAPT services. They get it developed through research monies aligned to an evaluation of its efficacy. The trouble is, they are incentivised and motivated to generate new research, not for the most part to build and run businesses. This means their ideas often remain within the walls of the institution and never see the light of day. Anyone who has run a digital company knows that the product may be the cornerstone of their business, but to make it successful they need a whole lot more. An open platform could help researchers make the output from their projects available for use beyond the confines of academic endeavour.

This open platform approach is not a new idea. Global management consultancy McKinsey argues that what they call an *open innovation platform*: "would serve as the basis for an ecosystem of digital-health-services innovation by certified third parties and could be steered by the respective health system.[30]" They acknowledge that the development of such a platform would create technical and regulatory challenges, as well as require close cooperation from a wide range of stakeholders, but they argue the benefits are worth the effort. A central NHS body could act as custodian of the ecosystem with responsibility for the platform itself along with governance, standards, certification and reimbursement. The process for companies, researchers and even NHS-led products to join the platform would be dynamic rather than locked for a set time period. Could this be part of the answer to a flourishing digital ecology?

This may be a great idea, it may be a bad idea and it may have some limited merit. As we have seen throughout this book, a hypothesis such as this must be tested through a user-centred design process and the contextual factors understood and accounted for. The balance between a national approach and local determination is always fraught. There is an imperative for the NHS to be bold when it comes to the actual transformative use of digital technologies to make a step change in care that benefits citizens and aligns with the underpinning principles of the NHS.

Bending the Curve ▪ **183**

This chapter has explored just a small part of NHS mental health provision in England. It is just part of the story. The wider story includes a wide range of secondary and inpatient mental health services. It also includes other types of digital interventions such as virtual reality exposure therapy for people with phobias and coaching chatbots. The digital ecology of secondary care mental health is relatively mature and the sector holds lessons for other parts of the healthcare system. However, even here we remain in the foothills of exploiting digital technologies at scale to make a real difference to the mental health of our nation.

Notes

1 https://www.annualreviews.org/doi/full/10.1146/annurev-publhealth-032013-182435#_i1
2 https://www.nuffieldfoundation.org/project/covid-19-social-study
3 https://www.bmj.com/content/369/bmj.m1994
4 https://www.covidsocialstudy.org/results
5 https://b6bdcb03-332c-4ff9-8b9d-28f9c957493a.filesusr.com/ugd/3d9db5_3e6767dd9f8a4987940e7e99678c3b83.pdf
6 https://www.mind.org.uk/news-campaigns/news/mental-health-charity-mind-finds-that-nearly-a-quarter-of-people-have-not-been-able-to-access-mental-health-services-in-the-last-two-weeks/
7 https://www.nuffieldfoundation.org/project/covid-19-social-study
8 https://www.health.org.uk/news-and-comment/blogs/emerging-evidence-on-covid-19s-impact-on-mental-health-and-health
9 https://cep.lse.ac.uk/pubs/download/special/depressionreport.pdf
10 https://www.babcp.com/What-is-CBT
11 https://www.nuffieldtrust.org.uk/resource/improving-access-to-psychological-therapies-iapt-programme
12 https://www.england.nhs.uk/mental-health/adults/iapt/
13 https://digital.nhs.uk/data-and-information/publications/statistical/psychological-therapies-report-on-the-use-of-iapt-services/june-2020-final-including-reports-on-the-iapt-pilots-and-quarter-1-data-2020-21/waiting-times
14 https://www.england.nhs.uk/wp-content/uploads/2020/05/iapt-manual-v4.pdf
15 https://www.nature.com/articles/s41746-020-0293-8
16 http://www.tara.tcd.ie/bitstream/handle/2262/91707/Published.Paper.pdf?sequence=1&isAllowed=y
17 https://www.nice.org.uk/advice/mib215/chapter/Expert-panel-conclusions
18 https://digital.nhs.uk/data-and-information/publications/statistical/psychological-therapies-report-on-the-use-of-iapt-services
19 https://www.theguardian.com/society/2021/jan/01/covid-antidepressant-use-at-all-time-high-as-access-to-counselling-in-england-plunges?CMP=Share_iOSApp_Other
20 https://www.theguardian.com/society/2020/aug/18/depression-in-british-adults-doubles-during-coronavirus-crisis
21 https://www.nuffieldtrust.org.uk/files/2017-01/into-the-red-nhs-finances-web-final.pdf
22 https://www.nuffieldtrust.org.uk/news-item/privatisation-in-the-english-nhs-fact-or-fiction

184 ■ *Towards a Digital Ecology*

23 https://novaramedia.com/2019/06/25/like-an-ae-run-by-virgin-active-physiotherapy-firm-awarded-86m-nhs-mental-health-contract/
24 https://www.crunchbase.com/organization/ieso-digital-health/company_financials [accessed 10 March 2021]
25 https://digital.nhs.uk/data-and-information/publications/statistical/psychological-therapies-report-on-the-use-of-iapt-services
26 https://appinventiv.com/blog/spotify-statistics-facts/
27 https://www.ethicalhealthcare.org.uk/blog/2019/3/2/why-an-open-health-platform-is-inevitable
28 https://www.businesswire.com/news/home/20201119006082/en/
29 https://opensafely.org/
30 https://www.mckinsey.com/industries/healthcare-systems-and-services/our-insights/how-healthcare-systems-can-become-digital-health-leaders#

Chapter 10

The Theatre of Tech – A Study in Solutionism

> If we don't find the strength and the courage to escape the silicon mentality that fuels much of the quest for technological perfection, we risk finding ourselves ... with lackluster (if not moribund) cultural institutions that don't take risks and only care about their financial bottom lines.
>
> Evgeny Morozov. To Save Everything Click Here. [Allen Lane, 2013]

> The NHS is one of the most trusted and well-loved institutions in the UK. It stewards our healthcare data, which is of immense social value. It has an on-the-ground workforce greater than any tech company on the planet, and an unrivalled relationship with the British public. No computing power or ad-revenue can create this for tech companies. Government, NHS leaders and tech-companies must realise this: the pandemic cannot become a free-for-all where panicked responses create easy access to precious NHS resource – the interests of the NHS, the patients and the public it serves must come first.
>
> Aidan Peppin, The Ada Lovelace Institute[1] (28 March 2020)

There is a fancy office in central London that I regularly visit for meetings. One of its more annoying features is a small iPad propped up at the reception desk. As I arrive through the revolving doors, I know the drill. The security guard waves me towards the white device sitting primly on the countertop where a receptionist would once have been. Instructions on the screen compel me to add my name and then pose for a headshot. Never quite sure why the photo is taken, where and for how long it will

DOI: 10.1201/9781032198798-10

186 ■ *Towards a Digital Ecology*

be stored, I usually dodge the camera, turning away as the camera flashes. No one seems to notice or even care.

This ritual is a classic example of technology used as a theatre. Let me explain. The notion comes from what security technologist, Bruce Schneier, has dubbed *security theatre*. According to Schneier, authorities have a tendency to put in place security measures in order to make people feel more secure without doing anything to actually improve their safety. In the months after the 9/11 terror attacks, National Guard troops were stationed in the US airport security with guns that had no bullets.

Security is both a feeling and a reality. "When people are scared, they need something done that will make them feel safe," explains Schneier, "even if it doesn't truly make them safer." Along with the public's desire to feel safe, "politicians naturally want to do something in response to a crisis, even if that something doesn't make any sense."[2] Finding signals to suggest that politicians are in control of scary situations is tempting to those in authority but run the risk of backfiring, as we shall see.

The wilful government fixation on a contact tracing app in the early days of the pandemic had all the hallmarks of theatre. The ins and outs of how the app would work (or not) were splattered across columns of newspaper print. Some began to argue that this frenetic discussion about every technical detail of the app was serving an insidious purpose, it was creating an impression that authorities had the pandemic in their control.[3] This front-stage performance was obscuring a back-stage reality of ineptitude and inadequacy. The real story of COVID-19, as we saw in Chapter 7, is the ravaging impact of inequality.[4] Put simply, the elevation of the contact tracing app in public discourse in those early days of the pandemic served to give the impression that the government was doing something. It was technology theatre at its most duplicitous.

Writing in the early days of the pandemic, Professor of Security Engineering at the University of Cambridge, Ross Anderson, called out the Government's app hyperbole. Situating the debate in a historical context, he argues that for decades the *rhetoric of terror* favoured by governments has facilitated over investment in security at the expense of putting cash into public health and disease prevention. Whilst it is terror attacks that hit the headlines, a pandemic has actually been at the top of the country's risk register for many years:

> We must call out bullshit when we see it, and must not give policymakers the false hope that techno-magic might let them avoid the hard decisions. Otherwise, we can serve best by keeping it out of the way. The response should not be driven by cryptographers but by epidemiologists.[5]

This chapter is a case study in tech-solutionism and theatre, that is technology looking for a problem to solve. Evgeny Morozov defines such solutionism as: "recasting all complex social situations as neatly defined problems with definite, computable solutions or as transparent and self-evident processes that can be easily optimised – if only the right algorithms are in place!"[6] Tech solutionism elevates and obscures at the same time, and it almost always creates unintended consequences. The story of the contact tracing app is a lesson in the dangers of technology used to obscure and obfuscate the real challenge at hand. It is a salutary lesson instructing us that we should be cautious when anyone claims that technology is the answer to a complex problem.

"This tech solutionist, you know everything can be solved through the tech, is kind of funny," observes Natalie Banner as we muse on the litany of health tech projects that have failed to hit the mark over the years. As the lead for the Wellcome Trust's' Understanding Patient Data programme, she knows better than most the consequences of becoming beguiled by the allure of quick-fix technology. "You know anyone working in the space for any length of time would have told you the same thing," she reflects, "that the tech is not going to solve what are fundamentally very human problems."

There's an App for That

"Take 1 minute each day and help fight the outbreak." This was the call to action from the C-19 COVID Symptom tracker[7] that I downloaded onto my phone in the early days of the pandemic.

Developed by doctors and scientists at King's College London and Guys and St Thomas NHS Foundation Trust, working in partnership with health science company ZOE Global Ltd, the not-for-profit initiative gathered symptom data for research purposes. The app was fairly non-intrusive, with a daily reminder to complete a set of simple symptom questions.

It was only in researching this chapter that I decided to check out the app's privacy[8] notice and discovered that the application tracks both my IP address and location. It also states it is unable to give a time limit for when my data will no longer be kept, although it reassures me this will be kept under regular review. I was surprised to discover that I had consented to my data being shared in the USA where GDPR rules do not apply; I wondered what the implications might be and what risks, if any, it may present. I came to the conclusion that I am pretty clueless.

We routinely leak data from our mobile phones as we go about our daily lives. Every time I use Citymapper to plan a journey or hail an Uber to get somewhere, I make a trade-off between convenience and privacy that those platforms compel me to make. Surveillance is a contemporary reality, and many of us are active and willing accomplices, in order that we might consume the goods and services we desire. Most of us are unaware or uncertain about what we share, how it is used and by whom. Even when we are aware, we mostly resign ourselves to sharing our data anyway because we feel helpless in the face of these data-hungry corporates.

Like many others, I initially found myself agreeable to increased surveillance during the crisis, motivated to contribute to helping researchers develop insights that may curb the pandemic's grip. The personal, societal and legal implications of

188 ■ *Towards a Digital Ecology*

digital technology and data felt somewhat intangible and remote against the urgent crisis in front of us. There was a degree of social pressure as well, with the secretary of state for health chiding us that it was our *civic duty* to allow the state to keep tabs on us during this public emergency.

Through the contact tracing app, we were coaxed into becoming co-actors in government efforts to stem the viral tide. What might once have seemed Orwellian, authorities knowing our every move, appeared to have side-stepped into our lives through the backdoor of our collective fear and angst. At the time, I decided that rather than download the app, I would sit back and wait to see how its theatrical performance played out. Some nine months later, I went to the iOS app store to belatedly download NHS COVID-19, the official NHS contact tracing app. With 276,310 ratings, giving the app 4.6/5, the developer information implores us to download it *Protect your loved ones. Please download the app.*

With media headlines such as *Coronavirus contact tracing apps were meant to save us. They won't.* as early as a month into the pandemic, sceptics and detractors were out in force from the get-go.[9] In those early days, many predicted that app notifications compelling us to self-isolate, having been in the proximity of someone with the virus, would become the new normal in our lives. Take this excerpt from a *Wired* article:

> This is our new normal. Contact tracing apps aren't here for the short-term. After the first waves of coronavirus have passed and the public inquiries into government responses have started, the apps will still be watching over us. On their current trajectory they will become essential parts of our daily lives. And it will continue to be this way until a vaccine for coronavirus arrives.[10]

The scenario envisaged by this journalist was never quite realised in reality and the app ended up playing a much smaller bit-part in the pandemic theatre than many predicted. This is despite the initial elevation of the app as the solution to the virus' spread. So what happened?

In those early days, technology was the big idea to solve the pandemic as it raged through our lives. In an open letter[11] to the government on 28 April 2020, the British Computer Society (BCS) it is clear that they, like everyone else, have the app front and centre of the pandemic response. The authors make the case that mass levels of testing must be put in place to work in tandem with the app. The app is centre stage. Grappling for something positive to tell the public, an app that could stop the virus in its tracks must have been a seductive idea. But the big idea turned out to be another sorry tale in a litany of tech-solutionist damp squibs. Beyond the theatre it created, this chapter lays bare the dangers of myopic tech-solutionism and do-something-itis. It has lessons way beyond the pandemic for anyone who is minded to think an app on its own can save the day when faced with the most perplexing problems.

The Theatre of Tech – A Study in Solutionism ■ 189

So why did I and so many others make a decision to resist government pleas to incorporate the app into our shared effort to respond to the virus? Whilst nowhere near the colossal spending disaster of NPfIT, this story shares many of its characteristics – big promises, chaotic delivery, civil society pushback, public distrust and a healthy dose of hubris. This is less a story about the technical ins and outs of the mobile app, plenty has been written by that. It is rather a reflection on the positioning of technology in the narrative of a disaster and what it can tell us about how we might better approach the use of technology in the sphere of public health and healthcare services.

Silicon Valley Style Hubris

Three types of digital technologies were announced to be under rapid development as the pandemic began to take its early course. Firstly, there were symptom tracking apps such as the one I downloaded; secondly were contact tracing apps aimed at identifying people who have been in contact with an infected person and asking them to self-isolate for two weeks; and lastly, digital immunity certificates for people to evidence they are free of the disease. All were touted as ways to flatten the pandemic out of its viral existence.

These high hopes pinned on technology put me in mind of an incident back in 2018 when a drama of a different flavour appeared in our newsfeeds. A group of 12 boys and their soccer coach had become wedged deep in caves in Thailand, whilst on a group expedition. The world looked on in horror and fascination as, over the course of 28 days, international efforts were galvanised to save them. Expert divers and engineers from around the world travelled to Thailand to help.

Somewhat bizarrely, Silicon Valley entrepreneur, Elon Musk, decided to weigh in and send a team of engineers with a purpose-built submarine to help them out. Perhaps predictably, the submarine turned out to be impractical and was left at the side of the cave "in case it might be useful in the future" as Musk and his team retreated. It was actually a low tech well-evidenced diving method that saved all 12 boys. Musk's tech solutionism was merely a sideshow in the drama in which established low tech methods saved the day.[12] Many saw this incident as an illustration of Silicon Valley arrogance.

The Covid tracing app, initially touted as the solution to our problems, has similarly become a side-show at the margins of the pandemic which has ultimately relied on low tech, track and trace efforts. This tendency towards tech-solutionism carries many risks and the potential for unintended consequences. There is a danger that we are led by what is possible rather than what is desirable. In other words, are we doing something just because we can? It appeared in those early days that technology offered the potential to stem the pandemic but the answer turned out to rely on much more than just an app.

190 ■ *Towards a Digital Ecology*

Do Something. Do Anything

On 24 April, the development of a NHS contact tracing app was announced by NHSX Chief Executive, Matthew Gould. In a blog post, he describes how users will be able to choose to allow the app to inform the NHS if they become unwell, and it will trigger an anonymous alert to other app users with whom the user has come into significant contact over the previous few days.

With a vaccine out of easy reach, politicians across the world jumped on contact tracing apps as a means to stem the spread of the pandemic. It seemed common sense that automating at least part of the laborious process of contact tracing would enhance efforts to stem the spread of the infection and cost a fraction of the number of human contact tracers.

It is fascinating how once-obscure practices became part of our everyday existence over the course of 2020. What was once a remote and unfamiliar public health activity has become a routine part of our lives. Contact tracing requires people with a positive COVID-19 test to be tracked and then the people they have had contact with to be tested and quarantined. Tracing doesn't just focus on people with the virus; it aims to get ahead of the disease by testing people who have come into contact with someone with the disease during the incubation period before they experience symptoms. If you only identify and isolate people with active symptoms, you will not stop the disease from spreading. Timing is everything.[13]

In a pre-digital era, the response to communicable disease pandemics has been painstaking in-person contact tracing which, whilst labour intensive, is an effective means of curbing infection. However, it has limitations. Firstly, it is a slow and time-consuming process; secondly, it relies on our memory to accurately recall where we have been and who we have had contact with. Finally, it requires governments to galvanise massive resources for it to be effective.

Keen to show they were making inroads into curbing the pandemic, governments around the world invested in contract tracing apps to speed and scale up this previously exclusively human process. But the best way to go about it and whether there was evidence that they would actually work was hotly contested. The fact that this approach relies on each of us having and carrying a smartphone, reliable internet access and to have downloaded the app appeared to have been overlooked in a flurry of activity somewhat reminiscent of Elon Musk's cave rescue attempt just a few years earlier.

For a contact app to be effective, we need to trust it to be accurate when it tells us that we have been in contact with an infected person, and we need to be sufficiently motivated to take the necessary steps to self-isolate. Reports suggested the app would have to be downloaded by 60% of the population to have any chance of it making a difference.[14]

However, straight away it was clear that this would be a challenge. Led by technologists, it appeared to have been overlooked that not everyone has a mobile phone. Those of us who do have a mobile phone, don't necessarily carry it with us at all times. The potential for the app to drain battery life would affect people

The Theatre of Tech – A Study in Solutionism ■ 191

with older and less powerful mobile phones.[15] Furthermore, it turned out that the Bluetooth signal from one phone to another is not bulletproof. If you and your next-door neighbour in your separate houses have a contact tracing app enabled on your phones, it is possible that they will indicate you have been in contact even though you have a brick wall between you.[16] Neither the technology nor our daily human activities turn out to be as reliable as people modelling how smartphone contact tracing apps would like them to be.

When we see a piece of theatre we must ask ourselves what is going on backstage that some would prefer remains out of sight. The contact tracing app served a purpose in the early days but latterly almost disappeared from public discourse. As I write this chapter, and with one of the highest death rates in the world, there are already calls for a public inquiry into the UK Government's handling of the pandemic response.[17]

We Don't Have an App for That

At this point, I want to take us back to the early days of the development of the contract tracing app, along with the frenzy that surrounded it. On 10 April, Apple and Google announced an unprecedented collaboration to develop a toolkit for app developers based on a decentralised system where data is communicated between people's phones and does not sit on a central database. "Google and Apple are announcing a joint effort to enable the use of Bluetooth technology to help governments and health agencies reduce the spread of the virus, with user privacy and security central to the design."[18]

Some governments built smartphone applications on this toolkit, whereas others embarked on a different route. The UK Government was one of those that initially attempted to develop a centralised system where data sits on a computer database so it could be analysed by epidemiologists and others. Their mind was on future preparedness and real-world data for research. This approach is arguably much less privacy-friendly, whereby data about our health, where we go, our movements and who we are in contact with is all collected by government departments.

With assurances of an ethical approach, NHSX was at pains to engage civil society institutions and the Information Commissioner's Office in the app's development. The NHS unit also committed to publishing key security and privacy designs along with the source code to ensure transparency. An Ethics Advisory Board was established to give oversight and feedback on the app as it developed. In April, the Board published an open letter to the government in which they gave *conditional* support to the app based on the information they had at that time.[19] The Board implored the Government:

> A trustworthy approach is crucial to the success of a CV19 app. The Government's perceived success or failure in this endeavour will have

192 ■ Towards a Digital Ecology

implications for future uses of data driven technology by government and public services for many years to come. Indeed, this is the time for the Government to demonstrate its ability to use technology for the public good, in an ethical way, and to build strong foundations of trust.

The letter concludes that the Government should avoid making commitments to citizens, in a desire to encourage take-up of the app, which are then reversed at a later date. Public trust, members of the board argue, is key. The symbolic properties of the contact tracing app were clear to see. Get this right and technology can be shown to augment and enhance properly resourced and proven track and trace activities. Get it wrong and the app becomes yet another debacle that sets back future efforts to use digital technologies in health and other public services.

Checks and Balances

As the newspaper headlines continued, I began to feel deeply uncomfortable about the trajectory of the contact tracing app having seen the consequences of damaged public trust by previous well-intentioned NHS initiatives. The care.data debacle,[20] in which the NHS had to abandon plans to bring together patient data for research and other purposes in the face of massive opposition, came to mind.

In a blog post for the Ada Lovelace Institute, Imogen Parker argues that if the government puts their weight behind a tool such as the contracting tracing app, it must live up to high standards or risk denting public confidence. Furthermore, "badging the contact tracing app as NHS brings blowback on the NHS, and it undermines faith in future tech tools that could prove lifesaving." Would this be an exemplar project that demonstrates how technology can be employed for public service or would it be another care.data. Only time would tell.

It wasn't long before further questions started to be raised about the app. Murmurings of disquiet began to surface, as urgency and an absence of red tape began to collide. Even creating the space to ask questions seemed like a luxury when people were dying in hospital beds and care homes every day. But those were important questions because an app that collects data about our everyday lives carries ramifications well into the future and beyond the pandemic haze.

Enter stage right, civil society. I for one am grateful that there we have organisations such as Amnesty International, alongside investigative journalists, who are in a position to dig into the issues on our behalf and hold governments to account. This is exactly what happened. A media-fuelled battle ensued between technologists, governments and civil society, each fighting a corner between a desire to curb the spread of the disease and resistance to unchecked surveillance, along with a concern about what all this might mean for public privacy beyond the pandemic.

In an open letter to the secretary of state for health and the NHSX chief executive, a group of self-declared *responsible technologists* argued against the use of novel

The Theatre of Tech – A Study in Solutionism ■ 193

and untested technologies. They point to the 22% of the UK population who do not have a smartphone which they suggest would make contact tracking both ineffective and at risk of reinforcing inequalities. Another group of 200 information security researchers and scientists produced a joint statement declaring they were *unnerved* by NHSX's plans and asked for reassurance that the app would not enable "data collection on the population, or on targeted sections of society, for surveillance."

Both the Ada Lovelace Institute, the Wellcome Trust's Understanding Patient Data Programme, the British Computer Society and others, quickly geared up to contest the hyperbolic dash to develop the contact tracing app. They sought to illuminate that which is problematic beneath the surface validity of this newest surveillance kid on the technology block.

In Love with Ada

The Ada Lovelace Institute is an independent research and deliberative body dedicated to ensuring that data and AI work for people and society. On 20 April, still relatively early on in the pandemic, they produced a rapid evidence review[21] on the technical and societal implications of the technologies under development.

The research institute argues for a proportionate and cautious approach that digs beneath the hype or surface plausibility of the app's effectiveness, to make informed and robust decisions about its use. They point to the absence of evidence to support the national deployment of the technical solution under development, and they argue that the success or failure of any technology would be contingent on public trust and confidence.

I interview Aidan, a researcher at the Ada Lovelace Institute, one Friday evening at the end of May 2020. We had first met earlier in the year when Aidan was a member of a panel I chaired at a conference on artificial intelligence and digital health. We begin our conversation reflecting on the seismic changes that have occurred since our previous encounter; we opine that if anyone had told us that we would be locked down in the grip of a havoc-wreaking pandemic, we would have barely believed them. A not unfamiliar refrain. Little did we know at that point, that the ill-fated contract tracing app endeavour would play such a diminutive part in public health efforts to stem the pandemic tide.

Aidan has an intriguing background, mixed as it is with a blend of cultural studies, arts, drama and science. When he tells me about his interest in the interaction of society and technology, I ask him to share what stories we are telling ourselves about the role of technology in the pandemic. "That technology will save us," quickly retorts Aidan with a wry smile. He goes on to explain why he believes this particular narrative is so problematic: "The trouble with a story like that, with stories in general, is that they highlight certain things and they obscure others."

For Aidan, this tech solutionist tale diminishes the possible risks, burdens and even damage that technology can do. He argues that this story situates technology

194 ■ *Towards a Digital Ecology*

outside of its social context "acting on its own and ignoring the fact that it is inherently social, it is made by people, it is deployed by people, it is affected by people, people use it." I add that maybe this is a convenient story for a government that is looking for easy answers and quick solutions. It's a case of magical thinking where technology sweeps in and saves us from hidden malevolent forces. Aidan does not disagree.

Centralised database options for contract tracing applications came under fire from Amnesty International as being the most invasive technology response to pandemic surveillance by governments around the world. Just to give an indication of how intrusive such applications have the potential to be, Bahrain's smartphone contract tracing app was connected to the "Are You at Home" television show. Amnesty reported how ten phone numbers from the country's contact tracing app were randomly picked every day, and the numbers were called to see if people were at home live on air during Ramadan. Prizes were given to those who were found to be obeying the stay-at-home rules. The authorities even published online sensitive personal information of suspected COVID-19 cases, such as people's health status, nationality, age, gender and travel history.[22]

Whilst such activities seem both outrageous and unimaginable in a UK context, the Bahrain example illustrates what is possible and the ways in which our data *can* be misused by governments in certain contexts. Once we have slipped down the slick slope of surveillance, it is almost impossible to scramble back up again. What seems innocent and well-intended has the potential to be used and exploited in any number of ways by those in power. Although the Bahrain example seems inconceivable here, it should be the canary in the mine for abuses of data and we should take concerns about civil liberties seriously, however remote they may seem.

During our conversation, Aidan explains that whilst he supports contacting tracing efforts, he has substantial concerns about the app:

> My personal biggest critique … is that assumptions for why contract tracing apps would work are based on mathematical models … they assume everyone interacts with the app in the same way, or the consequences of using the app are always the same, so I get a notification and I isolate for two weeks, job done.

Aidan is correct in his assertion that the underpinning model for the app was based on statistical models rather than real-world sensemaking. The case for a digital-first solution was made by scientists at the Big Data Institute, Nuffield Department of Medicine, at Oxford University.[23] They asked whether, from a mathematical point of view, it was possible to stop the epidemic: "we concluded that the epidemic can be stopped if contact tracing is sufficiently fast, efficient and scalable. We suggested that the best way to achieve this is by using a digital approach."

Their modelling concluded that at least around 60% of citizens would need to download and use the app for it to be effective. Aidan expresses frustration

The Theatre of Tech – A Study in Solutionism ■ 195

with the apparent absence of critical thinking about the inherent human and societal impacts:

> There are all of these social elements in that bit in between when the app tells you to self isolate and you self isolate … a whole world of social complexity that has been ignored and kinds of reduced what is a hugely social phenomena to a mathematical model and a series of tests.

Aidan points out that the 7 million people who do not use the internet would be immediately excluded from the data. Just because I walk around with my iPhone welded to my hand, does not mean this is the case for everyone. Digital contact tracing is based on the assumption that we all individually own a smartphone that we carry with us all the time. But what about those low-income families that may either not have or perhaps share a phone between them,[24] the 11 million people who don't know how to download an app and the 1.9 million people with no internet access?[25]

It's not just about who has a smartphone and how they used it. It's also about trust. The bottom line is that people not only have to trust the technology, they also have to trust the Government. Whilst there is relatively high trust in the NHS to look after our data in the right way, this drops dramatically when it comes to trust in our Government. Analysis by the Institute of government in 2019 found that whilst around 60% of us trust the NHS (and we trust our National Health Service more than any other institution) you can half that percentage when it comes to Government. Our governing class doesn't score much higher than insurance and credit card companies when it comes to our confidence in them to do the right thing with our data.

Give them an inch and they'll take a mile. This is the concern of many who believe that the compromises to our privacy that we make in crisis situations quickly become the everyday norm. They argue this new normal opens the door to further intrusions on our privacy. On 26 April, an article in the *Financial Times*[26] announced that global accountancy global professionals services company PwC planned to develop an employee contact tracing app to monitor the spread of COVID-19 in the workplace. To be effective, such a tool would require all employees to use it and so the article speculates it is unlikely to be voluntary. Tracking the activities of staff carries all sorts of trust, privacy and other implications that can be trampled over in a time of crisis. And is there any going back?

And then there is The Cummings Effect.[27] Whilst there is a *greater good* argument for downloading the app, there are few individual incentives, particularly for those who feel less vulnerable to the deadly effects of the virus. On May 20, a story broke in the media that senior prime minister aide Dominic Cummings had broken lockdown rules and travelled 420 kilometres to his family estate. To add insult to injury, his wife who travelled with him had suspected COVID-19. If it couldn't get any worse, he refused to apologise. Various public attitude surveys showed a subsequent marked decline in trust and confidence in the Government. People started to doubt the narrative that we are *all in it together*.

196 ■ *Towards a Digital Ecology*

With Dominic Cumming's incident still reverberating in the media and public opinion, Natalie is sceptical about the public's willingness to engage: "Certainly the events of the past week have radically undermined the sense of solidarity and "I will sacrifice some individual rights for the greater good" which is fundamentally what contact tracing needs to be able to do – you give up information that protects wider society."

Many will remember 2020 as a terrible year. The global pandemic was only one of a number of truly awful incidents during the year that many of us might wish we could have skipped. My conversation with Aidan takes place with the backdrop of the shocking murder on 25 May of George Floyd, an African American man in Minneapolis, at the hands of a white police officer, filmed live on mobile phones. We have this in our thoughts as we reflect on the deep levels of inequality the pandemic has rendered visible.

Particularly pernicious is the impact on people from black and minority ethnic communities who are four times more likely to die from the virus than their white counterparts.[28] Aidan has seen the consequences of systemic discrimination before:

> One of the things that we've seen in another work, with things like biometrics and surveillance technologies being used by the state or organisations, is that your past experience with institutions of power, and not just your individual, but your community's experience, totally affect how you feel about it.

We know that the pandemic has disproportionately affected people from black and minority ethnic communities and lower socio-economic backgrounds. There is a danger that tracing applications could increase social stigma and harassment of individuals, particularly if there is a risk of hacking and data being leaked.

When it comes to privacy and data, all of us will have heard others say or even might have said to ourselves that we have nothing to hide so what's the problem? "I've got nothing to fear is a privileged attitude to have," explains Aidan, "for the Black British community they can't afford to say 'I've got nothing to hide' … I've still got fear because I'll still get pulled over in my car at the very least." For Aidan, the contact tracing app increases the ability for the state, which historically has discriminated against minority communications, to extend and deepen its pernicious reach.

And what about the many other variables of human behaviour with an app that relies on self-reporting symptoms. I may be a died in the wool stoic who refuses to pay attention to COVID-19 symptoms; I may have COVID-19 but am free of any symptoms so I never even engage with the system; I may have symptoms but my livelihood depends on me working so I choose not to report them. Knowing all these possibilities, would you then choose to trust an app that told you to self-isolate for two weeks because you may have had contact with someone with the virus. I'm not sure I would.

The Theatre of Tech – A Study in Solutionism ■ 197

I wonder what this all means for the reliability of the data. There is a whole range of unintended consequences that can arise from incomplete and siloed data. With variable digital take-up both in geography and demographics, there is a risk that research based on the data that is collected, ignores the experiences of people with lower socio-economic status. Self-reporting relies on accurate disclosure and its quality is problematic given the novelty of COVID-19, the many asymptomatic cases and the similarity of symptoms to other common illnesses. If the proliferation of symptom checking apps does not contain common data fields, then the ability to aggregate data between them is limited and will result in fragmented insights.

A Masterclass in Mismanagement

Whatever the rights and wrongs of centralised versus distributed systems, there remained a big question about whether contact tracing apps are actually effective. In an article for the American website, The Hill,[29] researchers Bourdeaux, Gray and Grosz argue that contact tracing is an essentially human endeavour built on contextual knowledge and trust rather than simply a technological one: "Human contact tracers need to guide a rattled parent to think through who their child might have played with at a neighborhood potluck a two weeks ago or an undocumented immigrant find support and care should they fall ill."

Furthermore, contract tracers need to persuade people who may be infected to keep a 14-day quarantine. Whilst an app cannot do either of these things, they argue that it can augment and assist a human contract tracing programme if designed intentionally with and for them: "Human-centered tech can combine the power of data with the irreplaceable compassion of frontline contact tracers to help us keep COVID-19 at bay until we have a vaccine."

In an article in The Times on 13 May, Matt Hancock announced that the Isle of Wight rollout was going well, and the app would be launched in the next few weeks. Just a week later Boris Johnson, speaking during Prime Minister's Question Time, bullishly asserted that England would have a "world beating" test, track and trace operation by 1 June. Then it all went very quiet.

I asked friends what they knew and searched internet news feeds but to no avail. A trial of the contact tracing app on the Isle of Wight started out with lots of media attention that quickly fizzled to nothing. The Wired headline on 16 June: What's really happening with the NHS COVID-19 app trial? asked the same question that I and others were pondering.[30] The manual contact tracing programme finally got going on 28 May, but with 25,000 call centre army of contact tracers using phones and email to get in touch with people, the contract tracing app was conspicuously absent.

On the same day as the contact tracing scheme began in earnest, local news websites on the Isle of Wight reported that they had sought to find the answers to

198 ■ *Towards a Digital Ecology*

the unnerving silence from local public health officials and Government about the absence of the smartphone app. With no response to what they called questions with a legitimate public interest, they raised concerns that the absence of communication would only fuel misinformation around the app. It would appear from a further article on 23 June that their questions of public interest, despite promises to the contrary, were never actually answered.[31] Trust cannot be built and maintained when the shutters go down and an eerie silence ensues.

Wired 19 June magazine's headline: *The UK's contact tracing app fiasco is a master class in mismanagement*[32] pointed to the ignominious end that appeared to have befallen what was at the outset lauded as a pivotal component of the Government's plan to cut off the pandemic's viral lifeblood. It was then announced that its contact tracing app plans had been replaced by a much smaller project using the decentralised App and Google model and with no specific delivery date.

According to the *Financial Times*, 160 people had spent three months working 18-hour days and seven-day weeks on the app before it was abandoned.[33] What's more, the centralised app development cost £11.8 million of public money.[34] Beyond the money is also the wasted effort and an inevitable question about where better those efforts could have been targeted to have a positive impact on the spread of the pandemic. It remained unclear what would happen next.

An All-Party Parliamentary Group for Data Analytics (APGDA) panel discussion considered the technical alongside ethical issues challenges. One panel member, Ross Anderson, professor of Security Engineering at the Computer Laboratory within the University of Cambridge, called out the contact tracing app as a case of *do-something it is*, in which "action is demanded, and doing anything – regardless of effectiveness - is seen by policy makers as a superior option to doing nothing at all."[35] In a conversation with Natalie from Understanding Patient Data, she expresses her reservations: "The fact that it started off being so tech led was I think problematic … we all got a bit swept away with the app as this big shiny thing. The tech led approach distracted from the wider issues."

Natalie's concerns turn out to be well placed. In a Commons science and technology committee in June, Lord Bethnell, the minister responsible for the app, had to concede that people prefer being contacted by a human being with bad news rather than through a mobile app. It turns out yet again that failing to pay attention to human factors creates unintended consequences: "One of the things it has taught us is that it is the human contact that is the one most valued by people," observes Natalie "and in fact there is a danger of being too technological and relying too much on text and emails and alienating or freaking out people because you're telling them quite alarming news through quite casual communications."

In early July, the Government remained firm that a new track and trace smartphone app would be developed using the decentralised Apple and Google platforms. The US-based company Pivotal had reportedly been replaced by Swiss digital form Zuhlke,[36] and the *Financial Times* reported that NHSX officials were

The Theatre of Tech – A Study in Solutionism ■ **199**

taken with the idea of rebranding the app *PPE in your pocket*. This revamped version of the app began trials in the London Borough of Newham on 21 August. But beyond these basics, there was no sense of when it would be ready to add to the manual programme. What was once front and centre of the Government's attempts to reassure the public appeared to have become a footnote in the tragedy of the COVID-19 story.

The app was slowly but surely ignominiously downgraded from the central plank of the government's pandemic response to the *cherry on the cake* of the Test and Trace programme. Interrogated by the House of Lords' Science and Technology Committee, programme head Baroness Harding described the app in muted terms: "I think what we are building is a digitally assisted human service rather than something that is going to be purely digital."[37]

Once the hype had been blown away, this is probably how the app should have been conceived in the first place; an additional tool to augment proven and established track and track methods. A measured article in the scientific journal *Nature* in February 2021 assesses the role of contract tracing apps in government efforts to contain the pandemic across the globe. The authors conclude that results indicate that they can be useful, provided they have adequate political backing and are properly integrated into public health systems.[38]

The Beat of the Drum

At the cost of £35 million, seven months after it was announced, the contract tracing app arrived in the UK on 24 September 2020. It was quickly followed by a Government press release three days later that six million people had downloaded it on the first day and 460,000 QR code posters had been downloaded by businesses to give customers the option to check in to their premises using the app. With ten million downloads within three days of launch, the press release heralds an *overwhelming response* from the British public.

As of 28 October, the NHS COVID-19 app had been downloaded over 19.22 million times in both England and Wales according to the Minister of State for the Department of Health and Care.[39] With a population of 51.6 million (including children) this is around half the number required for the app to be effective according to experts.[40] Even this figure doesn't give the whole picture in so far as downloading and using an app are not the same thing. Statistics show that only around 30% of people who download an app, return to it more than 11 times.[41] Apps tend to have a low retention rate, and there's no reason to believe this would be any different for the contact tracing app.

An IPSOS Mori poll in November 2020, commissioned by the Health Foundation, found that just over half of us (61%) support the contract tracing app. People from professional backgrounds are more likely to be enthusiastic about the

200 ◾ *Towards a Digital Ecology*

app and those of us from black and minority ethnic backgrounds are far less likely to support it. The most common reasons for not downloading the app are not having a smartphone and worries about data privacy. Perhaps unsurprisingly, it is those most affected by health inequalities who are not able to access the app even if they were inclined to do so.[42]

The story of the app's lacklustre impact has all the familiar characteristics of previous failed NHS IT projects. It was a chaotically managed project, there were changes at the top, scope creep led to overspending, along with wasted effort and time.[43] Insider interviews with journalists back this picture up, talking of shifts in priorities and changing leadership all taking place alongside public claims that the project was progressing well.[44] This all took place against a backdrop of many people publicly telling the Government that the app was flawed and these criticisms, to all intents and purposes, ignored.[45]

However, whilst it is tempting to simply focus on incompetence and hubris when considering the downfall of the smartphone app, there is something equally worrying at play. This is a theme I return to throughout the book. It's a theme of who has the power. Ultimately, decisions about the fundamentals of smartphone contract tracing were not made by democratically accountable governments, however flawed they may be. They were instead made by two of the most mega-powerful private companies in the world, namely Apple and Google. Whether we agree or disagree with their approach is less material than the fact that governments, including the UK, were in their thrall. It was a huge demonstration of their power and illustrates how increasingly we are at their whim. We are reliant on their benevolence and fearful of their self-interest. The NHS project attempted to bypass it and failed. They allegedly tried to negotiate and influence the tech giants without success. "Our app won't work because Apple won't change their system,"[46] opined Matt Hancock.

So what does this tracing app travesty tell us, and what can we learn from it? I can't help but be struck by the distant drum that beats in the background of many of the digital health endeavours I recount in this book. It is the familiar beat of imperiousness on behalf of governments and bureaucrats rushing to the promise of the quick-fix tech solution at the expense of leaning into hard complex knotty problems.

It is the fact that all these problems turn out to be human at their very essence. Technological solutionism and magical thinking inevitably reduce complexity to simple ideas that, on the face of it, seem to make common sense, but are never enough. Worse still, they provide a temporary distraction to those looking for a simple fix. But in the long term, they fundamentally undermine the very real potential of technology, designed and developed in the right way, to help improve health and reduce inequalities.

As our conversation draws to a close, I ask Natalie for her opinion on my decision to delete the COVID-19 symptom tracking app: "I just think it's really unfortunate" she tells me: "because I think many people have done exactly what you've done, you started looking into it and then you've gone [sucks breath] which

The Theatre of Tech – A Study in Solutionism ■ 201

means that for any future ones you're going to think twice before downloading it." As Natalie intimates, all future progress and innovation are built on what has gone before but without public goodwill and trust: "[you] don't have anything to build up because you've already taken the crest and peak of public goodwill and chipped away at it."

Contact tracing and the contact tracing apps that support them have struggled across the globe. The UK is by no means alone, although it has fared worse than some. According to a feature in *Nature*, app-related efforts to stem the curb have faced similar issues including privacy concerns and eroded trust in public institutions. With a balanced perspective, the article suggests such apps are a useful part of an overall track and trace system but have been beleaguered by "a history of large-scale data breaches and privacy scandals in digital technologies."[47]

In an interim report from the National Audit Office on the test and trace scheme, the contact tracing app is hardly mentioned.[48] It has become barely a footnote in the wider story. The salutary lesson. There are no technology shortcuts. Tech theatre only distracted for so long. Invest in public health services.

What can we learn from the story of the contact tracing app that might help shape future initiatives and that is part of a nurturing digital ecology? We should anticipate and be open about anxieties that people are likely to have about the role of technologies within healthcare; we should involve people who will be affected by them from the outset to understand what will make the difference between whether they are used or left sitting in the app stores; we should embrace the expertise of civil society and actively involve them in deliberations and scrutiny in respect of design, development and use of technologies; and finally, we should conceptualise all aspects of technologies such as the contact tracing apps as part of wider social and political processes. This is a mature and responsible digital ecology where technology can flourish and add value to human systems and processes.

A Footnote

This book focuses squarely on the intensity of the first pandemic wave. However, there is a footnote to this story that provides an insight into concerns raised about public trust and the government keeping to its promises. I share it as a final reflection on the concerns raised by civil society and the media that the contact tracing app could open the door to increased surveillance and erosion of liberty. What seemed less important in the pandemic panic has salience in our lives as the heat subsides.

On 18 October, a story broke in the *Health Service Journal* that the police would be given access to information about people on a "case-by-case basis" to assess if a person has been told to self-isolate when they are failing to do so.[49] This was after it was made a legal requirement for people testing positive to coronavirus to isolate, with a fine starting at £1000 up to £10,000 for repeat offenders. All

202 ■ *Towards a Digital Ecology*

the fears expressed in the early days that people's data could be passed to authorities became a reality.

Privacy information on the Government's website[50] informs the readers that if an individual has been instructed to self-isolate by the NHS Test and Trace programme they will be contacted regularly by phone and text. If you do not respond to three attempts at contact, then your details can be passed on to the individual's local authority who can then pass on your details to the local police: "This may lead to enforcement action being taken against you, which could include you being fined." In reverse, if the police suspect an individual to be breaking self-isolation rules, they can request information from NHS Test and Trace.

Remember what Aidan from Ada Lovelace had to say about the app only working with public trust? When the *Health Service Journal* broke the story, it was Susan Michie, a professor of health psychology at University College London and member of the Government's Scientific Pandemic Insights Group on Behaviours who captured the mood in a series of tweets[51]:

> The evidence is strong that one of the key barriers to people downloading the app is distrust in how the Govt would use the data. And a key barrier to people not informing contact tracers of their contact is the same. This is a disastrous policy.

> The behavioural science group advising the Government has consistently said enable & support, don't punish & blame. Another example of the Govt not only ignoring scientific advice but going against it. And we are not asked about specific policies such as this. I wonder why not.

> Threatening to hand over #TestTraceIsolate data to police will discourage people from getting tested, giving contacts & downloading the app – disastrous in the middle of #Covid19UK that is out of control. This Govt is out of control – listen to the science!

At the beginning of this chapter, I recounted how I had downloaded the Covid Symptom Study app and then deleted it as I became concerned about privacy issues. It turns out that this app has become a surprise success of the pandemic, making its inventor, Tim Spector, something of a celebrity.[52] With over 4 million regular users, the data the app has generated was the first to identify that loss of smell is associated with virus symptoms and that children, young people present with very different symptoms than adults, and delirium is a common presentation in older people.

The app is perhaps an exercise in how, when you can build trust and confidence, a mobile app can be the gateway to vast amounts of data which in turn creates invaluable insight. It is an exercise in people making an active choice to volunteer their data for a common cause that has resulted in tangible benefits for all of us. Maybe it is a lesson in how to do this right. It opens up the possibility that there might be an alternative play to be written than in theatre of technology.

Notes

1 https://www.adalovelaceinstitute.org/data-driven-responses-to-coronavirus-are-only-as-good-as-the-trust-we-place-in-them/
2 https://www.schneier.com/essays/archives/2009/11/beyond_security_thea.html
3 https://www.cigionline.org/person/sean-mcdonald
4 https://www.cigionline.org/articles/technology-theatre
5 https://www.lightbluetouchpaper.org/2020/04/12/contact-tracing-in-the-real-world/
6 Morozov. 2018. p.5.
7 https://covid.joinzoe.com/about
8 https://covid.joinzoe.com/privacy-notice
9 https://www.wired.co.uk/article/contact-tracing-apps-coronavirus
10 https://www.wired.co.uk/article/contact-tracing-apps-coronavirus
11 https://www.bcs.org/media/6571/contact-tracing-apps.pdf
12 https://www.wired.com/story/elon-musk-thailand-cave-boys-rescue-engineering/
13 P. 9 https://ethics.harvard.edu/files/center-for-ethics/files/white_paper_5_outpacing_the_virus_final.pdf
14 https://www.wired.co.uk/article/contact-tracing-apps-coronavirus
15 https://www.bbc.co.uk/news/technology-52441428
16 https://arxiv.org/pdf/2005.11297/
17 https://www.ft.com/content/aa53173b-eb39-4055-b112-0001c1f6de1b
18 https://www.apple.com/newsroom/2020/04/apple-and-google-partner-on-covid-19-contact-tracing-technology/
19 https://nhsbsa-socialtracking.powerappsportals.com/EAB%20Letter%20to%20NHSx.pdf
20 https://www.bbc.co.uk/news/health-26259101
21 https://www.adalovelaceinstitute.org/wp-content/uploads/2020/04/Ada-Lovelace-Institute-Rapid-Evidence-Review-Exit-through-the-App-Store-April-2020-1.pdf
22 https://www.amnesty.org/en/latest/news/2020/06/bahrain-kuwait-norway-contact-tracing-apps-danger-for-privacy/
23 https://www.coronavirus-fraser-group.org/
24 https://arxiv.org/pdf/2005.11297/
25 https://www.goodthingsfoundation.org/news-and-blogs/news/leave-nobody-in-the-dark
26 https://www.ft.com/content/caeb250b-8d8b-4eaa-969c-62a8b58464aa
27 https://www.thelancet.com/journals/lancet/article/PIIS0140-6736(20)31690-1/fulltext
28 https://www.health.org.uk/news-and-comment/charts-and-infographics/same-pandemic-unequal-impacts
29 https://thehill.com/opinion/technology/493648-how-human-centered-technology-can-beat-covid-19-through-contact-tracing
30 https://www.wired.co.uk/article/contact-tracing-app-isle-of-wight-trial
31 https://onthewight.com/apple-and-google-deny-knowledge-of-uk-government-working-with-them-on-contact-tracing-app/
32 https://www.technologyreview.com/2020/06/19/1004190/uk-covid-contact-tracing-app-fiasco/amp/?__twitter_impression=true
33 https://www.ft.com/content/9446192a-aff1-4e95-93fb-a5adfbc7bbd5
34 https://www.digitalhealth.net/2020/06/nhs-contact-tracing-app-cost/
35 https://www.policyconnect.org.uk/appgda/news/how-data-responding-covid-19
36 https://www.ft.com/content/2fb504a3-fbc7-40a8-8996-f7dae596c831

204 ■ *Towards a Digital Ecology*

37 https://www.digitalhealth.net/2020/07/house-of-lords-committee-nhs-covid-19-roll-out-date/
38 https://www.nature.com/articles/d41586-021-00451-y
39 https://www.theyworkforyou.com/wrans/?id=2020-10-15.104209.h&s=covid-19+app#g104209.q0
40 https://www.ethnicity-facts-figures.service.gov.uk/uk-population-by-ethnicity/national-and-regional-populations/population-of-england-and-wales/latest
41 https://www.statista.com/statistics/751532/worldwide-application-user-retention-rate/
42 https://www.health.org.uk/publications/public-perceptions-of-health-and-social-care-in-light-of-covid-19-november-2020
43 https://www.technologyreview.com/2020/06/19/1004190/uk-covid-contact-tracing-app-fiasco/amp/?__twitter_impression=true
44 https://www.ft.com/content/9446192a-aff1-4e95-93fb-a5adfbc7bbd5
45 https://www.theverge.com/2020/5/5/21248288/uk-covid-19-contact-tracing-app-bluetooth-restrictions-apple-google
46 https://www.forbes.com/sites/zakdoffman/2020/06/19/how-apple-and-google-created-this-contact-tracing-disaster/#11cb43c77ca2
47 https://www.nature.com/articles/d41586-020-03518-4#ref-CR1
48 https://www.nao.org.uk/wp-content/uploads/2020/12/The-governments-approach-to-test-and-trace-in-England-interim-report.pdf
49 https://www.theguardian.com/world/2020/oct/17/police-get-access-to-people-told-of-self-isolate-by-nhs-test-and-trace
50 https://www.gov.uk/government/publications/coronavirus-covid-19-testing-privacy-information/testing-for-coronavirus-privacy-information-quick-read--2
51 https://twitter.com/SusanMichie/status/1317738648318640133?ref_src=twsrc%5Etfw%7Ctwcamp%5Etweetembed%7Ctwterm%5E1317738648318640133%7Ctwgr%5E%7Ctwcon%5Es1_&ref_url=https%3A%2F%2Fwww.digitalhealth.net%2F2020%2F10%2Fpolice-to-get-access-to-self-isolation-data-from-nhs-test-and-trace%2F accessed 13 January 2021
52 https://www.bmj.com/content/371/bmj.m3921

Chapter 11

We Get the Market We Deserve

In this country, we have a proud record of invention, but we lag behind in systematic uptake even of our own inventions.

Lord Darzi. High Quality Care for All: NHS Next Stage Review Final Report. London: Department of Health (2008)

How the Money Flows

It's all about how the money flows. One of the most fundamental challenges of digital health, which is rendered almost invisible by the frenetic activity of incubators, accelerators and the like, is the perplexing absence of a thriving marketplace. Selling to the NHS turns out to be a substantially more fraught process than might be imagined by an entrepreneur new to this sector. The digital sector is in poor health. Or as an industry colleague once described it, the NHS gets the market it deserves.

Back in 2011, the Department of Health and Social Care produced a plan for the NHS called *Innovation, Health and Wealth* (IHW) which tried to line up the health of the population with wealth created through innovation. However, over time it has become apparent that there is an ambiguous and misaligned relationship between the different stakeholders whose interests the Government sought to align. An official evaluation of the strategy points to competing values and norms whereby for example, the wealth agenda is meaningful to industry but less so to frontline NHS staff, where it is in the interests of industry to reduce what is seen by healthcare as a complex physical, emotional and social experience to a more simple and scalable

DOI: 10.1201/9781032198798-11

205

206 ■ *Towards a Digital Ecology*

consumer transaction. These are some of the tensions that come into play when we think of the marketplace of digital health.[1]

You might ask how and why a vibrant market is relevant to the healthcare system and if we should care at all. We should care. The NHS spends tons of money purchasing the equipment and infrastructure it needs to operate.[2] If healthcare is going to benefit from the sorts of digital technologies that are transforming other aspects of our lives, then it needs to be able to buy them, just like it needs to buy operating tables and MRI scanners. But digital is still a new and immature marketplace for the NHS and so the path to selling and buying is nowhere near established. That means we risk losing out as patients, citizens, health professionals and taxpayers.

When we imagine health services, it is likely that our minds conjure up our local GP, a kind nurse or the hospital ward. Our contact with the NHS is often when we are at our most vulnerable, when we are frightened and scared, where we have symptoms that concern us and are looking for reassurance that we are ok or treatment if we are ill. But behind the frontstage of care is the backstage of administration, logistics and finances. Like it or not, these are as important to the functioning of the NHS as doctors and nurses. That's why we need to wrap our heads around how the money flows if we are to fully assess the present and the future of an NHS enabled by digital technology.

This chapter digs into how the money moves in the NHS to help us understand how technologies get bought and sold. I've seen it from both sides – I've bought digital products from within the NHS, and I've sold them into the NHS. Neither is easy. I have always had this sneaking suspicion that the NHS is a terrible customer, but the reasons why this is the case have eluded me. Conversely, I know that startups are often wide-eyed and green about what they are letting themselves in for when they think they can develop a business and distribute their product with the NHS as their customer. They often learn the hard way that this is not the case. So what is going wrong?

Through conversations with some very smart people, I probe this conundrum from two vantage points – that of the NHS and how it moves money around the system and that of the entrepreneurs and innovators creating new technologies that *could* bring benefits to the healthcare system. I also consider when it makes sense for the NHS to build its own technology and when it does not. I have seen a lot of public money wasted on enthusiastic tech projects within NHS organisations that have never realised their value. I wonder how we can prevent this from happening.

I speak with Tom Whicher, who is a start-up founder making inroads into the NHS, to find out how he has gone about getting investment and how he and his team have persuaded the NHS to buy their products. I take a masterclass from people I trust to understand the devilish complexity of NHS finances. Lauren Bevan is a clinician who reinvented herself as an NHS head of finance and then left the NHS to work in tech. Having experienced the challenges from all sides, she coaches me through this tricky terrain. John Lee Allen gives me an investor perspective. Between them, they help me paint a picture of a digital marketplace in need of care and attention.

A Founder's Story – Fixing a Simple Problem

Before we get into working out how the money moves, I want to introduce you to Tom, who co-founded DrDoctor back in 2012. His company is solving a problem that we all recognise and understand. His story demonstrates that it is possible to build a business in the NHS, albeit that it is a rocky path to traverse.

I've known Tom since my early days of starting out in digital health. Our paths regularly cross at conferences and events. He is an all-round good guy and co-founder of one of the small number of start-ups that are successfully selling to the NHS. The simple idea germinated when Tom, an engineer by background, was doing a consultancy project in a hospital, where he witnessed first-hand the laborious analogue process that the hospital had for managing patient appointments.

We've all received that letter through the post with a hospital appointment, only to check our diary and see that the date has already been and gone. Tom explains:

> The thing that shocked me and surprised me was the fact that there wasn't any good patient facing technology at all. There were all these letters for appointments and often those letters were wrong or slightly out of date; and I was like, there has to be a better way of doing this. I thought surely we can use mobiles to improve accessing healthcare, and that was the starting premise.

He and his two co-founders played around with the idea of starting a company to make it easier for patients to access their appointments, and then over dinner in 2012 they finally decided to take the leap. They set about developing a technology for sending hospital appointment notifications by text message to patients and allowing them to accept, cancel or change that appointment. Their business proposition held the promise of ditching envelopes and stamps in favour of text messages, whilst reducing phone calls to booking centres.

With this deceptively simple idea, they bootstrapped their business, finding the money to get it going by using their own savings and even selling their cars. They got some grant money from a charity and then secured a bigger pot of money from a fund aimed at small businesses. Very early on, they were fortunate to get on to an incubator called Bethnal Green Ventures (BGV) which helped them take their idea and turn it into a concrete business proposition.

Many start-ups like Tom's do not have their origins from within the healthcare system. They are catapulted into a whole new set of acronyms and systems and processes they can't hope to understand. Tom believes that getting people outside

208 ■ *Towards a Digital Ecology*

healthcare innovating is important because they bring new thinking. But they find it hard to make sense of the NHS:

> To get them up to speed in understanding this like, special language that the NHS talks ... like most industries we basically speak a foreign language when you look at it from the outside in ... and it's important to get those people up to speed ... lots of great people with great ideas who need some help so they don't fall over at the first hurdle.

This is where incubators and accelerators come in, coaching and mentoring entrepreneurs in the peculiarities of the NHS and helping them develop a decent proposition.

Now, eight years on and DrDoctor is becoming an established business, building gradual success by staying focused on solving that very specific and granular challenge of getting patients to their appointments with as little friction as possible. As an offer to the NHS, Tom has struck gold because patients not turning up for appointments is very expensive: "DNAs (did not attends) are a billion pounds a year problem for the NHS," Tom tells me: "And by solving those discrete unsexy problems bit by bit in an incremental way, you end up building a platform which solves a need and which no one else has managed to solve before."

By finding a solution to a simple challenge and making savings to the NHS along the way, Tom has managed to build a business that works. He is emphatic that making the case for financial return on investment for any start-up is key:

> We always try and tie it back to the money, the great thing about money is that it's universal and everyone understands the value of the pound .... At the end of the day if you want a finance director to sign off a business case then you've got to show you are going to save money.

Tom's product is neat because it solves a transactional problem which can be relatively easily quantified. This is not the case for most digital technologies, especially those with a therapeutic application that has to be implemented in a multidimensional system. He is one of the lucky ones.

Tom's story belies a whole heap of complexity and any number of challenges along the way. It *is* possible to create a sustainable business model with the NHS as your customer, but I'm not sure how easy it is to create a *profitable* business. And it is hard graft. I recall a conversation with a digital health founder at a networking event in Mayfair some years ago, which stuck in my mind. Pulling at his receding hairline, he recounted how five years into his start-up, he would never have done it knowing what he knows now.

I have heard a similar story from the lips of many a founder. This is an all too familiar conversation. I am doubtful there is a substantial digital health business to be made when you have a comparatively small market, when the NHS is so

The Scissors of Doom

Tory politician, Nigel Lawson, once described the NHS as: "the closest thing the English people have to a religion." It is for this reason that political parties of all persuasions are keen to demonstrate they are pouring money into its coffers. But what about the reality? It is not a rosy picture. In desperate need of a cash injection, the lungs of the NHS are intubated, as it struggles with every breath.

Around half of NHS trusts are in the red.[3] This doesn't surprise me; for the 20 or so years that I worked in the NHS, it seemed that each year the money decreased whilst the work stacked up. Every year, I was instructed to cut my budget in what was euphemistically dubbed a cost improvement target. If I wanted to get cash to innovate, then I had to respond to grant opportunities from central NHS bodies – a short-term injection that came with a hidden price tag of onerous targets and reporting. Because budgets were reset each April, I would tend to protect my budget carefully throughout the year, only to furiously spend it in January before I lost it at the end of March. One-year budget cycles drive short-term thinking and opportunism.

Hard cash is one reason underlying the slow pace of technology adoption in the NHS. There is a stark misalignment between the promise of technology and the system's ability to capitalise upon it. A recent report from the National Audit Office lays bare the reality that there is insufficient money allocated at both national and local levels to fund digital transformation. The amount that NHS trusts spend on IT varies widely but collectively is less than 2% of overall expenditure. This compares badly to what experts believe should be closer to5%. That is a significant gap.

According to Richard Corbridge, an ex-CIO of a major NHS trust: "If you're sat at a board meeting in an acute trust and you're still having to defend 1% of the Trust budget to spend on digital solutions to bring transformation to the Trust, then there's something wrong." There simply isn't enough money being allocated to digital technology to make the changes promised by bureaucrats and policymakers. The most recent plan for the NHS, *The Long Term Plan*,[4] incorporates some positive signals about the role of digital, with a whole chapter dedicated to technology-enabled transformation.

But Richard is sceptical:

> When the Long Term Plan came out, everyone thought it would come with a long term budget as well. And a long term plan without a long term budget, I've always said isn't a plan then, it's an aspiration ... don't then judge the NHS when it can't achieve that if you've not spent money.

210 ▪ *Towards a Digital Ecology*

The National Audit Office report asserts that there is a "significant risk" that Trusts will be "unwilling or unable" to fund the £3 billion collectively required of them to achieve full digital transformation. There is a yawning chasm between the promise of technology and the cash available to deliver it.

Lauren describes NHS finances as the "scissors of doom" with costs going up on one axis and income going down on the other. As a chartered accountant and ex-head of finance and performance in an NHS trust, self-proclaimed dweeb Lauren is also a physiotherapist by profession and now works for a large tech company. I couldn't think of anyone better to give me a masterclass in how NHS budgets work when it comes to buying technology.

My first surprise is to learn that technology is often paid for through capital rather than revenue budgets. Capital budgets refer to money spent on assets such as buildings and infrastructure, including the backlog of maintenance and repairs to buildings and facilities, as well as equipment such as laptops and MRI scanners. Revenue budgets refer to the day-to-day costs of running services, including salaries and administration.

NHS trusts tend to innovate with digital when central bodies give them a dollop of cash in the shape of capital. Back in the day, capital could be used to buy hardware and licenses. But with a move towards software as a service and cloud, the need for data centres has gone and revenue is what is required to oil the wheels of digital tools and services. Revenue accommodates ongoing costs and not just a big bang in the shape of a one-off purchase. Revenue facilitates a more sustainable and adaptive approach to the use of technology over time, enabling NHS organisations to keep up with new technologies as they emerge. One-off capital injections turn out to be part of the problem.[5]

Another challenge with this way of financing technology spend is that capital budgets tend to go to the estates department, which is responsible for managing a backlog of any number of urgent repairs. It can be hard to justify a new software license when a nurse is asking for the damp patches in the ceiling on his ward to be fixed or there is a bucket to catch the drips from the leaky roof in the staff-room. According to figures from NHS Digital, the NHS has a collective estates backlog of £6.5 billion pounds, so to say capital budgets are under pressure is an understatement.

Financial pressures mean there is an all-round lack of cash to support innovation. The cash there in the system is unevenly distributed, with rural areas tending to have more of a deficit than metropolitan parts of the country. Organisations struggling with bigger deficits are more likely to focus on anything which looks like it can save money in the here and now, rather than investing in longer-term transformation. They are less keen to take a risk.[6]

To put financial pressures in perspective, the combined deficit of NHS trusts in 2018–19 was £827 million, with £10.9 billion in loans from the Department of Health and Social Care (DHSC) to trusts in financial difficulty. Problems in capital spend are stored up for the future, as money for investment in buildings and other

We Get the Market We Deserve ■ 211

long-term assets get moved over to spending on day-to-day services. It seems we are storing up problems for the future whilst trying to fix things in the present. In April 2020, the Government wrote off these internal debts between NHS trusts and the DHSC to the tune of £13 billion, easing pressure in the system which may make it easier for trusts to make the case for more investment in their estate in the future.[7]

When Rachel Dunscombe was a chief information officer for an enterprising acute NHS trust, she found workarounds to this capital headache. With insufficient funds to support her Trust on its digital journey, she worked out that she could buy a physical computer server with a capital budget and then rent out server space to the hospice down the road. She used the revenue from the hospice to invest in cloud capacity and software-as-a-service capability that would have otherwise been out of her reach. "So you had to create a micro economy that served your mismatch of data and revenue," explains Rachel. Whilst it helped her solve a problem, she is highly alert to the limitations of this sort of workaround: "It's not right, it doesn't scale, it takes you away from the day job, it takes cognitive load away from the NHS."

All NHS trusts have what are known as "cost improvement" (CIPs) targets, that is money that they have to take out of their budget every year. I remember that we weren't allowed to call them cuts in my NHS trust. Each year when I was asked to take out 5% of my budget, I felt like an impossible mountain to climb, but dutifully I would snip away by whatever tactic was to hand, be it replacing previous staff with more junior ones, leaving empty posts vacant or even cutting them completely. Working to annual budget cycles, it is hard for NHS trusts to invest in anything that might save them money eighteen months or two years down the line. Rather than being seen as an investment in making the NHS run safely and smoothly, IT departments similarly face CIPs, always having to look for ways to make money out of the system.

So how does the money move within the NHS? Put simply, there are commissioners and providers. Commissioners decide what services are needed and then invite providers to bid to deliver that work. They purchase a service and pay the successful provider to deliver that work through a contract. Some specialist services are commissioned nationally across the whole country, but most are commissioned at a local level through Clinical Commissioning Groups (CCGs), groups of GPs who come together to decide what is needed for the population they serve.

If you are a digital technology company, your customer may be the CCG or it may be the provider organisation whose services have been commissioned. It won't necessarily be the same in each locality. The system is now moving away from CCGs to regional commissioning arrangements through integrated care systems (ICSs). Whilst regional commissioning may make it easier to purchase at scale, it is still very early days. The system is in constant flux, with a never-ending slow motion ricochet between central control and local determination. If you're not part of the system, it can be hard to keep up.

In primary care, the picture is different again. All practices have an electronic patient record, and they have been required to offer patients access to online GP services since 2015.[8] Each CCG will have a number of GP practices in its patch and

212 ■ *Towards a Digital Ecology*

is responsible for procuring their IT services. The Department of Health and Care pays the bill directly, with IT services managed by the CCG on behalf of GP practices. Primary care services have an operating model, standards and a commissioning framework for technology.[9] It is more tightly prescribed with firmer technology foundations than secondary care.

Then there is the national tariff; a set of prices and rules issued each year by NHSE/I. Should you care to look, you can find the information online; but be warned, it is fiendishly complex with any number of exceptions and idiosyncrasies. Unlike me, Lauren loves this stuff and she explains to me why it is relevant to digital transformation. Put simply, the national tariff means that for the most part NHS trusts only get paid for the activity they deliver. As an example, and at risk of being macabre, if you arrive at A&E but you are already dead, then according to the 2019 national tariff, the hospital will be paid £73 to process your cadaver. Everything has a price tag. Who knew!

Lauren explains that this system of paying NHS trusts for the activity they deliver (that is care and treatment to you and me) means they find it harder to take a chunk of money and use it to do something different or innovative. They don't know how much money they are going to get because they don't know how much activity they will deliver. This in turn disincentives them to go out on a limb and take a risk doing something new.

Lauren instructs me in how hard it can be for NHS trusts to license software from small start-ups with neat products and good ideas: "This is where process becomes the enemy," she tells me, "because you probably have to do a business case to justify it, because there's known and unknown benefits and so for innovation it's really hard to know the return on investment.... so you have to rely on a forward thinking finance director to keep aside a pot of money [to pump prime innovation]."

Lauren describes the process that has to go on in an NHS organisation to firstly justify spending money on digital technology and then to access money to pay for it. As I write this chapter, I am working with a large mental health Trust on a business case for a new technology. The business case template is 43 pages long with any number of flowcharts and appendices. Even embarking on the process of putting together a proposition for a new technology purchase is a daunting and time-sapping endeavour. It requires motivation and steel.

The Elusive Return on Investment

Return on investment is a jargon phrase that simply means you have to show the value you are going to get for what you spend. "It used to be called invest to save money," Lauren tells me: "you see these great ideas but they never actually result in cash savings and some of them, because they divert activity out of the hospital, means there's a drop in income." Lauren is describing a common problem that can disincentivise innovation – if they buy a technology that keeps people out of

We Get the Market We Deserve ■ 213

hospital then they don't get paid. How services get commissioned has a material impact on what technologies a provider organisation will or won't buy.

Common sense tells us that it's a good thing to keep people out of the hospital and if we can do this through technology we should. But keeping people out of hospital means a decrease in activity which results in less income to the organisation. So the money you spend on the technology is an extra cost at the same time as you lose income. A double blow. Lauren explains further:

> Most of the NHS budget goes on staff and estate; not only do you not get a drop in staff, you still have to operate the buildings and you then have a drop in income because activity is done elsewhere.

Matthew, a hospital respiratory consultant picks up the story: "As a patient you don't care how many times you see me as a doctor. You want to see me as few times as possible. What you really care about is getting better." An enthusiastic adopter of technology, when Matthew and his team introduced virtual consultations they ended up with a financial headache they hadn't expected: "So we were in a situation, when we were doing virtual [clinics] which I was doing a lot of, and instead of getting around £200 for seeing a patient, we got £25."

He explains how the payment system disincentivises new ways of working:

> Of course that idea that if you go to a hospital manager and say I'd like to save the CCG lots of money, make the life of the patient more convenient, and by the way it's going to cost you almost the same amount [the tests still have to be done] but instead of £200 you're going to get £25, they look at you and ask what you've been smoking 'unless you want a 75% pay cut Matthew, this case isn't going to fly anywhere.'

Matthew is a critic of the way the money is organised between commissioners and providers: "One of the big disincentives is the tariff system and it's one of those ideas that sounds very good until you start digging into it." He argues that the way the money moves drives the wrong outcomes:

> My tendency is to be at the very moderate end of conservative politics, so I'm no socialist, but a free market, it just doesn't work in healthcare very well, and the Lansley reforms, which I thought were not a bad idea at first, didn't work in healthcare because they incentivise activity rather than outcome.

Lauren explains that there is a more recent move towards *block contracts* whereby NHS providers are given a chunk of money, usually on an annual basis, which means they get a timely and predictable budget that they can use relatively flexibly. This is similar to how GPs are paid using what is called a *capitation* payment system,

214 ■ *Towards a Digital Ecology*

whereby they receive a lump sum based on the number of patients in a target population, whether or not they actually treat them. In Lauren's view, block contracts give a bit more certainty which in turn create a bit more scope for innovation. This might be chink of light in the quest for NHS digitisation, and it may be the pandemic that has created it.

It would appear that COVID-19 has created an inflection point in how the money moves in the NHS. The national tariff was suspended in March 2020 for at least a year. Early signs suggest that the move to block contracts appears to be incentivising positive behaviour in the system with more emphasis on the collective over the siloed. The newly forming ICSs are expected to continue to work in this way, sharing opportunities and risks between organisations. Whilst the tariff incentivised everyone to focus on activity and do more stuff, the block contract facilitates the possibility that the system can reorganise budgets towards preventing ill health rather than just treating it. A digital ecology emphasises collaborative endeavours over the individual and seeks to create benefits across the collective whole.

Who Buys?

So why is understanding how money moves so important? Any entrepreneur with a compelling idea to develop a digital product for the NHS needs to understand how the money moves to work out if they can develop a viable proposition. What I take away from my conversation with Lauren is that companies need to appreciate that money is tight. Patients may love your technology but they do not hold the purse strings. You may have interest from a clinician, but it is the finance director that has the final say. The CIO is arguing the toss with the estates team who want to fix the hospital roof, and they are busy trying to keep the show on the road with basic IT infrastructure. Sometimes referred to as *technical debt*, the last thing they want is a novel technology that may create new costs and unintended downstream impacts on their systems.

So where does this leave start-ups and small companies with digital products that could make a difference in the NHS? This is fiendishly tricky terrain, and my advice is usually to find another market or at least not rely solely on the NHS as your customer.

Start-ups can do worse than try and work out early on if their product can save the NHS money. Known as making a *health economics case*, demonstrating that investing your technology will create savings somewhere else in the system, is hard to do but immensely valuable. Any finance director signing off a business case will find their enthusiasm piqued by a convincing case. But the reality is that most of the time there isn't a financial case to be made and improving quality and releasing staff time are the closest you will get.

We Get the Market We Deserve ■ 215

Understanding that the NHS is used to procuring tangible assets (physical items) and just hasn't fully got its head around buying intangible assets in the shape of software is the key. Any company needs to understand and navigate the scissors of doom if it is to stand a chance of success with the NHS as its customer.

But Does It Even Work?

Saving cash, or at the least saving clinicians' time is just part of the story when it comes to return on investment. In a highly evidence-driven sector, healthcare practitioners and managers want to know that a digital product is not only safe, secure and meets regulatory standards but that it will have the impact claimed by its inventor. I wish I could tell you that this is a straightforward issue, but how that evidence is generated proves to be mired in complexity, just like everything else.

Unlike the pharmaceutical sector, which has a clear process established over many decades, the digital sector is still working things out. There is a ton of regulatory compliance that needs to be met, along with the need to generate evidence. Digital health is dominated by start-ups and small companies, who either don't have the capacity or the wherewithal to create the evidence of cost and clinical effectiveness that the NHS demands. It is only in the last few years that NICE has developed a classification system for generating such evidence but when I speak to start-ups, they are often unaware of it.[10]

Randomised control trials (RCTs) are regarded as the best quality research, but they are costly, time-consuming and don't work well with technologies that move fast and iterate rapidly. It is not uncommon for companies to claim they are evidence based when in fact their technologies are merely *informed* by the evidence – it is not the same thing. This opacity runs the danger of undermining trust and building suspicion on the part of clinicians. In an editorial in *The Lancet*, the authors argue that without evidence, it is impossible to "differentiate efficacious digital products from commercial opportunism."[11]

Neelam Patel is the chief executive of MedCity, a not-for-profit organisation, that aims to stimulate digital health innovation between industry and academia. She tells me that an awareness of the role of evidence has massively increased over the last five years: "the challenge still remains however, how do you generate [evidence], how do you get the right data in the timeframe needed." Neelam observes that research still tends to be the domain of enthusiastic clinicians at a local or regional level "and then the evidence is critiqued, because unless it's invented here it's not good enough." The consequences for small start-ups are stark "then you end up in this constant turmoil of pilots and endless evidence generation." A small company needs sufficient investment or grant funding to keep afloat whilst evidence is being generated.

Neelam sees a light at the end of the tunnel, or at least some light in the tunnel, in the shape of central bodies working more closely together and the development

216 ■ *Towards a Digital Ecology*

by the National Institute for Health and Care Excellence (NICE) of a classification system for digital health evidence. However, leaving the European Union has had an impact on regulation such as that for medical devices. "It started off really complicated because there weren't any regulations, or any clear regulations, and then there started to be some clear regulations, and then Brexit happened, and then it started to get complicated again."

There are thousands upon thousands of health and well-being apps on the commercial app stores. How we go about choosing them tends to be influenced by rankings, ratings and number of downloads. But these indicators tell us nothing about how effective those apps actually are.[12] A recent *The Guardian* article exposed the fact that most health apps don't even meet basic evidence and regulatory requirements.[13] Snake oil appears to be in abundance on the app stores.

The NHS has its own apps library which curates those which have gone through a more rigorous review, but they are a tiny fraction of the overall number of apps on the commercial app stores. A new assessment framework called the Digital Technology Assessment Criteria is the latest attempt to provide a common set of standards that app developers should meet.[14] Having passed the assessment is often a criterion of NHS procurements for digital tools, but there has been an impasse whilst the new framework has been developed which means it has not been possible for companies to evidence that they meet the criteria.

The British National Formulary (BNF), which clinicians around the country use to decide which medicines to prescribe, was born out of the Second World War, precipitated by an urgent need for more economical use of drugs. A company called Organisation for the Review of Care and Health Applications (ORCHA) both assesses, validates and publishes apps, in an effort to solve the challenge of knowing which tools to trust. Liz Ashall-Payne, the founder and CEO of ORCHA, tells me clinicians increasingly use ORCHA app libraries as a BNF for digital tools, precipitated by the pandemic.

"The reality is," explains Liz, "with no regulation in app stores, changing regulations and standards introduced and apps continuously updating, clinicians need one single source where they can be confident that the current downloadable version of an app meets today's standards." Whilst clinicians have been trained to prescribe medication, this is not the case for digital health technologies. This would represent substantial changes to training and practice that are unlikely to come about any time soon. Such an idle pace is yet another barrier to creating a dynamic digital ecology.

The Dark Art of Procurement

As a patient and citizen, the word procurement may not be foremost in your mind when you think about the NHS. However, if you are a CIO or a digital health entrepreneur, then it is something you will wrestle with on a daily basis.

Understanding procurement is important because the NHS needs to buy all sorts of things so it can deliver care to patients. Whether it be mattresses for hospital wards or stethoscopes for doctors, the NHS is a big buyer of products and services. Each NHS trust has a procurement team dedicated to making sure it gets good value for the things that it buys and that the rules are obeyed to make sure taxpayers money is spent in the right way.

Lauren is not bashful when it comes to sharing her thoughts about the role of procurement in digital technology: "We've all been there," she says, "and I'm not knocking procurement people for the sake of it, but it's really process and not outcome driven." She describes the disconnect between what health practitioners want and what they end up getting:

> I've seen some really good specifications developed by clinicians setting out what they want, but then it goes into the procurement machine and it comes out completely different. And then you end up with a vendor who thinks they're providing something and a client who goes 'well we didn't want one of those' and then you as a vendor look awful because it looks like you've consumed public money and not delivered the goods.

Tom has a similar experience of what he calls the 'dark art' of poorly misunderstood procurement both on the side of the NHS buyer and the startup seller. In this experience, the procurement team is often: "several steps removed from the user and ends up buying based on a tick list of features rather than good user experience and a real understanding of their needs. These often-extensive lists of generic functional ingredients, detailing the expected capabilities of the software, somehow miss insight into the most important piece of the jigsaw – what the purchaser is actually seeking to achieve from deploying the digital technology. Imagine if a procurement not only expressed the end goal to be facilitated by the technology (for example, improving patient outcomes) but also provided baseline information about the current position and where they wanted to get to. We would shift gears from purely transactional to potentially transformative.

A recent government report concludes that procurement is weak in the public sector, with poor pre-market engagement, that is research and conversations with suppliers before a formal tendering process that would lead to having a better idea of what they want to buy.[15] This backs up Tom's experience:

> They'll shoot themselves in the foot by not talking to suppliers at certain points in the process when actually they should, not negotiating under the impression that they're not allowed to talk whereas they should be negotiating and therefore sometimes making poor purchasing decisions.

218 ■ *Towards a Digital Ecology*

A common absence of trust between NHS staff and companies means that the opportunity to collaborate is often lost.

Procurement teams are used to purchasing equipment and drugs, but digital technologies are more novel and buying them is a path less trodden. It is apparent that most NHS organisations don't understand sufficiently what is a fair price because they don't have enough comparisons to make, and when they are bringing in a company to develop a website or smartphone app, they have fewer points of reference. Lauren explains:

> So people don't want to sign stuff off for fear of the Daily Mail headlines and feeling like you've been taken for a ride. Lack of price and cost and value is stuff going out to tender and you think, well we could never do it for that.

Tom has a similar take on the appetite for the NHS to go out on a limb and buy an innovative solution to their problem:

> There is very little reward for taking risk, as a person who works in the system, why would I ever try something new because all that's likely to happen is that i'm going to get in trouble, there's no reward.

An absence of risk appetite is compounded by inertia when it comes to getting things done. Not only is the business case and procurement process painfully cumbersome, there is very little urgency in the system. When I ask Tom to tell me how long it takes to sign a contract with a new client he smiles: "I've got one client in my pipeline … It's been five years and I think they will buy from us for another six months months so it'll be six years by the time we close the deal."

Whilst that is at the extreme end of Tom's experience, there is typically a long lead-in time of around 18 months and any number of hoops to jump through. A small company is swimming against the tide of bureaucracy, and I've seen a number of start-ups fold because they just can't survive the length of time it takes to acquire an NHS customer. They simply run out of money. This in turn creates worry for NHS organisations purchasing digital systems from start-ups – what if they go bust and all the effort they have put in is wasted?

A survey of NHS digital leaders found great frustration amongst many CIOs when it comes to managing relationships with digital technology companies.[16] Participants reported suppliers were often slow to respond to their requests for new features and functions or to fix problems. The report notes the sometimes-limited resources of companies to react promptly to change requests. If you join the dots with a broken marketplace, it isn't impossible that many digital health companies (particularly start-ups) just don't have the revenue at a scale that means they can move fast to improve their products. Never-ending scope creeps, with NHS clients making requests for changes but without the cash to fund them, can be a challenge

We Get the Market We Deserve ■ 219

to a small company trying to balance the books. This is all symptomatic of a marketplace operating in life-support mode.

NHS bodies have tried to simplify procurement by creating frameworks whereby a company has to demonstrate it meets a certain level of compliance to get on. Local NHS organisations can then use the framework confident that the vendor has met certain standards and requirements. G Cloud is one of those frameworks which requires gargantuan effort to get on, but once you're there you have a route to being awarded a contract. Another framework is the Health and Social Care Apps Dynamic Purchasing System – a framework developed to include condition-specific apps across 25 categories with assurance provided through an accreditation process through ORCHA.

The drawback to frameworks for small companies is the effort they take to get on, the fact they often open up to entry periodically and the proliferation of frameworks developed by local NHS organisations. Frameworks make sense if they are consolidated into just a few at a national level, and they refresh regularly for new entrants. But any number of local frameworks pop up on a routine basis. Each time, a company has to decide if it can afford the time and effort to apply to get on.

A Government white paper on procurement (December 2020) recognises that the existing system, characterised by complexity and duplication, deters start-ups and small businesses from bidding for public sector contracts. It remains to be seen if proposals to simplify the regime will afford more innovation should they be approved and put in place.[17] The well-known reality of the situation, although you won't find this articulated in any procurement marketing material, is that companies don't sell through frameworks. It is often the case that an NHS organisation decides what it wants to buy and then finds a framework through which it can do it. Procurement is a theatre to demonstrate frontstage fairness, which belies a somewhat different backstage story.

The gulf of understanding is immense. Whilst procurement might feel like a dark art to start-ups, the digital sector feels like smoke and mirrors to the NHS. I have been approached by people working in charities and health research with expectations that developing a mobile application will cost anything from £5k to £500k and everything in between. We need to get better at transparency in the digital health sector so that companies can be better suppliers and NHS clients be better customers. We need to build trust on both sides, but system barriers get in the way.

There are some green shoots emerging that may help bring digital health procurement a spring-like step from the cold of winter. NHS procurement bosses have recognised the problem and techUK, the industry body for the sector, appears to be making inroads in lobbying for procurement frameworks to be streamlined and consolidated. The newly created ICSs mean that purchasing decisions are more likely to be made at a regional level rather than hyper-local level, meaning it is easier for start-ups and SMEs to at least know who to talk to.

However, none of these are immediate solutions, and experience suggests that the proof must be in the pudding. Tom's advice to an entrepreneur starting out in the digital health sector: "Yeah, be really patient, be bloodyminded and patient."

220 ■ *Towards a Digital Ecology*

Who Holds the Purse Strings?

Who holds the purse strings and ultimately, who is the buyer? Well, that's another layer of complexity.

The NHS logo is a sticking plaster that masks some 8,000 separate organisations all providing and commissioning primary, secondary and tertiary healthcare. The NHS is more of a franchise than a monolith. These organisations are currently grouping together to collaborate in regions known as ICSs, but the reality is that the configuration is in continual flux and subject to political and policy vagaries. There are currently 15 Academic Health Science Networks across England that are each responsible for the diffusion of innovation, and with a five-year licence to operate from NHS England, their shelf life is unknown.

After the disaster of NPfIT, there has been a steer from central towards regional organisation. This fragmentation has resulted in not only variation in digital readiness but also infrastructure and procurement expertise. In a recent report, the Care Quality Commission concluded that regional arrangements are highly variable in their maturity which has knock-on impacts for services themselves.[18] There is a bewildering myriad of access points for digital health companies, and getting to the right organisation who is interested in your product is a matter of luck more than design.

Without going down the rabbit hole of how the NHS organises itself, the broad point is that it is a minefield to navigate, particularly if you are a small start-up with limited resources. Many, but not all, NHS organisations have a chief information officer or Head of IT, but it may be the medical director or the entrepreneurial clinician in a specialist service who could be your friend and advocate. And just because that individual decides to back you and your idea does not mean they hold the purse strings or know how to navigate their organisation's purchasing systems. They are as constrained by institutional barriers as you are innocent of them. Neither of you knows what you are getting into.

For most entrepreneurs, it is luck and serendipity that leads them to a site to whom they can sell their innovation if they are lucky to find one at all. And the reality is that most sites will only be willing to pilot and test that innovation, maybe as a research project, to a small number of patients. It is not often they are willing to buy outright. The nurse you have been wooing over the last six months may not even have any budgetary control, and it is entirely likely they know next to nothing about the various departments within her organisation who will have an influence over what can or cannot happen. Ultimately, the finance director is often the person who needs to be convinced.

The Imperative Gap

With limited funds and a fast burn rate, start-ups do not have time to waste. But there is no similar imperative for the person on the NHS side of the fence, and they will have any number of competing demands for their attention and their budget.

In consumer digital products, there is generally a simple relationship – I have to satisfy the needs of the user, and they will pay for my product. Tom reinforces the point:

> If you're selling direct to consumer then the buyer is the user and they know what their needs are and they know what the job to be done is and so they can buy a product which perfectly solves that.

When I downloaded a transcribing app to help me write up interviews for this book, it was a simple process – it was only my need that had to be satisfied, I know my budget and I pay for it myself.

The user (often the patient) is not the same as the gatekeeper (the clinician) who is not the same as the payer (the service or organisation). The payer may be the organisation where the gatekeeper delivers the service (an NHS trust) or it may be the organisation that commissions and contracts the service (the integrated care system), and it may be different for the same product as it gets deployed in each different locality. It is a maze of labyrinthine proportions.

Who benefits and who pays is not a simple relationship either. And because it is so complicated, many well-meaning entrepreneurs who want to create value for the NHS end up going for more simple and straightforward markets - corporate employee wellness programmes, private healthcare or health insurers or even go to overseas markets such as the US where the payer system is more geared up to buy from them.

This means that the NHS fails to get the benefit and worse still, the private sector gets the benefit and outperforms the publicly funded NHS, putting more pressure on the NHS and benefitting private companies who can do something more impressive than their public sector counterparts. The benefits are too widely distributed in the system which creates overwhelming complexity. Trying to galvanise all the actors in the system to cooperate and purchase technology is no mean undertaking. And there is more often than not, an absence of an imperative to do it.

A Static Market

Markets have existed since ancient times. When I visit my local Saturday Street market, it is characterised by a cornucopia of stallholders who set up their stands along the street each week. It is the range of vendors and diversity of products that is the market's strength. Between them, they attract a critical mass of potential customers who make an event of this weekend activity. I may go there to buy dog treats, but I end up buying a doughnut and a pot plant as well. There is strength in numbers and variety.

Should you care to stand back and take a bird's eye view of the digital health marketplace, what you will see is a jaundiced landscape. According to Tussell, the

222 ■ *Towards a Digital Ecology*

top ten suppliers to the NHS earned twice as much as all SMEs combined in 2019. Even more surprising, 90% of suppliers worked with less than ten NHS trusts, suggesting that adoption and spread is not travelling all that far for many producers of digital health products and services.[19]

The sector is dominated by a small number of large electronic patient record companies whose products are the mission critical to the health services. The NHS cannot operate without them. These are the systems that form the backbone of clinical services, allowing clinicians to record, find and share patient data, schedule, book and organise. They are massively costly with never-ending contracts. To give you a sense of scale, Manchester University NHS Foundation Trust signed a 15-year contract worth £181m with American company Epic in 2020.[20] If start-ups are the market vendors, then electronic patient record providers are the supermarkets of the healthcare sector.

In primary care, two IT suppliers, EMIS and TPP, dominate the market, providing electronic patient records to 95% of GPs. NHS trusts can choose which IT systems they procure and so there is a vast array in place, with sometimes hundreds in one organisation, which makes information sharing very complicated. Trusts typically change their electronic patient record systems every 10–15 years, and it costs tens of millions of pounds to do so.

Let's pause for a moment to think about how the different digital products we use in our personal or work lives create benefits beyond each individual service we use. When I send an email in Gmail, I can append a document from Microsoft Word or hyperlink to a website on Yahoo. My banking app integrates with my accounting software, which in turn integrates with an app through which I can upload receipts and invoices. The synergies between all these different products mean I get benefits that are way above those I would get if I was to use each service separately. The value created *between* the different assets creates self-reinforcing loops that benefit both customers and vendors alike.[21]

This is not typically how it works in a healthcare IT system. As the dominant players in the market, electronic patient record companies aim to create and deliver the entire ecosystem rather than seeking synergies with others. They are the supermarkets that only sell own-brand products. They are motivated to keep all the data and all the activities within their ever-expanding behemoth of a product. Even for them, the challenge of creating interoperability between their systems and others is just too daunting.

NHS organisations are hostage to these company's castles, with high walls and moats, which keep smaller companies at bay. For a busy and stressed-out IT department, it is simpler to deal with one product than many. It is also the case that every deployment of a new technology carries the opportunity cost of clinical safety assessment and data protection impact assessments, to name but a few. All of this creates a statis in the marketplace. Start-ups can't create the self-reinforcing loops found in other sectors because the big vendors make it almost impossible for them to do so. Until we compel vendors to separate out the data from the application, so that the data does not belong to them, this situation will persist.

Rizwan, a consultant radiologist, describes how the impenetrable castle walls make it impossible for him to reap the benefits of smart ideas turned into products by clever start-ups. As a radiologist, the main system he works with is a Picture Archiving and Communications System (PACS) that stores and reports radiology examinations in a digital format. Rizwan describes the company that provides his PACS as a: "behemoth company that is far too big to do anything innovative."

On the occasion that he has unearthed promising start-ups who have an innovative solution to a radiology challenge, he more often than not finds that the big supplier has a less good version of it in their platform: "I can't persuade procurement to punt for this other solution," he opines: "they say, but you've got that solution in the [PACS] product and we've paid a fortune for it." For Rizwan, rolling contracts with these large suppliers may offer consistency and low risk, but they stifle innovation and provide a barrier to start-ups with fresh ideas from getting traction.

Richard is similarly no stranger to this problem:

> [IT] is actually very expensive and in particular when large organisations like the NHS procure IT, it becomes even more expensive because it takes twelve months to procure, you're precluding startups, new entrants, in so many ways because of the nature of payment, of contracting, of procurement rules … it just stops you working with the next bright thing that probably has a better solution to your problem and probably in partnership with you could deliver more benefit at a higher value over a shorter period of time.

Many of these large electronic patient record providers have partner programmes, whereby smaller companies can integrate with their services, allowing data to flow between them. In some cases, they create their own ecosystems, bringing niche digital vendors into their own walled marketplace.[22] Integrating with a large electronic patient record provider is not much fun for start-ups who have to, in principle, get on a partner programme for each vendor. This costs time and money, so who pays? If the company is working with an NHS trust who wants that integration to happen, then it is the NHS trust who is going to have to pay. The barriers are high and so are the opportunity costs.

A number of these companies are large US vendors, such as Epic and Cerner, for whom the UK is a tiny fraction of their billion-pound business. Not only is the NHS a small voice in their world but it has not made the conditions easy for them to lower the drawbridge even if they wanted to. The standards with which such vendors would have to comply to open up their systems are not yet in place. Even when international standards have been put in place, the NHS has created its own idiosyncratic versions, requiring global companies to re-engineer to meet their requirements. From a bird's eye view, it appears that the NHS is as much complicit in creating those castle walls as the vendors in guarding them.

224 ∎ *Towards a Digital Ecology*

Speaking off the record, the managing director of one of the large global electronic patient record companies explains to me that these big vendors are themselves bureaucratic beasts. They have large development teams with a massive roadmap of features and functions they are continually rolling out to their customers. What gets his attention first and foremost is change in legislation they have to comply with. This is closely followed by their contractual commitments to their clients. Anything that is nice to have is more than likely to fall out of the bottom. Opening up their systems to start-ups and small companies just doesn't make commercial sense.

Because the EPR landscape is so battened down, one of the most promising routes for a digital health start-up is to be bought out by them. It's one of the more likely exit opportunities in the sector. However, the big players need convincing that the company has a decent track record and confidence of future revenue. The digital health marketplace is in a hostage situation. As these intransigent issues become better understood, there is some hope that the abducted market may be freed in the form of various efforts from central NHS bodies to incentivise, coax and compel.

An Open Future

It is in a conversation with David Hancock that it becomes evident that green shoots are emerging in the spring of a digital ecology. David is a Healthcare Executive Adviser for a large technology provider and co-chair of INTEROpen, a group of NHS leaders and vendors advocating for improved interoperability between systems. "Standards in healthcare data and systems are like toothbrushes," he tells me, "everyone has one, but nobody is prepared to share."

However, clouds are making way for blue skies in the shape of a new standard for integration called HL7 FHIR. David believes that HL7 FHIR, at last, gives a comprehensive, universal, open standard that really is a standard and not just a guide, as previous healthcare interoperability standards have been. This means that systems really can begin to interoperate in a more straightforward way. With this more advanced interoperability comes a recognition from suppliers that without vendor lock-in from proprietary interoperability mechanisms, it actually makes the market bigger for all of them and gives them a greater opportunity. Companies can compete based on the value they bring rather than being excluded simply because they cannot interoperate. This maturing of the ecology simply makes the cake bigger for everyone and creates more of an appetite for integration between systems. "Though it's still emerging, this is the way the software market is going," explains David, "however, the NHS still has a tendency to make this much harder to do because it has always tried to mandate standards top-down rather than through collaboration."

For David, interoperability is more a social rather than a technical challenge: "we have a collective action dilemma," he tells me, "a situation in which all individuals would be better off cooperating but fail to do so because of conflicting interests which discourage joint action." Put simply, in order to successfully solve an interoperability problem, one organisation often has to do the work, incur costs and make changes to the way they work, but it is the receiving organisation that gets the benefit. Whilst there is good for the overall system, it is not good for the individual organisation that has to incur the cost and the change.

If NHS organisations can work together as a collective, whilst building mature relationships with digital health companies, everyone benefits. This is because the most promising opportunities to really make a difference in healthcare require changes across many healthcare organisations in a system. Siloed NHS organisations, each motivated by their own internal logic, are continually trapped by this dilemma of collective action. These epic challenges may be ameliorated through the emergence of ICSs, but they need to be nurtured and incentivised if they are to fully mature.

You Don't Win by Designing for Health Outcomes

"Using a venture model, a for profit model, and trying to combine that with the non-profit sector; I would say that is a challenge, because the way the venture capitalist is incentivised." John Lee Allen, the managing partner at Knightsbridge-based asset management company called RYSE, gives me a whirlwind introduction to the world of venture capital. "They're just trying, to put it simply, they've raised a fund, and you've got ten years to return as much money as possible to the investors, with the minimum amount of risk."

John is refreshingly direct, which I appreciate, because the sphere of investment in digital health has always been a bit of a mystery to me. With an impressive pedigree as a physician, research scientist and technology entrepreneur, John speaks to me from Switzerland where he is weathering the pandemic storm.

"Along the way, as I became more specialised, I was bumping into these areas where I thought healthcare could really catch up with the modern world." John recounts how he joined the NHS clinical entrepreneur programme which opened his eyes to a new world of possibility: "culturally there wasn't really an outlet [for innovation] … we have an outlet for research … but not really time for innovation, or anything that might be construed as a commercial activity." John became fascinated with the commercial aspects of digital health, how to build a business that is not only sustainable but successful and profitable.

Investors are a critical component of the digital health jigsaw puzzle.[23] They back companies by taking calculated risks, giving them cash to grow their business in return for recouping investment and generating returns. A typical investor aims to bring the company to an *exit* whereby they are acquired by a bigger company at a substantial profit or an initial public offering (IPO) whereby the company can sell shares to the public. Investors have a simple and transparent motivation – to maximise the wealth of shareholders – and so businesses must grow.

226 ■ *Towards a Digital Ecology*

Venture capital is a speculative and high-risk form of investment to small private companies with few tangible assets and made before they generate revenue[24]. Venture capitalists typically commit funds for up to ten years before an exit, and they have a wide portfolio based on the assumption that not all initiatives will succeed. Because the risks are so high, venture capitalists aim to make a lot of money from the small number of companies in their portfolio that are successful.

"They [venture capitalists] are betting on the fact that the [NHS] market will mature in the next ten years or so … they are subsidising it," explains John. "Ultimately the philosophy for venture investors is geared towards growth, of course you're looking to invest in profitability, but you're willing to delay profitability in order to help a company actually gain a foothold in the market." This is a long-term game: "If you invest in a fund, your capital is locked away for a decade, you can't change your mind a few years later, so you have to believe in it, otherwise you would never invest in that way."

Can the internal logic of venture capital square with that of the purpose and priorities of the NHS? In other sectors, the extractive nature of the digital economy, fuelled by dollar hungry shareholders, has been castigated for forcing companies to seek quick profits for shareholders at the expense of long-term innovation.[25] Put bluntly, the job of the digital health company, backed by investors, is to extract value from its customer in return for a product or service, to pay it up to its investors.

However, within the investor world, there are some that are more impact-focused than others. "How investors focus depends on where the money comes from." John explains that RYSE is impact-focused because their main investor is a charity. "We raise money from individuals, that's why we call it venture philanthropy, major donors, charities, big science centres, that sort of thing." John differentiates this model from investors that raise capital from pension funds that he explains are highly financially driven: "they wouldn't really care so much what we were doing … they just want to make returns in line with the risk, so they can guarantee the corporate pensions." For John, impact is an important facet of his motivation: "It would be a very empty existence if we were focusing [just on returns]."

Tom is unusual in that he *bootstrapped* his company, which means he and his co-founders self-funded their start-up rather than getting investment from others to get off the ground. However, this is a less common route for start-ups to take and isn't open to those without cash in the bank or friends and family willing to bankroll. The more typical route is to source investment.

Let's think about how it works in another industry. The typical model for a digital start-up is to disrupt an existing industry – just think of all those blockbuster stores on the high street where we used to rent videos on a Friday night replaced in a heartbeat by the flick of the remote to stream a film on Netflix along with an automated monthly payment from my bank which I barely pay attention to. But to scale a business like this across the globe requires big bucks. I am one of 193 million subscribers to the video streaming platform which secured a $2.5 million initial investment to get going. These are big figures.

Back in 2010 when Tom set up the DrDoctor, he and his co-founders felt that the healthcare market wasn't ready for this sort of investment:

> We didn't feel that at that point that the healthtech market was right for VC funding, we felt that there was still a lot of mindset change that needed to happen in the healthcare service before hospitals would be willing to adopt this sort of tech at scale.

Rather than take the high risk with the hope of high scale path, Tom and his team decided upon a more organic route to development: "We didn't want to build a business that disrupted the NHS in a negative way," he explains: "So I talk about this thing called gentle disruption, which is you work with the system to change it from the inside out rather than working against the system."

This approach is counter to a company attractive to VCs that achieves high growth by replacing people with automated processes – think of all the jobs in high street travel agents that have been replaced by global flight booking websites.[26] Tom and his team worked with rather than against the system:

> So that led us down the route of bootstrapping the business and through building really strong client relationships and the last building technology alongside our customers in a really agile way and growing organically which is what we've done over the last eight years.

His company has more recently raised a modest £3 million Series A investment to further develop their offer but underpinned by a firm bootstrapped base.

The types of problems digital health entrepreneurs want to solve must translate into lucrative markets, or there will be no investment. This is the reason Tom made a good call to bootstrap his business back in 2010 and which meant he could focus on solving a very specific problem that he had unearthed in that hospital. With an investor lens, where the clinical need lies, may not be where the money is to be made, and so priorities may become distorted and reshaped, and the founder's original purpose can get lost along the way:

> Whether the technology delivers its promises (or fails to do so) matters, but it remains, to a certain point, secondary to the value of the venture itself. The fate of most technology-based ventures is to be sold to an established firm when their economic value is the highest. Yet, the fact the technologies will not entirely fulfill their clinical promises is not problematic from the speculative logic of capital investment ... Overall, venture capital supports technologies that generate health gains by accident, not by design.[27]

228 ■ *Towards a Digital Ecology*

I have spoken to countless start-ups whose original proposition was for the NHS but who have looked to the insurance, occupational health or private healthcare sectors for customers because their proposition is just not investable when orientated towards our most loved public institution.

John has a similar point of view from an investment perspective:

> Sometimes startups aren't particularly well placed to work with huge organisations, and so when they're starting up, it's like, do we spend the next eighteen months trying to get this really large national contract, or do we actually focus on a smaller private healthcare provider, an insurance company which might take six months to close that contract.

The NHS brand is powerful and so investors are keen for start-ups to develop and test their products within publicly funded healthcare because that tells a powerful story both within the UK and abroad. But what that means in practice is efforts on behalf of NHS clinicians collaborating with start-ups whose products are unlikely to ever benefit publicly funded services. None of this is necessarily transparent, visible or even understood by those involved.

In order to maximise the chances of success, venture capitalists offer value-adding activities beyond their cash investment such as coaching, marketing and strategy.[28] This is important because a digital health innovation system that incorporates venture capitalists then shapes and influences the kinds of innovation that get introduced. Their equity in the business gives them authority over the company, and they may direct it in ways that maximise revenue but may only create marginal, if any, value to the healthcare system.

In a digital healthcare ecosystem, heavily reliant on venture capital, these tensions and limitations are not explicit. It is not commonly understood that just because a digital health product has attracted venture capital, it does not necessarily have intrinsic value for the healthcare system. Indeed, it may well add little or no value. Beyond this, investors have an orientation to pick off the simpler propositions, so the more complex challenges where greater systemic benefits could be achieved are the least likely to gain investment. Reliance on investor capital to get digital health companies off the ground contributes to a distorted misalignment of what they are willing to fund and what the system needs.

Just like any other company with shareholders, digital health companies are duty-bound to grow. Companies with venture capitalist investors who have taken a big risk on future profitability are even more concerned with growth. The rules of corporations have their origins hundreds of years back, but now they mesh with digital platforms: "A corporation is just a set of rules, and so is software. It's all code, and it doesn't care about people, our priorities, or our future unless we bother to program those concerns into it" (Rushkoff, 2016, p. 69).

The tide of venture capital may be changing course. In an article entitled *Why telemedicine startups might not be such a smart investment after all*,[29] the authors argue that beneath the hype, there is the real possibility that digital health companies may be hitting some systemic barriers. For example, companies, with video consultation products, face challenges from two types of incumbents – firstly, global consumer video platforms with deep pockets are adding features and functions that make them more usable in a clinical setting; secondly, the big electronic patient vendors see the demand and create their own video consultation product. The best those start-ups can hope for is to be bought out by the bigger vendors, but it is often just as easy for those vendors to develop the products themselves.

Despite all these challenges, John is upbeat about the future of digital health: "Generally investors have to be pretty optimistic, and the same with founders, you've got to be optimistic because there are so many ups and downs, and sometimes you're creating new markets and doing things that haven't been done before." The reality of the digital health marketplace is not an especially pretty one. Because it is so emergent, so hard to navigate and so hard to reimburse, the only people prepared to take a long-term bet are venture capitalists. Whatever the rights and wrongs, it looks like this approach is here to stay. John and I finish our conversation on a buoyant note: "It's great to hear about the next generation of technologies," he tells me, "but it's even greater to see things actually bringing impact to organisations, to the people they are trying to serve."

What Business Models Actually Work?

How can digital health companies cut through this complexity with a proposition that gives them a thriving business and a fair proposition to their NHS customer? They need to work out who should pay for digital health products and services, what evidence is good enough to justify reimbursement and what are the right models for payment.

The simplest option is for the user to pay for a mobile application. Most of the apps on my phone are free because they are just a convenient interface for me to interact with services I subscribe to (Netflix) or pay for in other ways (banking). It is fair to assume that where I have other free apps (Facebook) they are making money by trading my data with other companies (advertisers) for whom it has value. I may be prepared to trade my data with Twitter, but I may be more cautious about trading my health data. Either way, the transaction is often not visible or clear to the end user, making it a problematic model in anything other than a consumer environment.

Some apps have in-app purchases or a monthly fee. As a regular runner, I record my runs on Strava and upgrade to the paid-for version to get more features when training for a race. This model is a straightforward consumer relationship but it does not sit well in a public sector context. Firstly, requiring people to buy apps sits at odds with a free at the point of the demand healthcare system; secondly, it creates inequality between those who can afford and those who cannot; thirdly, the data

230 ■ *Towards a Digital Ecology*

is likely to sit siloed on the app itself, not allowing rich data to be shared with the clinician and their platforms. So what's the alternative?

The other option is for NHS organisations to buy or licence products and services which patients and/or clinicians then use. This is the model we are most interested in here, as it is the most fraught and complicated. The most common approach is for companies to license their product using a software as a service (SaaS) model, whereby they provide the full service (hosting, maintenance, development and so on) and charge a subscription based on a fee per patient or clinician per month. This is how we operate in other aspects of our lives through our subscriptions to Netflix, Apple TV, Spotify, pet insurance or any other number of examples.

Yet another approach is for a company to charge for the development of the software which then belongs to the client, and then they get a small revenue for hosting, maintenance and further development. This model is sometimes referred to as *time and materials* where the technology company is paid to do the work but doesn't own any of the intellectual property or code. This model relies on a company bidding for contracts to develop software and they need a regular pipeline of work to thrive. Once they have built one thing, they go on to the next.

Sometimes, the technology can have a life beyond its use in one context, if the NHS client requires it to be developed using open-source code and published on the internet, so others can use it. This approach is common in local government, where there is a drive towards developing shareable software that is actively shared between localities. It is less common in the NHS. One electronic patient record provider, IMS Maxims, prides itself on having an open-source model. The company's former Chief Executive, Shane Tickell, explains his rationale for taking an open-source approach: "when you open up your code, we all move forward together," he explains: "I don't care about anyone behind me coming up and taking my code, because I should be ahead of them. But if I'm not, then I can benefit from them." He believes that open source enables the sector to grow together, contributing to those elusive self-reinforcing loops.

A more emergent approach is sometimes called *value-based digital health*, whereby companies and NHS organisations share the risk and the benefit according to the value their technology delivers rather than the activity it generates.[30] The data created from the use of the product can be used to measure the value it creates (for example, improved outcomes or better-quality services) and then the value shared. Sometimes value and activity are combined, with an upfront fee to the vendor followed by a value-based fee dependent on successful outcomes 18 months or so down the line.

Whilst this appears a promising approach, we have seen throughout this book that the relationship between the intended benefit of technology and the benefit it realises in practice is influenced by many complex and interdependent factors. So for example, if technology fails to deliver benefit, this could as much be the fault of the service adopting the technology as the responsibility of the technology provider itself. This model places a huge risk on the start-up or company unless the parameters and responsibilities are very clearly defined, and the NHS trust is honest about its capability and capacity to realise the benefits of that technology. A realistic independent assessment of the trust's experience and ability to do the work to adopt a technology would be a fair trade-off for value-based payments, which would help a digital health company determine if it would be likely to see the rewards. All parties are clear about the journey ahead to create the value promised and hoped for.

Another challenge to this approach is the *distribution* of the budget across various health and care organisations within a region, creating silos. If you consider a digital technology that acts within a patient journey cutting across primary, secondary, community care and various social (and non-health services such as housing), trying to convince an acute NHS trust to pay for a solution that benefits someone else (for example, reducing the need for GP appointments) is near impossible. Another tricky factor is the pressure on most organisations, bound by short-term thinking in one-year budget cycles, to demonstrate benefit in a short space of time. In many cases, benefits from technology are uncertain or can manifest in the form of prevention or improvement over a longer period of time.

For many digital health start-ups and SMEs, the UK is just one marketplace, and they have their sights set on Europe, America, Asia and beyond. However, each country has its own reimbursement idiosyncrasies that need to be understood. A bird's eye view shows some small green shoots elsewhere that may hold promise at a more local level. For example, in 2020, a new law came into force in Germany that allows digital health products to be included in the nationwide reimbursement catalogue as long as they meet certain safety, data privacy and efficacy conditions.[31] In March 2020, the US government broadened the array of services and codes that are reimbursed and structured them so that telehealth services are reimbursed at the same rate as they would be in a face-to-face encounter as opposed to a reduced amount.[32] The newly emerging ICSs may provide some of the answers to this challenge by coordinating efforts at a regional level and creating the right platform infrastructure that allows data to be shared between systems.[33]

Maybe our preoccupation with trying to loosen the digital health marketplace will in the end be futile. There are greater forces at play that dwarf even the Epics and Cerners of the world. They come in the shape of global technology companies such as Apple, Google and Amazon. Through its health record platform, Apple is developing an ecosystem of digital health consumers, developers and researchers. Increasingly, it is connecting its platform to health providers, including Oxford University Hospitals NHS Foundation Trust and Milton Keynes University Hospital NHS Foundation Trust in the UK.[34] An expert in logistics, Amazon now has an online pharmacy in the US, and it is presumably only a matter of time before this extends to the UK. With every acquisition and development, the tech giants are further locking us into their ecosystems and extending their influence over the most sensitive parts of our lives.[35] We omit to pay attention at our peril.

Lessons Learned

What does all this mean for us as patients, the NHS as a buyer of digital products and start-ups as the innovators, developing new ways of doing things for the health-care system?

It pains me to say it but in the conversation I have with start-ups, I routinely encourage them to not have the NHS as the market they sell to. The complexity and slow pace will likely kill their business and only the most tenacious will survive and prosper. Whilst many an entrepreneur I have met is driven by a mission to help the NHS, they are too likely to be crushed by the very sector they are hell-bent on helping. In reality, they end up focusing on health insurance or private healthcare providers or even going overseas to sell their products. The NHS brand means that any company that has tested their product successfully in the UK health service has a strong basis for selling elsewhere. Too often the NHS fails to realise the value of digital products it has invested in testing because it doesn't then buy them.

But what about advice from someone who's been there? Tom is a busy man. Our interview is a scrambled 30-minute video call over lunch. As I let him get off to his next meeting, I ask him what advice he would give to an entrepreneur starting out in digital health:

> Absolutely number one – go and talk to as many people in the system as you can … one of the most amazing things in healthcare is that every-body who works in the system cares about the system so they are willing to have conversations.

Tom believes that it is through conversations with clinicians that you validate your idea and work out if it has legs before you commit to building anything.

His second piece of advice is to do your homework when it comes to really understanding the value you will bring to the system: "If you are intending selling it to the health service then make sure you understand how the ROI (return on invest-ment) case works because that's critical." His final words of wisdom are about getting the right support and business model: "Leverage the accelerators, because there's an enormous amount of support … make sure you leverage the funding opportunities available because you don't need to go down the traditional VC route … it means you can do more with less." Tom's advice is from a man who has managed to create a sustainable digital technology business in the NHS. He's worth listening to.

Although it may not seem immediately obvious, this chapter has brought in the marketplace as an essential characteristic of a flourishing digital ecology. Dominated by entrepreneurs and start-ups, and with regulation and evidence still not settled, this is a highly emergent habitat. Clinicians and the organisations they work in, understand the problems that technology could help solve because they experience those challenges every day. However, they need software developers, designers, tech-nologists and data scientists to create the solutions to those problems. This means

We Get the Market We Deserve ■ 233

the NHS needs to be able to work with, as well as buy products and services from those entrepreneurs, innovators and start-ups. We must nurture the marketplace as much as other vital components of the digital ecology in healthcare.

Notes

1 https://www.rand.org/pubs/research_reports/RR1143.html
2 https://www.instituteforgovernment.org.uk/explainers/nhs-procurement
3 https://fullfact.org/health/spending-english-nhs/
4 https://www.longtermplan.nhs.uk/publication/nhs-long-term-plan/
5 https://www.nuffieldtrust.org.uk/files/2019-05/digital-report-br1902-final.pdf
6 https://bmchealthservres.biomedcentral.com/articles/10.1186/s12913-019-4790-x
7 https://www.health.org.uk/publications/reports/what-the-13bn-debt-write-off-means-for-the-nhs
8 https://www.england.nhs.uk/digitaltechnology/digital-primary-care/
9 https://www.england.nhs.uk/digitaltechnology/digital-primary-care/securing-excellence-in-primary-care-digital-services/
10 https://www.nice.org.uk/about/what-we-do/our-programmes/evidence-standards-framework-for-digital-health-technologies
11 https://www.thelancet.com/action/showPdf?pii=S0140-6736%2818%2931562-9
12 https://s3.ca-central-1.amazonaws.com/assets.jmir.org/assets/preprints/preprint-27173-submitted.pdf
13 https://www.bbc.co.uk/news/technology-56083231
14 https://www.nhsx.nhs.uk/key-tools-and-info/digital-technology-assessment-criteria-dtac/
15 https://www.instituteforgovernment.org.uk/sites/default/files/publications/carillion-two-years-on.pdf
16 https://www.nuffieldtrust.org.uk/files/2019-05/digital-report-br1902-final.pdf
17 https://assets.publishing.service.gov.uk/government/uploads/system/uploads/attachment_data/file/943946/Transforming_public_procurement.pdf
18 https://www.cqc.org.uk/sites/default/files/20201016_stateofcare1920_fullreport.pdf
19 https://blog.tussell.com/nhs-spend-on-technology-has-increased-by-38-since-2017
20 https://www.thehtn.co.uk/2020/05/29/manchester-university-nhs-signs-181m-15-year-deal-with-epic/
21 https://leadingedgeforum.com/insights/the-counter-industrial-revolution/
22 https://in.finance.yahoo.com/news/silvercloud-health-now-part-epic-173000630.html?guce_referrer=aHR0cHM6Ly93d3cuZ29vZ2xlLmNvbS8&guce_referrer_sig=AQAAAEOMkVUI7PHG24qq5ee2KIppiL6eWETr3F4gxXV-aNHzOP9aPuNIgaqztwaOpHcP0d9zULTUrHl8G8gF_Yi7PYFTvDnR6W8xYO47LvcnH4XDkMdiDCkFs4JhEjWkzUcc06Zq3QXRtgIE4_wqmrf17tLHJBDVQRkkNfITyyksnSF&_guc_consent_skip=1610220747
23 http://europepmc.org/article/MED/28949463#free-full-text
24 https://www.google.com/url?q=https://pdfs.semanticscholar.org/f9c9/8699da59bae44a631c851c2fa563eecbe0fc.pdf&sa=D&ust=1587714241618000&usg=AFQjCNHR5WBmNk7bWXQxoZ7ZtyNTufQM5A
25 Rushkoff, 2016

234 ■ *Towards a Digital Ecology*

26 https://www.technologyreview.com/2020/06/17/1003318/why-venture-capital-doesnt-build-the-things-we-really-need/
27 https://journals.sagepub.com/doi/abs/10.1177/095148481667019
28 Lehoux, 2016
29 https://sifted.eu/articles/telemedicine-startups-problems/
30 https://www.mckinsey.com/industries/healthcare-systems-and-services/our-insights/how-healthcare-systems-can-become-digital-health-leaders#
31 https://www.mckinsey.com/industries/pharmaceuticals-and-medical-products/our-insights/the-european-path-to-reimbursement-for-digital-health-solutions
32 https://medcitynews.com/2020/10/digital-health-reimbursement-the-transforming-landscape/?rf=1
33 https://www.digitalhealth.net/2020/10/apple-launches-health-records-in-uk/
34 https://www.digitalhealth.net/2020/10/apple-launches-health-records-in-uk/
35 https://www.adalovelaceinstitute.org/wp-content/uploads/2020/11/The-data-will-see-you-now-Ada-Lovelace-Institute-Oct-2020.pdf

Chapter 12

Momentum – towards a Digital Ecology

> Rich futures are mapped by those with the energy to convene, the passion to learn from the widest variety of human imagination, paying attention, changing course, discovery and investing what the world demands of us all.
>
> *Unchartered: How to Map the Future Together* (Margaret Heffernan, Simon & Schuster, 2020)

I'd like to share an encounter that once troubled me but has come to make sense over the course of many conversations which have shaped this book. I recall sitting on a sofa, sipping a coffee, as I introduced myself to the chief information officer of my local Clinical Commissioning Group. I had just started out in digital health, and I was super optimistic and excited about the various digital projects I had initiated with clinical teams. We were going to transform care and it was digital that was going to make it happen.

I went to him hoping for support and encouragement, but all I got was a lukewarm response and a high degree of equivocation. He tried to be kind, but he told me he wasn't interested in stand-alone mobile apps and solutions to micro problems at the point of care. It turned out he had more fundamental things on his mind. Intransigent challenges of interoperability and the quandary of how to create a technology architecture for the city were uppermost in his thoughts. He was probably as irritated by my focus on what might be possible, as I was by his preoccupation with the basics.

DOI: 10.1201/9781032198798-12

236 ■ *Towards a Digital Ecology*

I set out to write a book about digital innovation, but I realised that none of it makes any sense without paying attention to the foundations. I didn't intend to travel back to NPfIT days, but it became apparent that the story of digital health was incomplete without it. It is clear that we have to cultivate two parallel realities in the NHS – creating the foundations on the one hand, whilst nurturing the emergent digital future that is developing in and around us, on the other.

The notion of *digital transformation* borrows its nomenclature from the world of business. Its cache has been tarnished as it has become a euphemism for budget cuts, whilst worshipping at the altar of the linear, predictable and technocratic. How we conceptualise the world matters. It shapes what we do and how we go about doing it. We might do better to draw on concepts from biology, emergence and living systems than the technocratic language of industry. A *digital ecology* is one in which the NHS adapts to its environment and cultivates the technologies which enhance, improve and extend its ability to achieve its core purpose. A digital ecology embraces the fact that change is an adaptive, emergent and social process.

COVID-19 is a side actor in this story. That microscopic virus created a public health, social and economic disaster of such seismic proportions that the NHS had to lean on digital technologies in order to function. It is because the healthcare system has found it so difficult to take advantage of technology in the past and because it was forced to during the pandemic, that it becomes a fascinating case study in what is possible under certain conditions. It seems unlikely that the NHS can truly innovate when it is in flight or fight mode. It mostly engaged in tactical responses borne out of necessity. Whilst this book has told a story of human endeavour in response to totemic challenges, the question remains as to what might come next for a creaking analogue system doing its best to incorporate digital tools of the contemporary world.

The virus quickly became a drudgery in all our lives, its novelty waned whilst its nefarious impacts deepened and spread. It is worth recalling the sense of panic and disbelief in those early days. One clinician described to me how he hit peak fear when the prime minister succumbed to the virus:

> I don't know why, but Boris Johnson being ill in hospital was a source of great anxiety … there was this vulnerability that if the country can't even save its prime minister, regardless of your politics … then we're all screwed.

He recalls how back in those early days the pandemic felt like Armageddon. It was a time of fear coupled with improvisation, as the NHS sought to fight for its own life just as it was for the lives of its patients.

I wonder how we might leverage and sustain some of the advances in attitudes towards and adoption of technology that did begin to shift during the pandemic. Whilst many of the technologies deployed had already been around for decades, it is not just their adoption but the recognition and acceptance of their importance to patient care that have seen a seismic shift. It might well be that it is *attitudes* towards

Momentum – towards a Digital Ecology ■ 237

technology, rather than the use of technology perse, that have seen the most profound metamorphosis.

Let's put aside talk of digital technology for a moment. We don't talk about the telephone as an enabler of clinical services. That is because it is an accepted and embedded technology. The telephone is invisible to us because it is interwoven into the fabric of our lives. No service, clinical or otherwise would have a conversation about whether it needed to have a telephone number or whether there was a strong evidence base for the use of a phone. We don't need a randomised control trial to know that the telephone is a really useful tool.

Internet-enabled technologies have insinuated themselves into our lives to such an extent that it seems curious to imagine life before them. I recall car journeys in pre-digital days where I would sit in the passenger seat with a bulky WH Smith's A–Z map, trying to work out the best route by tracing my finger across the page as my partner awaited instructions for the next turn. Cross words would invariably ensue as we missed a turn or hit a traffic jam with no idea whether it would last for minutes or hours.

Decades later, those fraught car journeys are a distant memory that seem almost quaint and comical. These days I input my destination into Google Maps and have an instant route, arrival time and redirection to the most efficient route, avoiding jams and delays. If I want to stop for petrol or take a detour to a cafe then I make use of all the data Google Maps pulls in from multiple sources to do anything from check opening times to reviewing the menu. It is only in typing this on my laptop that I have cause to reflect on the seismic change in behaviour, attitude and assumptions that has afforded. It is just part of how we do things. What if we effect this same change to the NHS, a service that underpins all of our lives from the moment we are born through to the end of our lives. Imagine what might be possible.

Increasingly, digital technologies will become invisible to us because they will become part of how clinical services operate. This is already the case for the humble email, which we accept as an inevitable aspect of working life. It is less so for Microsoft Teams which has only just touched clinical services at scale over the past year. Digital's novelty, for the time being, means it has an annoying habit of occupying the centre of our thinking rather than something in the background that helps us do the things we need to get done – book an appointment, get a prescription, communicate with each other, view test results, understand our health (or illness) and manage our health condition(s).

Let's imagine an NHS of the future, where health professionals have the right information at their fingertips to provide the best advice, treatment and care to us, no matter whether we turn up at a GP, a pharmacy or at A&E and whether it be in Chester or Cornwall. What if we have not only access to our health record, but we are custodians of our data, which we can add to and share with whomever we want. What if those systems were so simple and easy to use that anyone could use them without the blink of an eye, a self-regulating *digital ecology*?

Towards the North Star

This book was never supposed to be purely about technology. I have always been interested in how you take ideas and make good things happen in large complex systems. In writing this book, I realised that the story could not be told without understanding recent history and the burden of the failed programmes, with the shadow they have cast. I now want to revisit the aspects of digital that fascinates me – how we can use technology to enable meaningful and positive change for people and systems.

There is a big massive gaping risk that digital technologies become sticking plasters to a creaking system that no longer works for the 21st Century. To illustrate the gap, and the potential, I draw on Andy Wilkin's work, anticipating and imagining an NHS 10–15 years in the future. The purpose of doing so is to illustrate the danger of incremental digital innovation that merely bolts on complexity to an already byzantine system.

Andy tells me how he was brought in by the Royal Free charity to delve into what the future might hold:

> The ask was, could you look at all the major trends and how they are going to play out in healthcare, roll them forward ten to fifteen years, imagine they've all landed at scale, what could health and healthcare look like and how might that help us in providing some kind of north star.

He explains the intention of creating this north star to orientate the decisions that get made now:

> There's a sense in which you start with your legacy and bolt bits of technology on to your legacy thinking, hoping somehow that this magical integrated 21st Century will miraculously emerge out of it. And most people don't know what the hell they are doing, or what to prioritise. The idea of a long term vision is that it will enable different parts of the system to see where we are going collectively ... and then in our uncertainty, we can start to plan towards that direction.

Andy's report[1] begins by setting out the population challenge that the NHS finds itself facing – a substantial shift in the type of ill-health we experience from the days when the NHS was first conceived. It is now the case that 70% of total expenditure on health and care in England is associated with the treatment of 30% of the population with one long-term condition such as diabetes, chronic obstructive pulmonary disease, arthritis and hypertension. As advances in technology reshape our world, so do the illnesses and conditions we experience.

By 2040, nearly one in seven people will be over the age of 75.[2] The number of people with one or more of these types of conditions is projected to increase from

Momentum – towards a Digital Ecology ■ 239

15–18 million by 2025. Care for people with such conditions presently accounts for just over half of all GP appointments as well as around three-quarters of outpatient and A&E appointments. The King's Fund estimates that the average cost per year of treatment for a person with a single long-term condition is £1000 and up to £8000 for someone with three long-term conditions. The point I am making here is that the modern world, along with the challenges and health conditions we experience, is very different to the formative years of the NHS.

The next challenge identified in Andy's report is the way the NHS organises itself. Firstly, only a tiny proportion of the NHS budget (6%) goes on preventing health problems in the first place. Largely structured to optimise care based on siloed functional specialities, it works well for acute and episodic illness but is fragmented with multiple handoffs from speciality to speciality for people with long-term conditions. If you or I have Type 2 diabetes, COPD, clinical depression, we likely to experience highly fragmented and disjointed care.

People have to manage the complexity of the system and they (and their carers) are often the only people with the full picture of their own care. The nature of a long-term condition is such that it is a permanent feature of someone's life and they have to take the load of their daily care. This means their outcomes are as much (if not more) dependent on the daily patterns of their life than their time in the consultation room. When people find it hard to self-manage, their health problems increase and they come to depend more on services over time. The wider healthcare ecology is all out of whack.

Andy's report goes on to articulate what the north star might look like, A radical reinvention of healthcare focused on prevention, holistic support which recognises people have multiple health and social needs, aspirations and goals; a focus on coaching and supported self-management over treatment; a recognition that how people live their lives is deeply rooted in psychological, cultural, economic and social beliefs, values, norms, expectations and opportunities that stretch way beyond the traditional clinical gaze. This feels more like the self-regulating *healthcare ecology* that could be cultivated and nurtured with digital tools doing some of the heavy lifting in the background.

A holistic approach to improving the health and well-being of the nation is an important part of reducing the personal and societal costs associated with managing chronic disease. Most of us drift into chronic disease over time. Prevention and active support for people to flourish needs a much more integrated and nuanced approach that addresses both individual and systemic causes. The social and environmental factors at the heart of health mean that a population and place-based approach on regional geographies will facilitate orchestration of the most effective collection of supporting interventions.

For Andy, this north star of integrated, holistic care will be enabled by emerging innovations such as personalised medicine, biosensors, wearables, the Internet of Things, communications, robotics and artificial intelligence. But all of these technologies will need to point towards this bigger vision as much as fixing things in the

240 ■ *Towards a Digital Ecology*

present, and the NHS will need to reorientate itself towards this new constellation if it is to harness the promise of emerging technologies in any meaningful way.

For me, the current phraseology of *healthy lifestyles* and *behaviour change* has an implicitly embedded judginess. If we don't optimise our health, then we have failed as citizens. Using the language of ecology, we can start to think of nurture and cultivation, helping each other grow and flourish. I wonder if this small conceptual shift might enable us to think about our health and well-being less as reductive moving parts and more as a holistic and integrated whole. Good health is as much about having a job, a sense of purpose and community, somewhere safe to live and a decent income, as much as it is about good quality health services. A systems approach to healthcare pays attention to the factors that influence ill health and employs policy and legislation to minimise the everyday stresses of our environment.[3]

As my conversation with Andy draws to a close, I ask him to share his final thoughts about how digital technologies can be employed for the NHS to save itself:

> If we're thinking in the old paradigm, there's a sense in which technology gives us more powerful tools to enact the old [ways of doing things]. If we come with a different orientation about how we solve the upstream issues of healthcare and how we more holistically support people because we know if we holistically support them they can look after themselves and that reduces demand, if we think in that paradigm, we can think about which technology is important and how do we deploy it.

For Andy, the north star is critical:

> [We need] an orientation towards problem solving that brings creativity to bear on how we think about deploying digital. This risk otherwise is that we are just using digital to double down on our old models and using digital as a go faster stripe to do that.

Right here is a call to action. If we are to take this more emergent approach, then we will pay attention to inequality, we will create foundations of trust, and we will tend the digital health marketplace so that entrepreneurs and innovators can help us cultivate the digital Shangri La. Everything starts to fall into place.

Entrepreneurs of the Future

It is in conversation with entrepreneurial clinicians and patients that I feel a sense of optimism about the future. Sandy Wright is a junior doctor who I began mentoring when he joined the NHS Clinical Entrepreneur's Programme a number of years ago. He is a new breed of clinician who is not content to follow the conventional route

Momentum – towards a Digital Ecology ■ 241

ascribed to his profession. Having run his own start-up, Sandy tells me that he's always had an entrepreneurial urge to try out different things.

For Sandy, the CEP helped him find like-minded people who he hadn't previously realised existed: Medicine is a hard career and it's not an easy path and it is a very set and established career path. Once you're in it, it's very easy to progress from one year to the next in a very structured way, explains Sandy, "and for a lot of people that's not what they want to do, they want to try to do different things." For him, the Clinical Entrepreneur's Programme exposed him to ideas, knowledge and a community that gave him the confidence to innovate, "the license to start pushing the boundaries of what you are doing whether it is in the boundaries of an established healthcare system or beyond."

Sandy's orientation is encouraging because he intuitively gets that we are dealing with relational processes and social change:

> We tend to think about digital health as purely technical, like it's a piece of technology, but it's not because when you deploy a piece of software ... there's a social aspect to it as well ... because by deploying a new piece of technology, you are fundamentally changing the way people work; when you deploy a new digital solution there is always going to be an element of repair work to remodel the way people incorporate it into their working lives.

When you try and do something with the north star in mind, it becomes apparent what a challenge this can be.

"There's a lot of expectation that you can deploy something and scale it rapidly across the ecosystem," says Sandy, reflecting on the naivety of many entrepreneurs starting out in digital health,

> a lot of startups in healthcare think they can do that ... and I wonder if a lot of money gets raised on that premise; but my worry is that, particularly in an industry like healthcare, although people think in the UK we have the NHS so things are fairly homogeneous, I don't think that is the case, I think it's very different across the country and ... it's much harder than people think.

> Sandy understands the paradigm shift described by Andy in his work for the Royal Free: "we need to think about how we move healthcare from something that is reactive to something that can be more proactive,"

> Covid has shone a light on that, because a lot of the people who have been most affected had pre-existing medical conditions and the health of the population has never been more in the limelight ... and there are

242 ■ *Towards a Digital Ecology*

obviously socio-economic factors that play into that. But I think digital health to promote self-care, because that could have such an effect on downstream healthcare usage, should be a clear focus.

Having spent time as a clinical fellow for a digital health company, Sandy switched his clinical multidisciplinary team to one that comprised user researchers and software developers. He found himself working on projects with a global reach and got to learn about how digital products are developed. More recently he has been accepted onto a Masters course on artificial intelligence in healthcare at University College London. With a blend of clinical expertise and digital sector know-how, he is developing into one of the next generation of specialists in the field. Sandy is an important part of a future digital ecology, spanning sector boundaries and bringing dynamism into this emerging field.

"One thing I"m worried about," says Sandy, as we conclude our conversation:

> Covid has completely stretched the NHS to breaking point, but digital has enabled it to continue some sort of business as usual in some respects. But I worry about accessibility and the equality aspect of increased use of digital health. It kind of relies on people having access to laptops, smartphones ... or people who don't have English as a first language, access to healthcare through these digital means might be harder than going in to somewhere in person.

Sandy's final reflection is salient to a core theme within this book, a call to create a digital ecology that binds us together rather than rifts us apart: "I don't think we've really thought about the impact it might have on how people access healthcare and my worry is that if we blindly proceed with the digital healthcare agenda, that it could lead to worsening health inequalities."

The Characteristics of a Digital Ecology

Let me pause for a moment to start to describe the characteristics of a digital ecology.

It is possible to create a digital ecology in the NHS. It will not be linear. It will be complex. Our approach to a digital ecology should be to not only recognise and tolerate emergence but embrace it. A strategy is something that more often than not sits in a PDF within a forgotten folder on an unnavigable intranet. An ecology takes a strategic approach to digital that blends the tactical and the visionary, the here-and-now with the possible. It works with assets and relies on relationships. It measures the right things.

Ecology is a self-regulating system made up of many different parts. It recognises the uniquely personal whilst being fiercely rigorous when it comes to standards. Its governance is reflexive, and it continually asks itself what is nurturing the ecology

Momentum – towards a Digital Ecology ■ 243

and what has ceased to support it. A digital ecology is not fearful about letting go of those things that no longer add value and correcting things when it needs to refocus. A digital ecology is a protected space and set of practices where people within a system can assemble to generate meaning together. This happens at the scale of the human and is fearlessly inclusive. Diversity is a feature of a digital ecology. It embraces the unusual suspects from disparate communities and disciplines. We need entrepreneurs as much as we need data analysts and ethicists.

A digital ecology will best sustain itself within a policy environment that sets direction but does not seek to determine how things are done. A digital ecology generates knowledge about what works and seeks to build on those things which make it healthy and vibrant. A digital ecology weeds out the practices that create a stranglehold and suffocate its emergent metamorphosis. We seek to understand what digital displaces and inquire as to whether we are happy with what we lose as well as what we gain.

A digital ecology is a metaphor that embraces emergence and eschews the reductive nomenclature of Taylorism. A digital ecology is thoughtful and rejects the careless introduction of technology as a sticking plaster to age-old problems. It is less factory and more habitat. It rejects the stick of targets and generates its own cadence and rhythms to uncover those characteristics that make it healthy and strong. It is not random. It is carefully co-designed by using tools that facilitate cooperation and collaboration. It has agility and it is continuously learning.

A digital ecology is in a permanent state of discovery. It has an appetite for the unexpected. It has its eye on potential threats and seeks to understand how it can learn from them and even absorb them. A digital ecology absorbs and discharges the core NHS principles that bind us in a collective social contract – a comprehensive service, available to all; based on clinical need, not ability to pay; the highest standards of excellence and professionalism; patients at the heart of everything; working across organisational boundaries; providing the best value for taxpayers' money; accountable to the public, communities and patients that it serves.

I expand on the metaphor of a digital ecology to provide a counterpoint. The way in which we currently conceptualise the labour of digital adoption is mired in normative and reductive technocratic language, efficiency, targets, cuts and effectiveness. You get what you put in. How we frame digital matters. The pandemic showed us if we didn't know it already that our fates are inextricably intertwined. A digital ecology assumes this to be fact and clasps it to its chest as an advantage rather than a handicap. A digital ecology is fair, and it binds people together.

Creating Curiosity

Mechanical ventilation is a breathing machine that enables the body to continue to breathe through artificial assistance. This form of ventilation is commonplace for patients in intensive care with the coronavirus, a disease that affects the lungs and

244 ■ *Towards a Digital Ecology*

airways. These mechanical ventilators are actually quite crude, they act as bellows, forcing air in and out of your lungs and require the patient to be heavily sedated while they are in use.

During the course of the pandemic, the NHS had its own version of life system support, to keep its blood pumping and its vital organs functioning, as the virus sought to devastate its ability to deliver universal services. With digital technologies playing a critical role, enabling clinical services to move from mostly in-person delivery to largely remote and online, the NHS was given an artificial stimulus of its own. I wonder what questions we might ask to help us transition from the ventilator to a place of recuperation and growth, towards a future horizon.

One evening, pondering over how I should approach this final chapter, a distant memory came to mind. Many years ago, when responsible for various corporate NHS services, I arranged an away day for my senior team. I liked to spend time with them, away from the hustle and bustle of everyday working life, to step back, reflect and plan. It struck me that this is what this chapter should be about – taking a step back and imaging the future, free from the ties of our current existence.

On one occasion, we brought in Wayne, a colleague from the organisational development team to help run the day for us. One of the exercises he asked us to perform has always stuck with me. It was so simple but so powerful in its effects. Each of us was tasked with taking it in turns to describe a work problem or dilemma that was on our minds. As we listened intently to each person describe their challenge, Wayne asked us to conjure up powerful questions that might help the individual to consider it from a different angle. We were prohibited from offering solutions, and the problem holder was not allowed to respond to the questions that we took in turn to ask. Each of us was instructed to simply make a note of the questions and take them away to consider at a later date.

I loved that this exercise drew us away from a desire to jump in on the one hand or even dismiss ideas on the other. I revelled in the fact that it was predicated on a belief that each of us could solve our challenges if we had help to consider them in a new light. I enjoyed that it was reflective and facilitated deep thinking.

Who knows where Wayne is now and if he even remembers doing that exercise with myself and my team? Either way, it leads me to consider what sort of questions we should be asking ourselves in considering the conundrum of a largely analogue NHS that needs to find a way of operating successfully in a digital era. I don't have every answer to how we nurture a digital ecology, but I do think curiosity about the sorts of questions we might ask may free up our minds to open up that paradigm shift.

It has become clear over the course of this book that adoption of digital technology is not a simple challenge. When we're dealing with complexity, our standard approaches of Prince 2 project management, committees and subcommittees, improvement tools and techniques don't seem quite up to the task. Dealing with complexity requires us to lean into the messiness, start somewhere and build from there.

Momentum – towards a Digital Ecology ■ 245

That starting point, the spec of agency and energy in a system, the small spark that can be fanned to a flame, will be different in every context. Uniformity and replicability will not help us here. The tools we have depended on to deal with things that are complicated will only impede our progress in a complex world.

Someone who isn't frightened to lean into complexity is Myron Rogers, and I am fortunate enough to interview him one chilly February morning over Google Meet. Myron tells me he has worked with the NHS as a management consultant for decades. An advocate of systems theory, he has been at the vanguard of bringing this discipline to the healthcare system: "And it's really good, after thirty five years, people now have the language of it, but they're still not doing it," he says with a wry smile.

Myron explains that people often ask him why complex change is so hard. It is a curiosity that when individuals can make a change, it is not always the case that systems can do the same. "The profound explanation," Myron tells me, "is that systems are emergent phenomena and once a system creates certain types of patterns of relating to itself, everything that happens goes through that screen and gets changed back into what it already was." Myron goes on to elucidate that people try to fix the current problem but the current problem is unfixable "everything that comes its way is going to take and turn back into itself."

Myron developed his Five Maxims© (2010, 2018) as a map for embracing complexity and working with it. Those maxims assert that people own what they help create; real change happens in real work; those who do the work, do the change; connect the system to more of itself; start anywhere, follow everywhere. Another maxim of Myron's is that the process you use to get to the future is the future you get. He is simply saying that how you get there is as important as arriving at the destination you have chosen.

All the bones in my body and several decades of experience tell me this orientation makes such good sense. But it is counter to the hyper-rational digital discourse of adoption, spread and scale. We saw in Chapter 6 how we ignore context and culture at our peril. This is an art as much as a science, and it has relationships at its heart. We have three possible horizons ahead of us – our current horizon where we hold on to the tools and practices of the past and the present, a future state in which we imagine a desirable destination and a middle horizon where we understand our current state whilst tending to the green shoots of the future. Using tools such as *three horizons* enable us to think creatively about our present and our future at the same time.[4]

In Chapter 9, we heard about public deliberation as a technique for exploring complex issues and arriving at a consensus between ordinary members of the public. The good news is that this approach is just one of many tools and techniques available to us. Design thinking which we explored in Chapter 7 gets us some of the ways there, but it too is reductive when it comes to big, messy contested problems. Myron's approach to living and learning systems has ecology at its heart. By asking expansive questions, through cultivating relationships, by

246 ■ *Towards a Digital Ecology*

tending to the soil, we can start to reorientate ourselves to a digital ecology of the future.

Here are some powerful questions to help us consider how we best nurture a digital ecology. They are a place to start rather than an exhaustive list. They are contingent upon context. Treat them simply as provocations to stimulate your thinking and ideation.

What matters to people in your digital ecology? Do you truly understand what each of you cares about most of all?

How can you collectively create a compelling vision of the horizon before you?

Who is included and who is left out of that vista ahead of you?

How can you engage with the unusual suspects to co-create the future?

What are the skills and attributes you need for the road ahead?

Who holds power, and how can you better share it?

Do you have the means to explore, discover – generating a deep and nuanced understanding of the challenges you are endeavouring to decipher?

How can you create space to experiment and an appetite to take risks?

How can you make your conversations and explorations diverse and inclusive?

Are you creating sufficient space for people to pause, breathe, reflect and plan together?

Is your approach underpinned by deep trust and an emphasis on the relational?

What does an inclusive future look, sound and feel like?

How and what are you learning from this emergent process?

What if you were to galvanise the assets in your system and build out from there?

How can you release data from silos so that it can be used (with the right permissions) for real-world evidence and to plan services for populations?

Are you nurturing a thriving marketplace that allows entrepreneurs to help you solve the challenge of the future?

Do you understand your current infrastructure well enough so you can work with and from what you already have?

What approaches and methods can you make use of that help you practically move forward in ways that enable you to lean into complexity and make sense of it?

And finally, what stories can you tell yourself about your digital ecology that facilitates it to thrive, grow and prosper?

Notes

1 https://www.researchgate.net/publication/333653217_10-15_Year_Vision_for_the_Future_of_Public_Healthcare_in_a_technology_enabled_21st_Century
2 https://bmchealthservres.biomedcentral.com/articles/10.1186/s12913-019-4790-x
3 Capra & Luisi, The Systems View of Life, 2014, p. 337.
4 https://www.internationalfuturesforum.com/three-horizons

Index

A

Accelerated Access Collaborative (AAC), 95
Aanestad, Margunn, 87
abortion, 144
accountancy, 195
accreditation, 219
Accurx, 55
Ada Lovelace Institute, 137n28, 148, 159–61,
     185, 192–93, 202
Adam and the Ants, 180
Alec, 49–50, 69
algorithms, 31, 127, 140, 148, 154, 167, 186
Allen Lane, 185
All Party Group for Data Analytics APGDA,
     136, 198, 203n35
altruism, 157
Amazon, 41, 85, 93, 144, 147–48, 160n16, 231
    Alexa, 148
America, 60, 76, 231
Amnesty International, 192, 194, 203
anchor institutions135
Anderson, Ross, 186, 198
antidepressant, 175
anxiety, 64–5, 132, 150, 165, 167–68, 236
app, 5, 11–2, 24, 27–8, 41, 45, 105, 123, 144,
     187–202
app-based, 178
appgda, 203
Apple, 144, 191, 198, 200, 203, 230–31,
     234n33–34
armageddon, 236
arthritis, 43, 238
Artificial Intelligence (AI), 6, 9, 14, 17, 46–7,
     62, 102, 126–7, 136, 154, 196, 198,
     239, 242
Ashall-Payne, Liz, 216
Asia, 231

asthma, 18, 31, 34, 99
austerity, 117
Azodo, Ijeoma, 130

B

Bahrain, 194, 203n22
BAME, 114, 116, 127–30
Banner, Natalie, 142–43, 159, 187, 196, 198,
     200–1
BBC, ix, 33n33, 126, 137n20, 145, 160n8,
     203n15, 233n13
Benn, Rachel, 117, 120–23, 131–33, 136, 211
Berners-Lee, Tim, 157
Bethell, Lord James, 36, 198
Bethnal Green, 206
Bethnal Green Ventures (BGV), 205, 207
Bevan, Lauren, 206
Big Data Institute, 194
biology, 107, 109, 111, 236
biometrics, 196
biosensors, 239
Birmingham, 18, 63, 115
Blackberry, 76
Blair, Tony, 19, 167
Bluetooth, 191
Boston, 70, 177
Bourdeaux, Margaret, 197
Brexit, 216
British Computer Society, 20, 26, 188, 193
British Medical Association (BMA), 17, 60, 91
British Medical Journal (BMJ), 21
British National Formulary (BNF), 216
Brown, Jonny, 50–4
Bryant, Beverley, 36, 38, 55, 57
BuddyApp, 74
byzantine, 1, 23, 91, 104, 238

247

248 ■ *Index*

C

California, 76
Cambridge, University of, 186, 198
cancer 9, 59, 69, 77, 93, 124
Cantwell-Smith, Brian, 127
Capra, Fritjof, 246
carbon, 54
Care Quality Commission, 21, 28, 84, 220
Caudle, Heather, 130
cephalgia, 68
Cerner, 5, 223, 231
charities, 120, 123, 131–32, 158, 164, 179, 219,
     226
charity, 31, 107, 118
chatbots, 183
Chester, 237
chief information officer, 6, 19, 30, 36, 40, 46,
     66, 69, 81, 94, 106–7, 145, 147, 211,
     220, 235
China ix, 1, 3, 38
Christmas, 170
chronic fatigue, 92
chronic health condition, 77, 122
CCC, 9, 64, 69, 77, 88, 92, 122, 238–39
CIO, 6, 7, 25, 27–8, 32, 56, 66, 103, 134, 145,
     214, 216, 218
CIOs, 7, 25, 27, 134, 145, 218
CIPs (Cost Improvement targets), 211
Citizen-Led, 74
Citizens Summit, 156
Citymapper, 187
civil society, 83, 132–33, 135–36, 155, 159,
     189, 191–92, 201
clap for carers, 37
Cleveland, 70
clinical
     care, 39, 65, 70, 79
     entrepreneurs, 27, 46
     systems, 5–6, 18, 31, 54
     practice 8, 101
     staff, 9, 24, 86, 101, 110
     teams, 24, 95,107, 235
clinical commissioning groups (CCGs), 26, 50,
     54, 211, 235
clinical entrepreneur programme, 88, 225
closed-loop, 85, 141
cloud, 40, 108, 219
cloud-based, 148
CNIO, 129
Cognitive Behaviour Therapy (CBT), 167–72,
     176, 181

command-and-control, 153
Commons, House of, 15
community, 54, 120, 128, 231
computer, 20, 26, 188, 193, 211
Conservative, 7, 21, 213
consumerism, 114, 117
contact tracing, 8, 11–2, 36, 186–99, 201–2,
     206
contact-based, 175
contagion, 9, 38, 43, 154
Cooper, Anne, 22, 25, 75, 101–2, 110
COPD, 20, 42, 239
Corbridge, Richard, 209
Cornwall, 237
coronary, 20
coronavirus, 3, 35, 58, 60, 71, 73, 83–4, 143,
     188, 243
COVID, ix, x, 4, 37–8, 40, 43–4, 54–5, 111,
     131, 133, 135, 137, 177, 187, 189,
     202–3, 241–42
COVID X, 83
co-working, 111
CPAP, 84
criminals, 146
Crohn's, 75, 78
Croydon, 42–3
crunchbase, 184
cryptographers, 186
crystal, 9
CSV, 42
cultural, 84, 103, 185, 193, 239
Cummings, Dominic, 143, 155, 195–96
cyber, 22, 43, 145, 147
cyberattacks, 145–47
cybercrime, 146–47
cybersecurity, 145–47

D

Daily Mail, The, 103, 143, 218
Darlington Amy's, 150–4
Darzi, Lord, 205
data, 10, 25–6, 31–2, 36, 46, 48–51, 67, 78–9,
     85, 112, 117, 119, 121, 125–27,
     139–40, 142, 144, 146, 148–59,
     175, 179–82, 185, 187–88, 191–98,
     200–2, 210–11, 215, 222–24,
     229–33, 237, 243, 246
DataKind, 158
Davies, Roz, 75, 80–1, 117–18, 134–35
DeepMind, 144
Denyer-Bewick, Rich, 113

Index ■ 249

depression, 118, 144, 165, 167–68, 174–75, 181, 239
design, 97–100, 111, 182, 201, 245
desktop, 43, 96, 119
DevicesDotNow, 132
Dhesi, Anoop, 50
Department of Health and Social Care (DHSC), 28–9, 36, 134, 148, 199, 205, 210–12
Department for International Trade, 48
diabetes, 20, 43, 74, 78, 84–5, 116–18, 122, 137, 157, 238–39
digital, 1–3, 5–32, 35–8, 41–2, 45–6, 48–52, 54–9, 65, 67–71, 73–8, 80–2, 85–8, 92–102, 106–15, 117–26, 128–31, 133–37, 143–44, 146, 148, 150, 157–59, 163–84, 188–89, 192–95, 197–201, 205–12, 214–33, 235–46
digital adoption, 1, 3, 8, 12–3, 15, 17–8, 22, 30, 36, 40, 42, 46, 49, 55–7, 60–3, 77, 93–5, 102, 106, 109, 111, 163, 168, 174, 178–79, 209, 222, 236, 243–44
digital age, 2, 9, 11, 13, 75, 78, 108
digital-first, 122, 125, 176–77, 179, 194
Digital health, 33–4, 58, 71, 137, 160, 203–4, 234
DigitalHealthFuturist, 4
Doffman, Zak, 204n46
DrDoctor, 207–8, 227
drugs, 152, 167, 216, 218
Dunscombe, Rachel, 27, 37, 107, 157, 211
Durham, 143
dystopian, 149

E

eBay, 76
ecological, 87–8, 108–9, 163, 173
economic, 35, 77, 114–15, 122, 135, 168, 170, 227, 236, 239
economy, 19, 226
ecosystem, 169–71, 180, 182, 222, 228, 231, 241
eHealth, 120
EHRs, 102
electricity, 15–8, 32, 119
electronic, 5–6, 10, 16–7, 19–20, 23, 32, 46, 102, 119, 125, 139–40, 157, 169–70, 182, 211, 222–24, 229–30
email, 22, 40–1, 45, 54, 66, 115, 119, 122–23, 131, 133, 146, 222, 237
EMIS, 222
empathy, 79, 98, 107

encrypted, 145
engineering, 80, 97, 107, 186, 198
England, 3, 6, 8, 16, 21–2, 26, 28–30, 33, 42, 45–6, 49–50, 58–9, 71, 76, 78–9, 83–4, 116, 122, 129, 142, 157, 160, 175, 179, 183, 197, 199, 220, 233, 238
English, 5, 115, 117, 133, 209, 242
entrepreneur, 10, 46, 88, 169, 189, 205, 214, 216, 219, 225, 232
entrepreneurialism, 38
entrepreneurs, 7, 11, 27, 30, 32, 39, 92, 94–5, 167, 206, 208, 220–21, 227, 232–33, 240–41, 243, 246
environmental, 35, 79, 239
epidemic, 194
epidemiologists, 83, 186, 191
EPR, 5, 170–71, 224
equality, 13, 51, 242
ethics, 142, 158, 191, 203
ethnic, 88, 114, 127–28, 130, 196, 200
ethnicity, 115–16, 127, 152
ethnography, 98–9
Europe, 38, 126, 155, 172, 231
euros, 179
Evans, Andy, 106–8, 147
evidence-based, 101, 167, 169
evidence-driven, 215

F

Facebook, 6, 23, 33, 81, 88, 144, 148–49, 154, 169, 173, 229
face-mask, 10
Facetime, 62, 66–7
face-to-face, 10, 39, 41, 55–6, 60–1, 118, 123–24, 169, 172–75, 178, 231
farming, 19, 60
fax, 2
Federation of Informatics Professionals, The (FEDIP), 26
Fisher, Becks, 69
Fitbit, 149
Floyd, George, 196
foot-and-mouth disease, 19, 32
football, 22, 103
Forbes, 204n46
Ford, Henry, 171
forensic, 179
foundation, 26, 39, 69, 107, 111, 117, 132, 137–38, 144, 170, 187, 199, 222, 231
Foundation's, 80

250 ■ *Index*

G

Gates, Bill, 19
Global Digital Exemplar Programme GDE, 29–30
GDPR, 143, 187
gender, 126–28, 152, 194
genetic, 142, 158
genomics, 157
Germany, 231
Gibson, William, 4
glaucoma, 127
Goldacre, Ben, 158
Google, 20, 57, 63, 82–3, 144, 191, 198, 200, 231, 233, 237, 245
    Gmail, 222
Google Hangouts, 63, 82, 97
Gould, Matthew, 17, 45, 190
government, 2–3, 7–8, 10, 12, 18, 23, 27, 30–1, 33, 51, 83, 91, 99, 102, 112, 115, 120, 122, 125, 133, 135–37, 148, 155, 159–60, 164, 167–68, 185–86, 188–89, 191–92, 194–95, 198–202, 204–5, 211, 217, 219, 230–31, 233
government's, 49, 65, 133, 135, 170, 186, 191, 198–99, 202
GPs, 7, 9, 49, 60, 62, 65, 100, 157, 168, 211, 213, 222
Gray, Mary L, 197
Greeks, 126
Greenhalgh, Trish, 60, 67, 93
greenhouse gases, 59
grief, 164
Grosz, Barbara, 197
Guardian, The, 23, 216
Guys and St Thomas NHS Foundation Trust, 39, 111, 150, 187

H

Hackney, 64
Hancock, Matthew, 27–8, 197, 200
Hancock, David, 224
Harding, Baroness, 199
harassment, 196
hard-code, 2
Harvard, 203n13
headache, 128, 147, 168, 211, 213
health, 1–8, 10–2, 14, 16–8, 20–4, 26–33, 36–7, 42–3, 49–50, 54–7, 61, 64, 69–71, 73–4, 76–80, 82–4, 86–8, 91–5, 97, 102–3, 105–28, 130, 133–34, 136–44, 146, 148–60, 163–70, 172–79, 181–83, 186–95, 198–208, 210, 212, 214–22, 224–33, 235–42
healthcare, 1–3, 5–7, 9–13, 15, 17–8, 20–7, 30, 35, 39–40, 49, 58, 60, 64, 68, 75, 78–9, 82, 87–8, 92, 94–5, 97, 99–103, 106–10, 112, 114, 116–17, 119, 122, 125–27, 129, 139–43, 145–48, 151, 153–55, 157–60, 171, 178–79, 181, 183, 185, 189, 201, 205–8, 213, 215, 220–22, 224–25, 227–29, 232–33, 236, 238–42, 245–46
Health and Social Care Information Centre (HSCIC), 142
Health Foundry, 111
heatwave, 60
Heffernan, Margaret, 235
Helsinki, 76
heterogeneity, 16
Hill, The, 197
Hillier, Meg, 16
history, 19, 126
HIV, 144
HL7 FHIR, 224
homeschooling, 119
hospital-based, 8, 59
housing, 114, 122, 164, 231
Human-centered, 197
human-centred, 97–102, 109
humanity, 1, 67–8, 108
Humby, Clive, 142
Hunt, Jeremy, 23
hyperaesthesia, 68
hypertension, 238
hypoxia, 44

I

IAPT, 167–77, 170, 179–83
IAPTUS, 169–71, 175, 180
ICU 4
IESO, 171, 179
ieso-digital-health, 184
Imperial College London, 25, 150
IMS Maxims, 230
inclusivity, 124, 129
incubators, 205, 208
independent, 57, 95
inequality, 2, 10, 41, 114–17, 123, 126–30, 133–36, 158, 186, 196, 229, 240
inhalers, 18, 31
Innovation, Health and Welfare Plan (IHW), 205

Index ■ 251

insomnia, 68
Instagram, 119, 150
Integrated Care Systems (ICSs), 17, 211, 214, 219–20, 225, 231
international, 48, 148, 189, 192, 194, 223
internet, 62, 92, 119–21, 123, 130, 133, 144, 148, 175, 177, 190, 195, 197, 230, 239
internet-based, 169
internet-enabled, 175, 179, 237
interoperability, 10, 17, 19, 30–1, 46, 139–40, 157, 169, 222, 224–25, 235
intransigence, 101
iOS, 188
Iowa, 60
ipad, 24, 123, 185
iPhone, 103, 195
Ipsos Mori, 152, 161, 199
ischool, 137
Isle of Wight, 197
iTunes App store, 46, 188

J

jargon, 98, 103, 212
Johns Hopkins University, 3, 143
Johnson, Boris, 197, 236
journalists, 192, 200
journals, 65, 71, 137, 160–61, 203, 234
judiciary, 33–4
junior doctors, 9, 61, 240

K

Kardashian, Kim, 116
Kellner-Rogers, Myron, 79, 80, 86, 91, 245
  Five Maxims, 80, 230, 245
Kent, University of, 33n23, 112n9
Kettering Hospital, 39, 58n7, 71n25
kinaesthetic, 99
King's College Hospital, 66
King's College, London, 187
King's Fund, 136, 239
Kinnear, Andy, 19, 26, 56
Knight, Matthew, 37, 43
Knightsbridge, 225

L

Labour Party 7, 15, 91, 167
Lancet, The, 65, 68, 122, 127, 146, 154, 203, 215

language, 13, 93, 101, 108–9, 133, 208, 236, 240, 242–43, 245
Lansley, Andrew, 21–2, 179, 213
laptop (s), 36, 51, 62, 83, 115–16, 119, 135, 143, 145, 181, 210, 237, 242
Law of Inverse Care, 121–22
Lawson, Nigel, 209
Layard, Richard, 167–68
LCHREs, 30
Leading Edge Forum, 108, 14n4, 112n10, 233n21
Lee-Allen, John, 185, 206, 225–29
Leeds, 37, 92, 111, 120–21, 128
legislation, 224, 240
Lewis, Dana, 84, 89n13
LHCREs, 29
Liberal Democrats, 7
LinkedIn, 37
literacy, 10, 120, 122, 130, 174, 178
lockdown, 1, 20, 37, 52, 56, 63, 81, 115, 119, 131, 143, 154, 165, 175–76, 195
London School of Economics (LSE), 167, 183n9
London, 15, 36, 40, 43, 66, 83, 143, 150, 152, 154, 165, 166
London, 152
London North West, University of, 66
Loosemore, Tom, 2
Lords, House of, 199
Luisi, Pier Luigi, 246n3
lungs, 44, 91, 209, 243–44

M

Macbook, 41
Madness, 180
Malik, Rizwan, 46–8, 106–7, 223
mammogram, 141
managerialism, 108
Manchester, University of, 222, 233
Manuel-Barkin, Carolyn, 97–8
marketplace, 12, 28, 84, 170, 181, 205–7, 218–19, 221–24, 229, 231–33, 240, 246
Marmot, Michael, 114
Massachusetts, 70
maternity, 176
Mayden, 170–71
Mayfair, 208
McDonald, Joe
McDonald, Sean, 19, 203n3
McKechnie, Sheila, 80

252 ■ Index

Mckinsey Company, 28, 130, 137–38, 182, 184, 234n32
MedCity, 215
medcitynews, 234
medconfidential, 155, 160
medConfidential's, 155
medical-tech, 78
medicine, 4, 15, 17, 49, 78, 86, 101, 107, 157, 194, 239, 241
MedTech, 95
Mental health, 5, 12, 16, 74, 92, 103, 105, 132, 134, 149, 163–70, 173, 175–77, 179, 183, 212
mentoring, 208, 240
Mercedes, 83
mHabitat, 80, 87, 109, 163
Michie, Susan, 202, 204n51
Microsoft (MS), 19, 42, 222
   Teams, 40, 56, 237
Midlands, 69, 147
Mills, Tamara, 31, 34n49
Milton Keynes, 231
MIND, 183n6
mindfulness, 132
Minneapolis, 196
MIT Technology Review, 48
MIT Sloane Management Review, 111
mobile, 1, 6, 24, 47, 51, 54, 74, 81, 95–6, 103–4, 114, 125, 136, 146, 163, 165, 167, 171, 177, 181, 187, 189–91, 196, 198, 202, 219, 229, 235
mobiles, 207
Morozov, Evgeny, 185–86, 203n6
MRI, 12, 145, 206, 210
Mumoactive, 74
music, 155, 180–81
Musk, Elon, 189

N

NASSS, 61, 93–4, 102, 109
National Audit Office, 49, 33n17–18, 58n22, 210, 204n47
National Cyber Security Centre, 147, 160n15
National Geographic, 64, 71n20
National Guard, 186
National Institute for Clinical Excellence (NICE), 167, 174, 216
National Programme for IT (NPfIT), 10, 19–20, 23, 24, 27, 29, 57, 87–8, 139, 142, 189, 220, 236

National Voices, 63, 71n17
natives, 119
neoliberal, 170
nephrology, 61
Netflix, 9, 36, 226, 229–30
Nevada, 27
Newcastle, 31
Newham, London Borough of, 199
New Scientist, 160
New York Times, 148, 160n20
NHS, ix, x, 1–13, 15–33, 36–40, 42, 44, 46–52, 54, 56–60, 62, 64–71, 76–84, 86, 88, 91–3, 95–7, 99–104, 106–13, 116–19, 121–23, 125–26, 128–30, 133–37, 139–48, 150–51, 153, 155, 158, 160, 163, 169–71, 173–85, 187–88, 190–92, 195, 197, 199–200, 202, 205–33, 236–45
   administration, 5
   administrators, 37, 53, 70, 106, 181
   budget, 2, 19, 32, 209, 211, 213, 220–21, 236, 239
   bureaucracy, 48, 78–9, 218
   cash-strapped, 95, 209
   commitment, 23, 60, 96
   committee, 15–7, 20, 28, 30, 32, 80, 94, 99, 104, 198–99, 244
   competition, 21–2
   costs, 19, 21–2, 32, 48, 95, 108, 140, 168, 172, 174, 210, 214, 222–23, 225, 239
   debts, 211
   culture, 2, 11, 28, 36, 39–40, 69, 78–9, 92, 99, 102–4, 106–7, 109–11, 117, 134, 143, 153, 245
   demographics, 6, 135, 197
   ecology, 2–3, 9, 13, 32, 54, 56–7, 86, 92, 100, 102, 111–12, 159, 179, 182–83, 201, 214, 216, 224, 232–33, 235–37, 239, 242–44, 246
   employment, 114, 116, 119–20, 124
   estate, 16–7, 40, 213
   expenditure, 209, 238
   finances, 22, 119, 130, 206, 210
   flora, 12, 163
   framework, 51, 61, 93, 102, 109, 181, 216, 219
   funding, 3, 16, 29–30, 53, 62, 95, 130–32, 179, 215, 227, 232
   future, 20, 24, 39, 56, 63, 69, 102, 107, 144, 163, 192, 206, 229, 237–38, 242

Index ■ 253

hierarchy, 9, 78–9, 86, 103
hospitals, 5, 8, 10, 16, 41, 43–4, 49, 54, 56, 59, 76, 116, 139, 145, 227, 231
inequalities, 36, 65, 84, 114, 121–23, 127, 129, 133, 159, 193, 200, 242
infrastructure, 6, 16, 19–20, 24, 27, 42, 49–50, 56–7, 62, 70, 87–8, 145–46, 169, 206, 210, 214, 220, 231, 246
innovation, 2, 5, 9–11, 27, 29–30, 36–7, 46–8, 57, 60–1, 73–4, 76–9, 83–6, 93, 95–6, 100, 102–10, 117, 126, 144, 148, 154, 156, 158, 166, 169, 172, 181–82, 201, 205, 210, 212, 214–15, 219–20, 223, 225–26, 228, 236, 238
innovations, 17, 27, 31–2, 43, 47, 77, 95, 109, 178, 239
investment, 41, 56, 84, 96–7, 106, 110, 126, 145, 167, 179, 186, 206, 208, 210–12, 215, 225–28, 232
leaders, 7–8, 20, 27, 37, 129–30, 185, 218, 224
legacy, 8, 16–7, 20, 28, 32, 36, 49, 77–8, 102, 238
management, 21, 40, 47, 50, 87–8, 104–7, 111, 118, 149, 153, 182, 225, 244–45
money, 12, 19, 21, 24, 29, 38, 51, 53, 55, 81, 88, 95–7, 100, 103, 105, 115–17, 168, 174, 198, 205–14, 217–18, 223, 225–27, 229, 241, 243
morale, 8, 32, 104
partnership, 32, 52, 77, 81, 83–4, 135, 144, 187, 223
pressure, 36, 40, 44, 57, 164, 169, 188, 210–11, 221, 231
procurement, 12, 24, 51, 53–4, 62, 216–20, 223, 233
professionalism, 26, 243
relationships, 13, 53, 56, 69, 83–4, 111, 225, 227, 242, 245
reorganisation, 17, 21–2, 29–30
revenue, 179, 210, 218, 224, 228, 230
restructure, 17, 22, 30
shareholders, 225–26, 228
silos, 49–50, 87, 108, 157, 231, 246
solutions, 8, 27, 36–7, 53, 74, 82, 88, 102, 111, 115, 117, 140, 149, 172, 174, 178, 186, 194, 209, 219, 232, 235, 244
Spine, 6, 20

stakeholders, 7, 96, 142, 182
standards, 17, 26–7, 29–30, 81, 86–7, 99, 157, 181–82, 192, 212, 215–16, 219, 223–24, 242–43
statistics, 44, 59, 199, 204
summary care record, 18, 32n12
suppliers, 9, 15, 19, 81–2, 88, 174, 217–19, 222–24
support, 5–6, 10, 19–21, 26, 37, 43, 47–8, 50, 52, 62, 70, 73, 81–2, 92–3, 95–6, 99–100, 102, 107, 109–10, 115, 118–19, 121–22, 125, 127, 130–34, 136, 140, 142, 151, 164, 166, 172–73, 178, 191, 193, 197, 199–202, 210–11, 232, 235, 239–40, 243–44
survey, 218
targets, 13, 54, 56, 70, 79, 88, 101, 103, 108, 169–70, 209, 211, 243
teams, 24, 40, 52, 70, 88, 95, 99–100, 106–7, 109, 128–29, 158, 177, 179, 218, 224, 235
transformation, 2, 7–12, 15–6, 19–25, 27–32, 35–6, 45, 48, 50–2, 68–70, 80–1, 85–6, 88, 111–12, 117, 125, 209–10, 212, 236
transparency, 152, 155–56, 158, 175, 181, 191, 219
treatment, 4, 6, 9–11, 18, 20–1, 26, 43–4, 54, 59, 65, 70, 105, 107, 140, 150, 168–69, 173–76, 178, 206, 212, 237–39
trusts, 6, 16, 22, 26, 29–30, 36, 40, 49–53, 57, 67, 73, 78, 100, 104, 111, 120, 145–46, 169, 179, 187, 209–12, 222
information centre, 160n10
underfunding, 3, 36, 167
value, 10, 221
vendors, 7, 103, 171, 221–22, 224, 229
vision, 40, 100, 238–39, 246
website, 39, 133–34, 148
waiting time, 21, 36, 78, 84–6, 168–69, 17, 183n15
workforce, 7, 14n13, 24–6, 38–9, 47, 70, 91, 118, 128, 176–77, 180, 185
workload, 17, 45, 51, 102
NHSE, 28, 50–1, 212
NHSX, 17, 27–30, 44–5, 58, 60, 67, 79, 129, 181, 190–93, 198, 233
Nicholson, David, 21
Nintendo Wii, 76
Nobel Prize, 156

254 ■ Index

non-NHS, 111
non-profit, 225
non-verbal, 64
Norfolk and Waveney, 50, 58n23
Norman, James, 28, 82–3
not-for-profit, 179, 187, 215
Numan, Gary, 180
Nuffield Foundation, 183n2, n7
Nuffield Trust, 14n13, 32–4, 71n22, 81, 89n8,
    n12, 95, 112n1, n2, 179, 183n11,
    194, 233n5
nursing, 25, 101, 110, 129
Nursing Times, 112

O

occupational, 25, 106, 149, 228
One London, 149, 151, 153–7
Open Data Institute, 83, 158
Open Democracy and Amnesty, 155
open-source, 66–7, 83, 85, 230
ophthalmology, 127
Organisation for the Review of Care and Health
    Applications (ORCHA), 216, 219
Orwellian, 121, 149, 188
Oslo, University of, 87
outpatient, 8–9, 43, 50–2, 59–61, 66, 134, 141,
    175, 239
Oxford, University of, 60, 93, 194, 231
oximeter, 44, 46
oxygen, 35, 44, 46
O'Connell, Mark, 116

P

pager, 41, 95
Palantir, 155
pancreas, 85
pandemic, 1, 3, 7–13, 21, 28–30, 35–43,
    45–7, 49–51, 53, 56–7, 59–61, 63–5,
    67–70, 81–4, 93, 111–12, 115–17,
    119, 124, 126, 129–32, 134–36, 143,
    146–47, 152, 154–55, 159, 163–65,
    172, 175–77, 179, 182, 185–94, 196,
    198–99, 201–2, 214, 216, 225, 236,
    243–44
pandemic-era, 19
pandemic-fuelled, 44
paper-based, 31
parliament, 32
parliamentary, 15–7, 28, 30, 36, 136, 198
Partridge, Sir Nick, 142

Patel, Neelam, 215
Patel, Sonia, 66–7
paternalism, 9, 78–9
Patient Administration System (PAS), 5
patient-centred, 69, 84
patient-driven, 77
patient-led, 76, 78, 88
patients, 2, 5–9, 11, 16–8, 20–1, 23, 26, 30,
    32, 36–9, 41–6, 49–52, 54–6, 60–7,
    69–70, 74–8, 84–6, 88, 94, 96–102,
    105–6, 108, 127, 130, 134, 136,
    141, 144, 146, 150, 157, 163, 168,
    170–73, 175–81, 185, 206–8, 211,
    214, 217, 220, 230, 232, 236, 240,
    243
    technology-empowered, 20
pay-as-you-go, 119
pensions, 134, 226
Peppin, Aidan, 185, 193–96, 202
Perez, Caroline Criado, 125–26, 137
personalisation, 107
person-centred, 134
Picture Archiving and Communications System
    PACS, 223
phenotyping, 148
philanthropy, 226
philosophy, 78–9, 127, 135, 142, 226
police, 149, 196, 201–2
Plas, Annemarie, 37
policymakers, 2, 7, 21, 136, 186, 209
politics, 58, 136, 160, 213, 236
pollution, 31
population, 6, 10, 18, 26, 44, 49, 54, 79, 84,
    119, 123, 128, 139–40, 152–54, 164,
    169, 181, 190, 193, 199, 205, 211,
    214, 238–39, 241
post-Covid, 47, 62–3
post-pandemic, 56, 65, 133
poverty, 10, 113–14, 116, 119–20, 122, 126,
    134
PowerPoint, 16
PPE, ix, 41, 70, 83, 126, 199
pragmatism, 37–8
pre-Covid, 55
prejudice, 129
pre-pandemic, 60–1
prescriptions, 6, 81, 123, 125, 131
Price-Forbes, Alec, 49
private-sector, 163, 179
privatisation, 21
productivity, 57, 114, 170
pseudo-science, 114

Index ■ 255

psychiatry, 164, 178
psychology, 202
Psychologist, The, 89n1
PTSD, 176
pulmonary, 132, 238
purpose-built, 67, 189
Pricewaterhouse Cooopers (PwC), 195

Q

quarantine, 197
Quere, 48

R

racism, 116, 127
Radiohead, 113–14
radiology, 46–8, 70, 223
Ramadan, 194
Range Rover, 27
ransomware, 145
Randomised Controlled Trials (RCTs), 173,
    175, 215
real-time, 175
real-world, 126, 147, 152, 181, 191
regional, 17, 50, 52, 55, 129, 141, 154, 181,
    211, 215, 219–20, 231, 239
regulatory, 76, 86, 182, 215–16
remote working, 8, 21, 36, 39–41, 45–6, 50,
    54–5, 60–6, 68–70, 83, 129, 135,
    152, 173, 175–78, 188, 190, 244
renal, 41
research, 10–1, 17, 20–1, 57, 60, 64, 74, 81,
    87, 93, 95–6, 98, 100, 111–12,
    114, 117–18, 120–21, 126–27, 139,
    142–44, 150–52, 154, 156–58,
    164–65, 173–74, 177–78, 181–82,
    187, 191–93, 197, 215, 217, 219–20,
    225, 233
research-based, 175
researchgate, 246
Resolution Foundation, The, 58n12
respiratory, 3, 37, 44, 99
robotics, 6, 9, 24, 38, 239
Rogers, Everett, 60–1
Rogers, Myron, see Kellner-Rogers, Myron
Royal Society of Medicine, 4
Royal College of Emergency Medicine, 17
Royal College of Physicians, 62, 70n2, 71n4
Royal College of Psychiatrists (RCPysch), 68, 164
Royal Free Hospital, London, 134–44, 241
    charity, 238

Foundation Trust, 107
Royal Society of Arts, 14n11
Rushkoff, Douglas, 228, 233n25
RYSE, 225–26

S

Salford Royal NHS Foundation Trust, 111
Samaritans, 165–67
sarcasm, 166
scandals, 201
scans, 47, 93, 127, 178
scepticism, 8, 134
sceptics, 188
Schneier, Bruce, 186, 203
school, 31, 167
science, 15, 26, 71, 109, 112, 127, 140, 145,
    157–58, 169, 187, 193, 198–99, 202,
    220, 226, 245
Science Direct, 112n11
scientific, 135, 202
sci-fi, 42
scorecard, 155
Scotland, 50, 53
secondary care, 13, 31, 50, 61, 71, 142, 163–64,
    168, 178, 183, 212, 220, 231
Secretary of State for Health, 8, 21, 23–4, 27,
    30, 148, 188, 192
Secretary of State for Culture, 28
security, 22, 43, 142, 145–47, 185–86, 191,
    193, 198, 203
self-assessments, 8, 36
self-care, 176, 242
self-isolate, 10, 42, 188–90, 196, 201–2
self-isolating, 47
self-isolation, 202
self-management, 31, 92, 99, 105, 239
self-optimisation, 170
self-quarantine, 36
self-reporting, 196–97
self-tracking, 141
sensors, 6, 146
sensory, 69
sepsis, 77
serendipity, 170, 220
service-manual, 112
sex-disaggregate, 126
Shah, Sam, 79, 117, 128
shame, 63, 69
Shangri-La, 240
ShCR (shared care records), 29
Sheffield, 84

256 ■ *Index*

shell-shocked, 112
shield, 39, 49
shielding, 47, 49
short-term, 102, 188, 209, 231
Shuri, 88, 130
signals, 186, 209
Silicon Valley, 3, 23, 122, 166, 185, 189
Simon & Schuster, 235
Skype, 62
Slack, 82–4
smartphone, 2, 31, 41, 46, 92, 96, 119–20,
  122–23, 140–41, 147, 173, 178, 181,
  190–91, 193–95, 198, 200, 218, 242
smartwatch, 141, 147
SMEs, 66, 129, 135, 170, 219, 222, 231
Snapchat, 119
Social Integration APPG, 136n1, 138n37, 138n38
Social Metrics Commission, 136n5
society, 2, 4, 7, 10, 20, 26, 58, 83, 113–14, 122,
  128–29, 132–33, 135–36, 139, 155,
  159, 167–68, 183, 188–89, 191–93,
  196, 201
socio-economic, 116, 135, 152, 196–97, 242
socio-technical, 87
software, 4, 11, 47, 51, 61–2, 66, 85–7, 92,
  98–9, 105, 108, 145–46, 148, 158,
  171, 210, 212, 215, 217, 222, 224,
  228, 230, 232, 241–42
software-as-a-service (SAAS), 211, 230
solidarity, 37, 157–59, 196
sourdough, 115
Spain, ix
specialist(s), 26, 40, 65, 79, 81, 97, 99, 117,
  157, 211, 220, 242
sport, 85, 134
Spotify, 100, 180–81, 184n26, 230
spreadsheet(s), 6, 42, 49–50
standardisation, 17, 32, 105, 107, 140
Stanford Center for Digital Health, 77
Stanford Medical Tech Conference, 78
start-up(s), 7, 12, 23, 30, 32, 74, 76, 96, 103, 119,
  127–29, 135, 144, 148–9, 168–70,
  181, 206–7, 208, 214–15, 218–220,
  223–24, 226, 228–33, 240–41
steroids, 51
stethoscopes, 217
Stevens, Simon, 134
stoma, 75–6
stomach, 141
Stone, Emma, 117, 121–25, 134–35
Strava, 229

Streams App, 144
students, 61, 70
subscription, 180, 230
suicide, 149, 166
summary care record, 18, 32n12
supermarket, 10, 140, 222
supply-driven, 30, 95
surgery, 24, 31, 36, 41, 54, 118, 136
surveillance, 86, 141, 149, 187, 192–94, 196,
  201
sustainability, 32, 61, 93–4, 179
swimming, 93
switchboard, 41
Switzerland, 225

T

tablet, 120, 122, 132
taxation, 1
taxpayers, 18, 115, 206, 217, 243
Taylorism, 13, 243
Taylorist, 105
technology
  adoption, 12, 15, 55, 168, 209
  companies, 79, 140, 144, 149, 155, 185,
    211, 218, 230
  infrastructure, 169
  innovation, 74
  in the NHS, 1–5, 7–8, 11–3, 15–7, 19–25,
    27, 29–33, 36, 38–9, 41, 43–51, 55–7,
    60–3, 66–9, 74–5, 79–80, 83–8,
    91–102, 105–7, 109, 116–18, 121,
    128, 130, 136, 140, 144, 146, 149, 155,
    157, 159–60, 163, 165–66, 168–69,
    173–74, 178, 180, 186–89, 191–95,
    198–203, 206–7, 209–14, 216–18,
    221–22, 224–25, 227, 230–32,
    235–38, 240–41, 243–44, 246n1
  untested 12, 193
technology-enabled 17, 209
Technology Review, The 203n32, 204n43,
  234n26
tech-savvy 43
tech-solutionism, 166, 186, 188–89
techUK, 36, 83, 219
telecommunications, 62
Telegraph, The, 154
telehealth 6, 8, 21, 36, 177–78, 231
telemedicine 6, 228, 234n29
telephone 3, 21, 43–6, 49, 55, 57, 60–2, 65, 68,
  166, 172, 237

Index ■ 257

telephonic 68
television 36, 194
tennis 166
terminology, 87
tertiary care, 220
Tesco Clubcard, 142
test, 147, 190, 197, 199, 201–2
TestTraceIsolate, 202
text, 60, 66, 85, 92, 102, 145, 198, 202, 207
text-and-telephone-consultations, 71
therapeutics, 6
Times Newspaper, The, 147, 160n16, 197
Think Tank Institute for Public Policy
think tanks, 164
Tickell, Shane, 230
TikTok, 36
Tomlinson, Jonathon, 64
Topol Eric, 24
Topol Review, The, 33n34
Toronto, University of, 127, 137n26
Torous, John, 177–8
tracers, 42, 190, 197, 202
tracker, 147
Trade Union Congress (TUC), 126, 137n21
transactional, 64, 69–70, 99, 108, 125, 208, 217
transplants, 77
TransUnion Database, 133
trauma, 64, 70
triage, 5, 48
Tudor Hart, Julian, 122
tweets, 4–5, 66–7, 111, 155, 166, 172–73
Twister, 26
Twitter, 4, 66–7, 82, 85, 93, 118, 129, 155, 166, 172–73, 203–4, 229

U

Uber, 187
ukbiobank, 161
underrepresentation, 127
UK, xi, 1–2, 12–30, 48, 57, 66–7, 70–1, 73, 76–7, 83, 95, 112, 118–19, 128, 133, 136, 143–44, 149, 155, 158–161, 165, 167, 191–94, 198–204, 219, 223, 228, 231–35, 241
Universal Credit, 113, 119–22
Universal College Hospital (UCH), 83
University College London, (UCL), 58n17, n18, 83, 165, 242
Understanding Patient Data (UPD), 136, 142, 159n3, 187, 193, 198

USA, 187
Utilitarian, 170
user-centred, 11, 97, 100, 182

V

vaccination, 158
vaccine, 188, 190, 197
value-based, 230
ventilator, 4, 67, 243, 244
venture capital, 12, 225–26, 228–29
venture-capital-backed, 55
Verge, The, 204n45
vertigo, 68
Viagra, 126
video, 21, 175
   calls, 40, 45, 131, 143
   camera, 65
   chat, 115
   communications, 9
   conference, 36
   conversation, 93
   consultations, 6, 9, 41, 45, 50–1, 53–5, 60–6, 69–70, 111, 171–2, 229
   platforms, 229
   streaming, 226
virtual
   clinics, 65, 213
   coffee morning, 132
   consultation, 62, 213
   meetings, 40, 64
   teams, 43, 70
   reality, 4, 6, 183
   wards, 42–5, 64
virus, 1, 3–5, 19, 36–8, 42, 44, 50, 66, 69, 115–16, 119, 132, 145–46, 165, 177, 188–91, 195–96, 202, 236, 244
voluntary sector, 81, 195

W

Wachter, Bob, 15, 23–4, 29, 33n28, 91, 102, 106, 112n7
Walkman, 180
WannaCry, 145–47, 150
wealth creation, 2
wearable, 4, 6, 11, 86, 146, 178, 239
web
   applications, 146
   server, 157
   systems, 171

258 ■ *Index*

web-based, 8, 36, 92
webcam, 41, 51, 62, 115
webinar, 37, 131,176
welfare, 119, 131
well-being, 2, 49, 74, 114, 120–4, 132, 146, 149, 159, 164, 216, 239–40
Wellcome Trust, 142, 187, 193
wellness programmes, 221
WhatsApp, 7, 22, 54, 62, 81–2, 115, 125, 154
Wheatley, Margaret. J, 91
Whicher, Tom, 206
white noise, 8
white paper
  government, 219
WH Smih's, 237
widget
  interoperability, 169
  smartphone, 140
Wi-Fi, 20
  zones, 131
wiki, 83
Wikipedia, 32n13, 83, 136n3, 160n24
Wilkinson, Sarah, 28
Wilkin, Andy, 238–41
Williamson, Sir Archibald, 15–6
Windows XP, 43

Wired Magazine, 14n6, 67, 71n24, 89n9, 188, 197–98, 203n9, n10, n12, n14
women's health, 126
Wright, Sandy Sandy, 240–42
World Health Organisation (WHO), 3
World Wide Web, 1, 157
Wuhan, 3

X

x-ray, 6, 41,47–8, 127

Y

Yahoo, 222, 233
York, 1
Youtube, 33n15, 37, 43–4, 58n17, 75–6, 89

Z

ZOE Global LTD, 187
ZOE COVID Study, 203n7, 203n8
Zoom, 56, 61, 64, 68, 71n17, 107, 116, 119, 124, 128–29, 131–32, 155
zombies, 129
  apocalypse, 42
Zuhlke, 198

Printed in the United States
by Baker & Taylor Publisher Services